PRINCIPLES OF OBSTETRICS AND GYNECOLOGY FOR NURSES

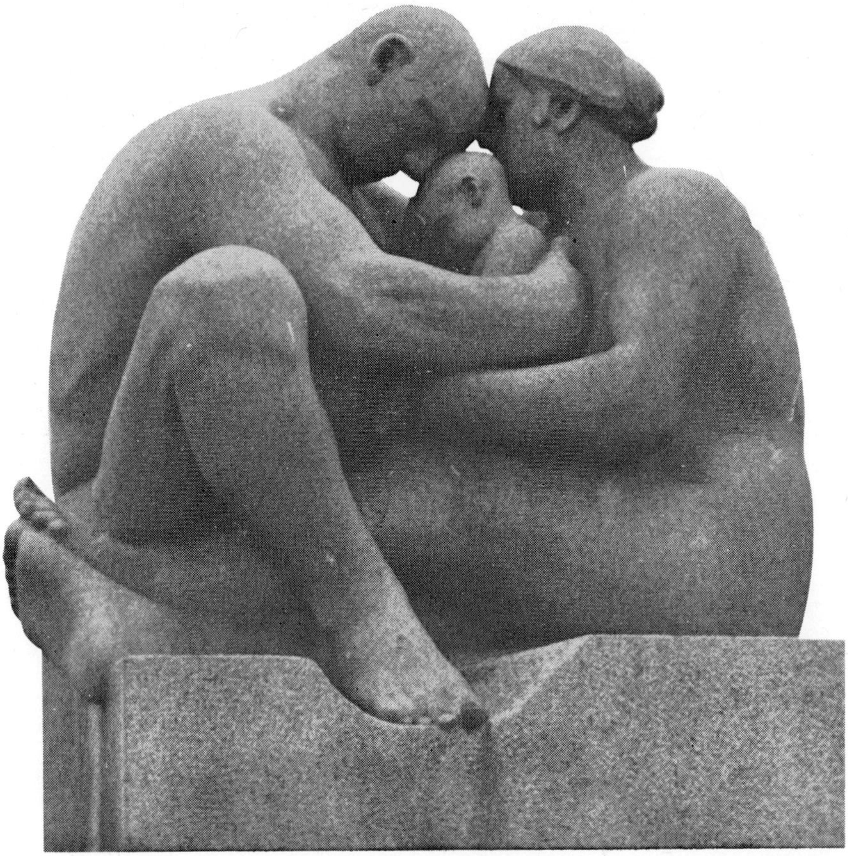

Vigeland's *Creation*

PRINCIPLES OF OBSTETRICS AND GYNECOLOGY FOR NURSES

JOSEPHINE IORIO, R.N., B.S., M.A.

Associate Professor of Nursing,
Seton Hall University School of Nursing,
South Orange, New Jersey

SECOND EDITION

With 171 illustrations

THE C. V. MOSBY COMPANY

Saint Louis 1971

SECOND EDITION

Printed in the United States of America

Standard Book Number 8016-2336-7

Library of Congress Catalog Card Number 71-146224

Distributed in Great Britain by Henry Kimpton, London

Dedicated to my father Giuseppe
and in loving memory of my mother Giovannina
who inspired me to write this book

FOREWORD

Josephine Iorio has written a book for nurses that has filled a long overdue need for the everyday clinician. She has successfully crossed the bridge of good maternity and gynecological care to good family-centered care with an all-in-one design.

Jo lives and breathes family-centered care, so why not write about it? This she has done in her second edition of *Principles of Obstetrics and Gynecology for Nurses.*

The second edition is highly updated with inclusion of scientific advances of such topics as phototherapy for premature infants and psychological factors involved in parenthood.

Jo Iorio believes that education of expectant parents gives rise to a more meaningful experience for them and their family, and this is well documented in her book.

Scientific advances and technicalities are easily absorbed and fall into the action pattern of the clinician, but sensitivity to the basic underlying problems of parents is a challenge. An understanding of this is made easy in the book through Jo's unmatched communication skills and her courage to include both parents in all phases of the maternity cycle. This gives the reader a family-centered approach that is here to stay.

This second edition of *Principles of Obstetrics and Gynecology for Nurses* is an important book for every nurse practitioner and student.

Sister M. Canice Fitzpatrick,
R.N., B.S., M.A.

Obstetrical Supervisor and Director of Parent Education, Holy Name Hospital, Teaneck, New Jersey

PREFACE

Obstetrics and gynecology are so closely related that it is fitting that a textbook be written considering both fields. Good practice in obstetrics includes gynecology, since many gynecologic problems are directly or closely related to obstetrics. It is because of my strong convictions of this interrelationship that this text was written.

Although this book is written primarily for basic nursing students, it will not provide the step-by-step procedures in nursing care. This book is designed to provide for creative thinking by students as they plan for the care of families during the reproductive years. It will be especially helpful in the application of scientific principles gleaned from the biologic and physical sciences. Physiologic and psychologic implications are stressed throughout, with emphasis on nursing care. Graduate nurses will profit from its new principle-centered approach.

The material is presented sequentially, from reproduction in general to the menopause. Deviations from the normal will be treated throughout the text as they relate to specific obstetric and gynecologic problems that are most common.

This book is a result of my teaching experiences in helping students think through nursing problems. Their stimulating and thought-provoking discussions inspired me to write it. I do not contend that this text is entirely inclusive, yet I do believe it will meet the needs of nurses as they care for parents during the childbearing years.

I would especially like to thank Sister M. Evelyn, C.S.J., administrator, Sister M. Canice, C.S.J., supervisor of the maternity unit, Dr. Peter Beaugard, Chief of Obstetrics, Dr. Peter J. Bonanno, Chief of Gynecology, and Dr. Elizabeth Perry, anesthetist, at Holy Name Hospital in Teaneck, New Jersey, for their cooperation in the preparation of this text. To the staff of doctors and nurses—Donald Rock, M.D., James Fox, M.D., David Landers, M.D., Ann Reardon, R.N., Mary Schaffroth, R.N., Leona Lauchaire, R.N., Barbara Dorney, R.N., Rita Fulcher, R.N., Mary McMahon, R.N.—who believe in and practice family-centered care,

I feel privileged to have worked with you. You will always be an inspiration to nursing students of Seton Hall University.

Sincere gratitude is expressed to Stanley Mosiello for the excellent photography, and to Shirley Baty for the splendid illustrations. Many thanks to Stanley and Louise Mosiello for sharing the birth of their second child, Laura; and to Steve and Angelina Hrnciar for the postdelivery photographs of their fifth child, Kimberly. Kimberly's sister Jennifer appeared in the first edition.

Josephine Iorio

CONTENTS

UNIT III DEVIATIONS FROM THE NORMAL MATERNITY CYCLE

UNIT IV INTERPREGNANCY PERIOD

UNIT V MISCELLANEOUS

UNIT I REPRODUCTION

The security and elevation of the family and of family life are the prime objects of all civilization, and the ultimate ends of all industry.

Charles W. Eliot

CHAPTER 1

THE NURSE AND THE FAMILY

NURSE'S ROLE

The objectives and goals in maternity nursing are family-centered since alterations in family size affect each member. The nurse's role in working with families incorporates knowledge in the biologic, social, and behavioral sciences. As an integral part of the health team, she collaborates with the physician, the nutritionist, the social worker, the public health nurse, and auxiliary personnel. Her knowledge of community resources is essential in providing complete health care. Knowledge gleaned from the sciences is utilized in assessing, planning, implementing, and evaluating health care.

The professional nurse perceives education for childbearing as a component of total care. She is aware of the importance of early medical supervision as a determining factor in fostering a safe labor and delivery. She makes referrals for continued health supervision, recognizing that the health of the mother influences the care given to the children. The childbearing period is a time when an introduction to health services can have far-reaching beneficial effects on the entire family.

THE FAMILY

The basic unit structure in our society is the family. Young people are products of their environment, and they perceive their role as parents in retrospect of their own family units. American families are moderate in size, averaging two to four children. Statistics reveal that there is more planning for children and that 15% of all marriages are barren.

Marriage involves the union of two persons who love each other. Love was designed to be a two-in-one relationship between man and woman. The greatest act of love is creation; therefore marriage is love-giving as well as life-giving.

The biologic union of man and woman in sexual intercourse is a reciprocal giving of oneself in which each partner is enriched and rewarded. It is a maturing process in which a young woman becomes a wife and mother, and a young man becomes a husband and father. What each brings to marriage biologically and emotionally determines the equilibrium and tempo within the family unit.

Marital patterns are changing in the United States. People marry younger than formerly, and there are now marriages of people of varying cultural, social and religious backgrounds. The average American woman has completed child-bearing at approximately 30 years of age. There are great changes in the stability of marriages, the sizes of families, the wife-mother and husband-father role, and various childbearing practices.

The health status each partner brings to marriage is of primary concern in predicting strong and healthy family units. Women have many questions about their reproductive systems, and premarital examinations are a common practice 6 weeks prior to marriage.

Community agencies offering services to young people include: private agencies such as marriage counseling services, family guidance centers, preparation for parenthood classes, social welfare agencies, prenatal clinics, family planning services, child health clinics, and public health services. Numerous religious groups are now making available to their people lectures, conferences, and discussions on preparation for marriage and responsible parenthood. Periodic group discussions for parents are helpful since they provide opportunity for the sharing of like experiences, knowledge of normal growth and development patterns, and support with common problems of sibling rivalry, illness in the child, etc.

Psychologic impact of pregnancy on the family

The family is a complex interactional system, and the impact of pregnancy affects all its members. The physical and emotional maturity of marital partners strengthens family stability. Adolescent couples who are still struggling for self-identity may find the intimacy of married life difficult. For the young couple for whom marriage is a result of pregnancy, tensions are greater. Economic and social adjustments result in added stress. An unhappy, tense couple cannot do a good job of mothering or fathering an infant. In a marriage where love and maturity exist, pregnancy is less stressful.

Maternal care

Optimum maternal care affords a state of physical, mental, and social well-being and the maintenance of this state prior to planned conception, during pregnancy, and throughout the postpartum period for the entire family.

Optimum maternal care incorporates two generations: the mother and the child. The maternal health continuum begins with the conception of a female child and ends with delivery of her last child. Conception of each of her female children will mark the beginning of another maternal health continuum. Each phase of such a continuum can be divided into two major divisions, the preconceptual period and the postconceptual period. The latter may be further subdivided into prenatal, intrapartum, and postpartum periods.

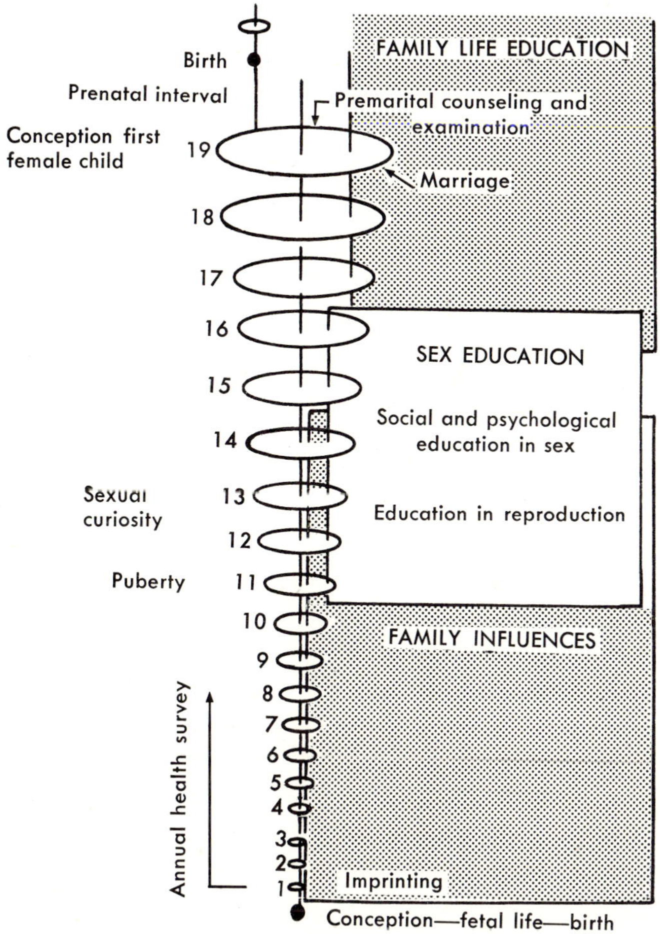

Fig. 1-1. Maternal health spiral.

SELECTED REFERENCES

Bell, N., and Vogel, E. F.: A modern introduction to the family, New York, 1960, Free Press of Glencoe, Inc.

Carroll, G. H.: First time parents, Child and Family, p. 13, Spring, 1965.

Duvall, E. M.: Family development, Philadelphia, 1962, J. B. Lippincott Co.

Freedman, R.: The growth of American families in Maternity Center Association, Meeting the childbearing needs of families in a changing world, Report of a Work Conference, New York, 1962.

Gibert, H.: Love in marriage, New York, 1964, Hawthorne Books, Inc.

Haire, J., and Haire, D.: Implementing family-centered maternity care with a central nursery, ICEA Supplies Center, 208 Dittly Bldg., Bellevue, Wash. 98004.

Hennel, M. F. C.: Maternity nursing in practice, Nurs. Clin. N. Amer. **3:**289, 1968.

Hosford, E.: The maternity cycle—a time of challenge, Bull. Amer. Coll. Nurse Midwifery **12:**45, May, 1967.

Hutton, I. G.: The sex technique in marriage, New York, 1961, Emerson Books, Inc.

King, E.: The pregnant father, Bull. Amer. Coll. Nurse Midwifery **13:**19, February, 1968.

Lynch, W. A.: Marriage manual for Catholics, New York, 1964, Indent Press.

Morris, M. L.: Teen age marriages, Child and Family, p. 49, Spring, 1963.

Moss, J. J.: Teenage marriage cross national trends and sociological factors in the decision of when to marry, J. Marriage and Family **27**:239, 1965.

Naismith, G.: The premarital examination—its importance to both the man and woman, Today's Health **42**:50, April, 1964.

Peckham, B. M.: Optimum maternal care, Obstet. Gynec. **33**:6, June, 1969.

Riker, A., and Riker, C.: The role of man and woman in marriage, Marriage **45**:6, July, 1963.

Simmons, L. W.: Effects of changing culture on childbearing and family life in Maternity Center Association, Meeting the childbearing needs of families in a changing world, Report of a Work Conference, New York, 1962.

Simmons, L. W.: Culture changes and family life, Child and Family, p. 79, Summer, 1963.

Simon, N. M.: Psychologic and social factors in family formation, Child and Family, p. 62, Winter, 1964.

Thomas, J. B.: Introduction to human embryology, Philadelphia, 1968, Lea & Febiger.

Treat, D. B.: Understanding the expectant father, Child and Family, p. 16, Spring, 1964.

Weidenbach, E.: Family-centered maternity nursing, New York, 1967, G. P. Putnam's Sons.

Wooden, H.: Family centered maternity care, Hosp. Top. **40**:69, April, 1962.

Wooden, H.: The family centered approach to maternity care, Nurs. Forum **1**:60, Spring, 1962.

Questions for study

1. Visit health facilities in your community related to maternal, newborn nursing. What is the nurse's role?
2. In your immediate family group identify the role played by family members. How do members in your extended family, grandparents, aunts, and uncles, interact with your immediate family? Do the roles of family members change when crisis situations such as marriage, new siblings, or family separations occur?
3. What facilities in your community are available in preparation for marriage and a family? What are the goals and services offered by each? Evaluate these services in light of your particular community need.

CHAPTER 2

REPRODUCTION PROCESS

The story of reproduction is said to be the greatest story ever told—it appears in the greatest book ever written, the Holy Bible. According to Genesis, "On the fifth day God created the universe and man was formed to His likeness. God then saw that man could not live alone, so he created woman from the rib of man. This explains why a man leaves his father and mother and cleaves to his wife till they become one flesh. Man then called his wife Eve meaning 'life' since woman is the mother of all living persons. And so did life go on with man and woman procreating as God has willed it!"

From generation to generation the process of reproduction has awed scientist, scholar, and poet alike. Man has attempted for centuries to explain reproduction in many ways, through mysticism, religious beliefs, and biologic and scientific research. Aristotle, with his simple observation of a baby chick, perhaps could be credited with the beginning of man's search, since his thinking discarded superstitious beliefs and focused attention on the human power of observation. Not until the minute cells involved in reproduction were first seen by Hamm and Leeuwenhoek in 1677 and not until the ovarian follicle was described by de Graaf in 1672 did the field of embryology come to be known. Many unexplained mysteries about reproduction arose with the knowledge that a female germ cell united with a male germ cell was responsible for the formation of a new individual. Since internal and external factors affect the growing embryo, research and study in the nineteenth and twentieth centuries are concerned with factors that influence and regulate development.

Reproduction is a process by which new life is generated. It occurs in all organisms—without it, perpetuation of the species would not exist. The reproductive cycle in the female begins with the menarche and terminates with the menopause; in the male the reproductive cycle begins with adolescence and goes on indefinitely into senescence. It is necessary, therefore, to start this discussion from the very beginning. How are the reproductive organs developed in the tiny male and female embryos? How do these quiescent organs mature at puberty? What are the reproductive years really like? What happens when the reproductive period has passed in the male and the female?

What is the responsibility of the nurse to the family during these years? A healthy infant, child, and adolescent will bring to marriage healthy germ plasm. Healthy germ plasm will produce healthy citizens, and on this the health of a nation depends!

TYPES OF REPRODUCTION

Asexual reproduction

In plants and in members of the animal kingdom lacking a backbone (invertebrates), reproduction is accomplished by the following methods:

1. Fission, in which there is a division into two equal parts such as occurs in bacteria or in single-celled animals.
2. Fragmentation, in which there is growth from stem fragments, such as occurs when, for example, ivy roots as a result of being immersed in water.
3. Budding, in which there is a small protrusion from the parent plant, which is common in plant life. Asexual reproduction does not involve union of two organisms possessing diversified germ cells.

Sexual reproduction

Sexual reproduction, the process by which vertebrates reproduce, involves the union of germ cells (Fig. 2-1), an egg *(ovum)* from the female and a sperm

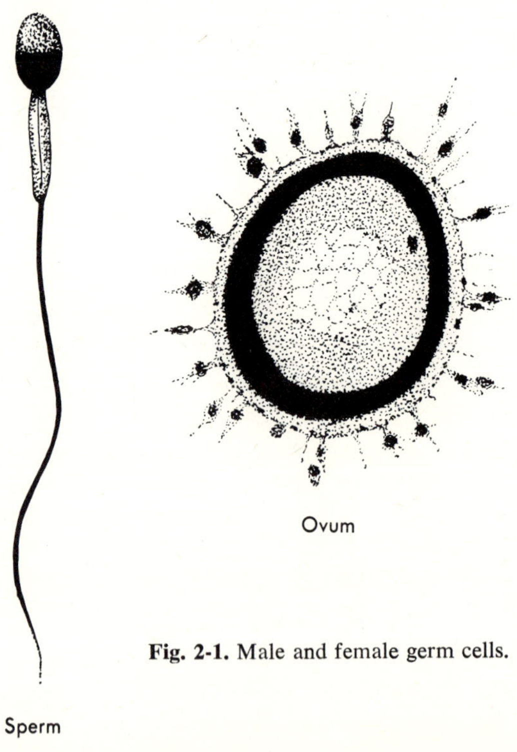

Fig. 2-1. Male and female germ cells.

(spermatozoon) from the male. Fertilization occurs when both of these germ cells unite. Once fertilized, the sperm and the ovum together become a zygote. It is only after fertilization that new life takes form.

NEW LIFE

Environment for survival of new life

The environment in which new life grows is vital to its very existence. In some aquatic and semiaquatic plants and animals, both the male and the female germ cells are deposited in water, where they meet, fuse, and develop with no care from the parents. In fish and frogs the female deposits the eggs, and the male then ejects his sperm over them. Following fertilization, the eggs nest themselves among the aquatic plant life, where they grow and develop with the parents protecting them from predators. In some species, such as the Surinam toad, the father smears the fertilized egg mass over the mother's back, and there protects it until the eggs develop into tadpoles. Conversely, the fertilized eggs of the sea horse are carried and protected by the male in an underlying belly pouch until they are able to maintain themselves.

Reptiles, birds, and mammals carry their unborn young within the body of the female. This is necessary for protection since these animals mate and reproduce on land or in trees. During sexual union the deposition of the male germ cell into the body of the female is made possible by the differences in the anatomy of both sexes. It is feasible that fertilization takes place within the body cavity of the female, since it is the female who is anatomically equipped to house and protect the developing offspring.

Life before birth

The period in which new life grows and develops within the body of the mother is known as the period of gestation or the prenatal period. It differs greatly among mammals, being as short as 21 days in the mouse and as long as 20 to 21 months in the elephant. Some mammals have a short period of gestation and deliver their young in a rather incompletely developed state—for example, the opossum and the kangaroo carry their incompletely developed young in a pouch containing nipples, where they may be fed and protected until development is completed. However, most mammals, like human beings, deliver well-developed young and have mammary glands with which to feed them following birth. The gestation period in human beings is approximately 280 days or 40 weeks.

REPRODUCTIVE ORGANS

Early embryonic development of reproductive organs

In the very early stages, human development is similar to that of other mammals. Each system develops at a specific time in the embryo, making for much order and preciseness. Disturbances in either the order or the preciseness, be it external or internal, result in imperfections.

Development of the reproductive organs begins during the fifth or sixth week of prenatal life. At first the sexes are identical, commonly known as the "indifferent period." The embryo possesses a pair of sex glands (gonads), a double set of ducts, and a genital tubercle (external protuberance) completely enclosed within genital ridges. The lateral parts of these ridges later become second kidney tubules that are beginnings of the excretory system. Thus it is apparent that the excretory and reproductive systems are closely related not only embryologically but also anatomically, which explains the frequency with which organisms from one system invade the other. In the sixth week the genital ridges begin to bulge and eventually become the ovaries and testes.

During the sixth week of gestation, a pair of ducts develops in both sexes. In the female the genital ridges form grooves, and the edges meet to form tubes. The uppermost ends remain open, expand, and form the fringed edges of the fallopian tube. The upper end of each duct becomes the oviduct, and the lower portions unite to form the uterus and the upper third of the vagina. In the male no special ducts are formed, but rather the second kidney tubules become the urethra, which later transports the urine and the sperm. The development of the third kidney allows the second kidney tubules to become the efferent ductules, which lead from the testes into the epididymis.

The mammary glands are formed ventrally in mammals and appear at the

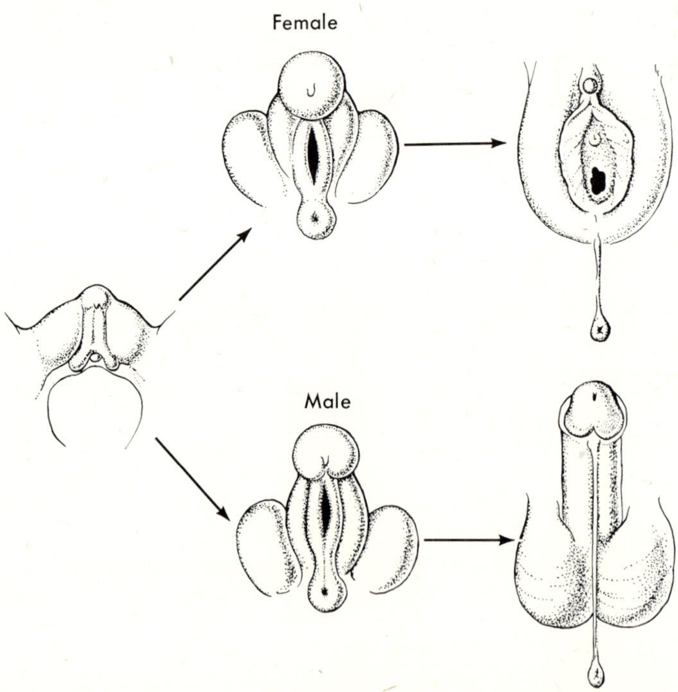

Fig. 2-2. Embryology of the female and male external genitalia.

sixth prenatal week in both sexes. At the time of birth the glands are found on the ventral wall of the thorax and are discernible by two small nipples.

At the sixth prenatal week the external genitalia resemble a protuberance in the midline of the ventral side of the body between the umbilical cord and the tail. As development of the internal organs progresses, the external genitalia take form (Fig. 2-2). While there is an increasing protuberance in the structures of the male, there is a decreasing recessiveness of the female structures. The sex of an embryo, then, is not possibly discernible before the twelfth week of prenatal life.

Reproductive organs at birth

At birth the reproductive organs are well developed. Little change occurs in them until the time of puberty. A knowledge of anatomy and physiology of the male and female reproductive organs is essential to the understanding of the changes at puberty.

SELECTED REFERENCES

Balinsky, B. I.: An introduction to embryology, Philadelphia, 1960, W. B. Saunders Co.

Barnes, A. C.: Intrauterine development, Philadelphia, 1968, Lea & Febiger.

Eastman, N. J., and Hellman, L. M.: Williams obstetrics, ed. 13, New York, 1966, Appleton-Century & Appleton-Century-Crofts.

Huffman, J. W.: The gynecology of childhood and adolescence, Philadelphia, 1968, W. B. Saunders Co.

Martin, P. C.: Human development, New York, 1960, The Ronald Press Co.

Questions for study

1. Define reproduction. What is its ultimate purpose?
2. Define asexual and sexual reproduction.
3. What are the essentials during the prenatal period for survival of new life?
4. Describe the embryonic development of the reproductive organs in the male and female.
5. When is sexuality discernible during the prenatal period?

CHAPTER 3

ANATOMY AND PHYSIOLOGY OF THE REPRODUCTIVE ORGANS

MALE REPRODUCTIVE ORGANS

The external genitalia in the male (Fig. 3-1) consists of the penis and the scrotum. The penis is composed of columns of erectile or cavernous tissue, separately enclosed by fibrous coverings held together by a covering of skin. It hangs downward directly in front of the symphysis pubis. The tip of the penis (glans penis) contains a small opening, the urethral orifice. The glans penis is sensitive because of its many nerve endings. It is covered by a foreskin. Smegma, a whitish cheesy material, is commonly found around the glans penis beneath the foreskin. If the foreskin is too tight to permit cleansing, circumcision (removal of the foreskin) is commonly performed to prevent irritation. In the Jewish faith, circumcision of all male infants 7 days after birth is an important religious ritual called a berith.

The penis has two functions: (1) it is the male organ of copulation by which sperm is introduced into the vagina, and (2) it transports urine from the bladder to the outside of the body.

As a copulatory organ the penis must be erect and rigid, as opposed to its usual flaccid state. Since it is a sensitive organ, it can become erect in a matter of seconds in response to physical and psychic erotic stimulation. The mechanism for erection involves engorgement of the vascular beds of the corpora cavernosa and the corpus spongiosum of the three erectile columns of the penis. With erection, copulation and ejaculation are accomplished. After ejaculation the penis returns to its flaccid state.

Emission and ejaculation may be described simply. Under the control of the sympathetic nerve fibers, the smooth muscle of the ductus deferens, seminal vesicles, and prostate contracts, forcing the semen into the prostatic urethra. At the same time the sphincter vesicae muscle contracts to close the internal urethral orifice, which prevents sperm from being ejaculated into the bladder. Emissions

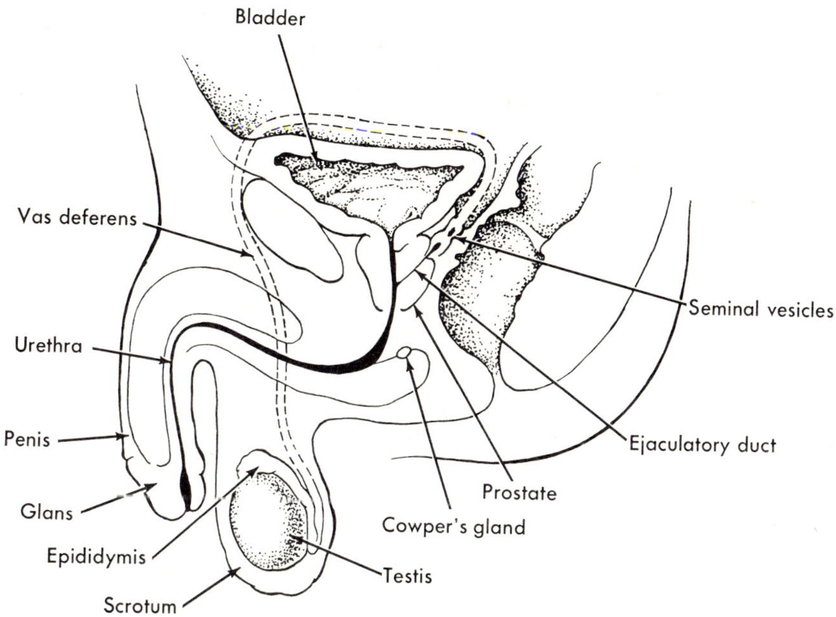

Fig. 3-1. Male reproductive organs.

and ejaculation are forceful pulsating contractions of the ischiocavernosus and bulbospongiosus muscles under parasympathetic stimulation. The semen is then forced under pressure through the urethral meatus.

The scrotum is a saclike appendage suspended from the perineum. It contains testes, or testicles, two ovoid bodies composed of seminiferous tubules that are suspended by a spermatic cord. Spermatozoa are produced in the seminiferous tubules in large number from puberty to old age. The testes are suspended in the scrotum to protect them from the extremely high temperature within the abdominal cavity. In early fetal life or shortly after birth the testes move downward into the scrotum. Failure of the testes to descend is known as cryptorchidism. Since sperm production would be impaired (resulting in sterility), endocrine therapy or surgical intervention would be indicated if descension does not occur before puberty.

At the base of each testis is a mass of convoluted tubules known as the epididymis. These tubules continue to form the vas deferens (ductus deferens) and together with the nerves, lymphatics, and blood vessels form the spermatic cord. The cord then passes through the inguinal canal, upward and backward between the fundus of the bladder, and meets the cord from the opposite testicle. At the base of the prostate gland, which surrounds the base of the bladder, the spermatic cord becomes narrowed and is joined by the seminal vesicles to form the ejaculatory duct.

Once the spermatozoa mature at puberty, they are propelled from the tubules to the epididymis and through the spermatic cord. As the spermatozoa approach the seminal vesicles, they mix with the secretions from the prostate gland, the seminal vesicles, and the bulbourethral (Cowper's) glands and are ejaculated through the urethra. During seminal emission only sperm is transported through the urethra.

The semen or seminal fluid is a mixture of spermatozoa and secretions of the epididymis, seminal vesicles, and bulbourethral and urethral glands. These secretions maintain a safe environment for the life of the sperm. The secretions aid in motility and provide nourishment—their alkalinity neutralizes the acid environment of the urethra, protecting the sperm. Semen is colorless, gelatinous, and contains several hundred million sperm cells in 6 to 8 ml. of seminal fluid. Spermatic fluid also contains an enzyme, hyaluronidase, which facilitates penetration of the ovum by the sperm.

FEMALE REPRODUCTIVE ORGANS

External genitalia

The external genitalia in the female (Fig. 3-2) include the mons veneris, the labia minora, the labia majora, the vagina, the clitoris, the urethra, and the

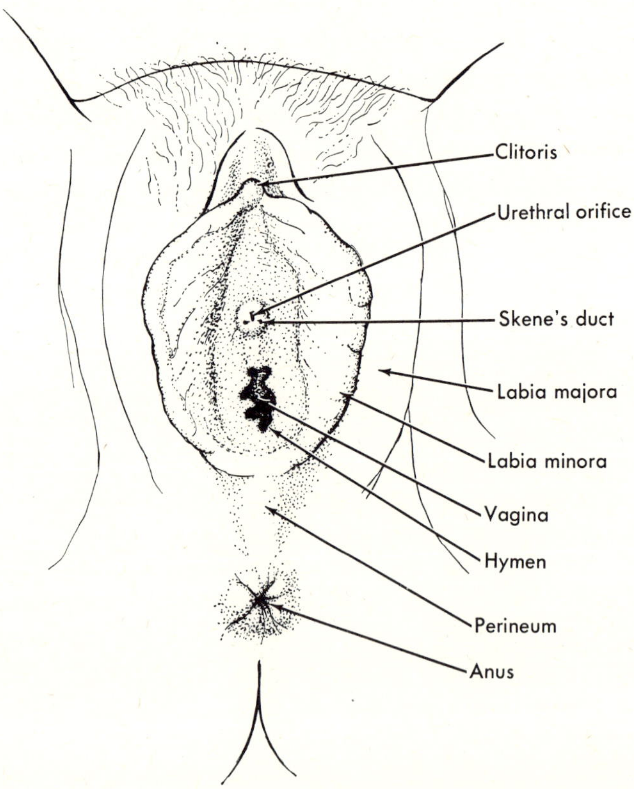

Fig. 3-2. External female genitalia.

perineum. The external genitalia (called also the vulva or the pudendum) are protective in function and sensitive to touch. The size and shape of the vulva differ among women.

The mons veneris is a pad of fatty tissue covered with hair and is located directly above the symphysis. The hair pattern is significant in determining hormonal levels, since it differs greatly in the male and female. An upward triangular hair growth toward the umbilicus designates androgenic activity. Extending downward alongside both thighs are two fatty layers of tissue covered with hair known as the labia majora; their innermost flaps are the labia minora. Both these structures are rich in nerve and blood supply, making them quite sensitive.

At the extreme upper end (directly beneath the mons veneris) where the labia meet is a fold of sensitive erectile tissue, the clitoris. The clitoris is analogous to the penis and becomes erect during sexual excitability.

Directly below the clitoris is a small fold of mucous membrane. As the folds are surveyed closely, there is a small opening leading into the urethra, the urinary meatus. On either side of the meatus, practically invisible to the naked eye, are two small glands known as Skene's glands. These glands are sensitive and become easily infected, particularly with the gonococcus.

Below the urinary meatus is the vagina. The vaginal opening is partially covered by a membrane known as the hymen. This membrane is perforated at the time of sexual union, yet the opening varies in size from a pinpoint to one that admits the tip of one or two fingers.

Even in young women before coitus occurs, there is a small opening allowing for passage of secretions and the menstrual flow. The vagina is a musculomembranous canal extending to the uterus—the bladder lies anteriorly, the rectum posteriorly. Its tissue is composed of many rugae (folds) that possess an ability for great distention and dilatation. At the lateral distal walls of the vagina are found the Bartholin glands, which secrete a lubricating substance during sexual excitement. At times these glands become infected. The vagina has three functions: (1) it is the canal through which the menstrual flow escapes; (2) it is the female organ of sexual union; and (3) it serves as the birth canal at the time of delivery.

The upper end of the vagina ends in a blind vault since the cervix of the uterus projects into the vaginal canal. The blind vault is known as the fornix and is divided into anterior, posterior, and lateral fornices. The vagina is attached higher in the posterior wall of the cervix, making the posterior fornix deeper than the anterior fornix. It is through the thin walls of the fornices that other pelvic organs can be palpated on pelvic examination. It is also through perforations of the posterior fornix that the peritoneal cavity can be easily explored. The vagina, although abundant in blood and lymph supply, is lacking in nerve supply, making it an insensitive organ. It is kept lubricated by secretions from the uterus and has an acid environment.

The perineum consists of muscles (Fig. 3-3) and fascia supporting the pelvic structures. The muscles can be divided into the urogenital and the pelvic diaphragm

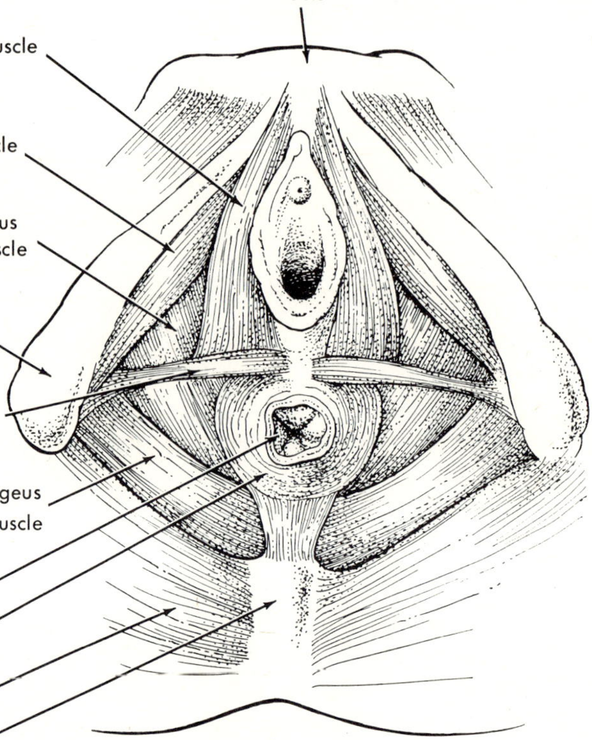

Fig. 3-3. Muscles of the perineum.

muscles. The urogenital muscles are the deep transverse perineal muscles, such as the muscle constricting the urethra. The pelvic diaphragm muscles are the coccygeus and the levator ani muscles. The levator ani muscles consist of the iliococcygeus, the pubococcygeus, and the puborectalis, which support the pelvic structures and through which pass the urethra, the vagina, and the rectum. These muscles aid in constricting the vagina and the rectum. Between the vagina and the anus there are three muscles that reinforce the pelvic floor and are sometimes incised or lacerated during delivery: the bulbocavernosus, the transverse, and the external sphincter of the anus.

Internal genitalia

The internal genitalia in the female (Fig. 3-4) include the uterus, the fallopian tubes, and the ovaries.

The uterus is a muscular organ in the pelvic cavity with the bladder lying directly anteriorly and the rectum lying posteriorly. There are three distinct layers: (1) the innermost layer known as the endometrium (shed during menstrual flow), (2) the middle muscular layer known as the myometrium, and (3) the outer layer

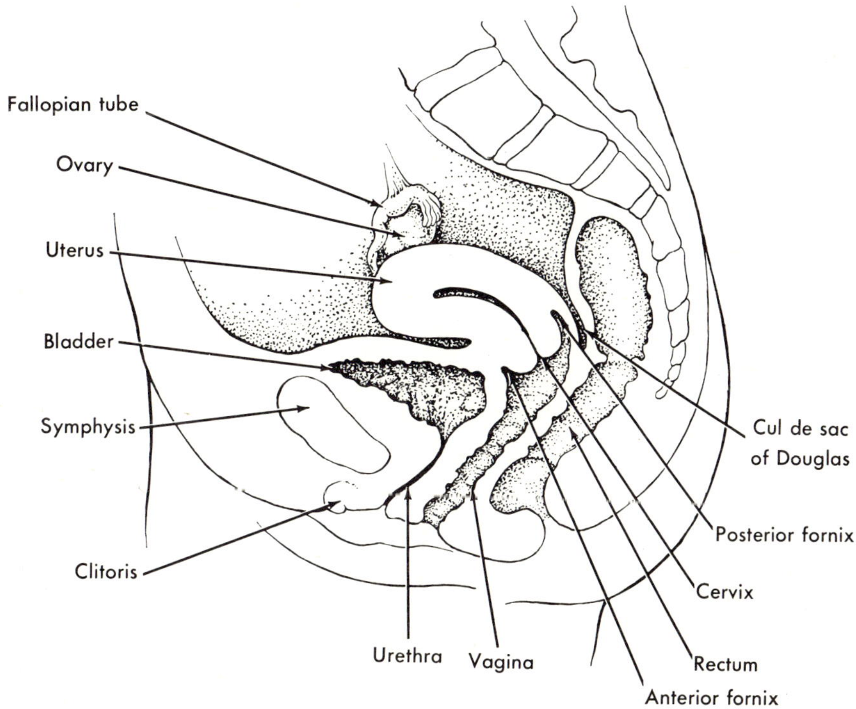

Fig. 3-4. Internal female genitalia.

known as the perimetrium. The uterus is partially covered by peritoneum anteriorly, since its lower portion is united to the posterior wall of the bladder. The posterior wall of the uterus is directly covered with peritoneum, and its lower portion forms the anterior portion of the cul-de-sac of Douglas (a blind pouch).

The uterus is composed of nonstriated or smooth muscle. It is divided into two unequal parts, the upper triangular portion, the corpus, and the lower cylindric portion, the cervix. At the lateral top portion of the corpus are the insertions of the fallopian tubes, one on either side. That portion of the uterus extending above the tubes is the fundus. The muscle fibers in the fundus lie in a crisscross fashion and have the power of great retractability and contractability. The muscles of the lower uterine isthmus and of the cervix are circular in structure, making effacement and dilatation feasible (Fig. 3-5). The blood supply to the uterus is derived principally from the uterine arteries (branches of the hypogastric arteries) and to a lesser extent from the ovarian arteries (branches of the aorta) (Fig. 3-6). The nerve supply to the uterus is derived principally from the sympathetic nervous system and also from the parasympathetic and cerebrospinal nervous systems. The uterus in adults measures 2½ inches in length, 1¼ inches in width, and ¾ inch in thickness, and it weighs about 2½ ounces.

The cervix is long and cylindric, having an internal os (opening into the isth-

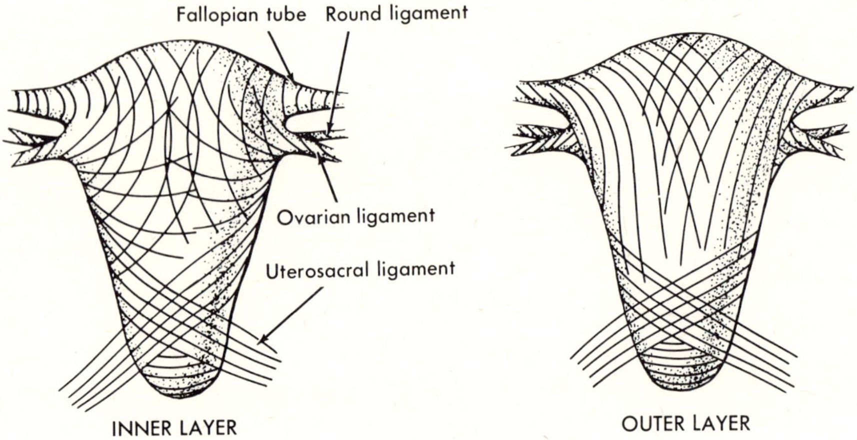

Fig. 3-5. Musculature of the uterus.

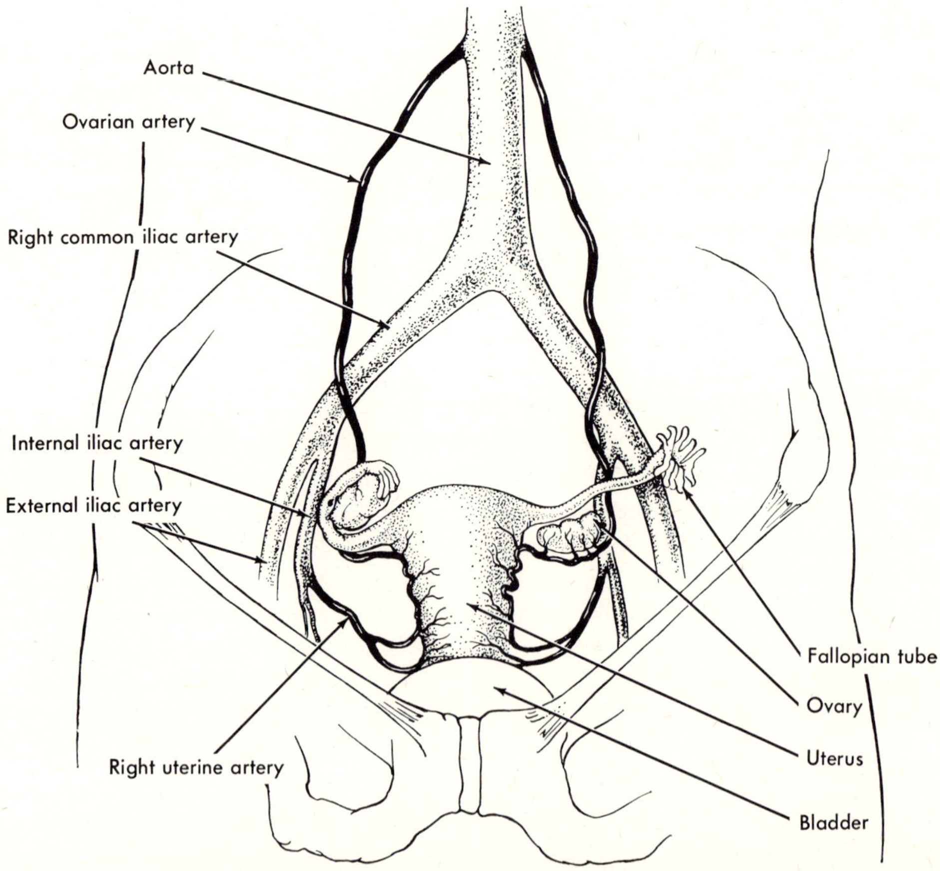

Fig. 3-6. Blood supply to the uterus.

mus) and an external os (opening into the vagina). The muscles within the cervix are circular and have the ability to dilate. The tissue in the vaginal canal is continuous with the epithelium of the cervix up to the internal os. Beyond the internal os the cervical canal is composed of glandular epithelium, which serves as a lubricant aiding in sperm motility.

The broad ligaments are winglike structures attached to the lateral walls of the uterus; they divide the pelvic cavity into anterior and posterior portions. The round ligaments are on either side of the uterus, just beneath the insertion of the tubes, extending upward and outward. They traverse the inguinal canal and terminate in the labia majora. The uterosacral ligaments extend from the posterior and upper portion of the cervix and are inserted into the fascia of the second and third sacral vertebrae. It is apparent that although the ligaments act as supports and anchors, the uterus is movable and not fixed within the pelvic cavity.

The uterus has three functions: (1) it prepares itself monthly for reception of the fertilized ovum—if the ovum has not been fertilized, menstruation occurs; (2) during pregnancy it is an efficient home for the baby; and (3) during labor its muscles contract, aiding in propelling the baby through the birth canal.

The fallopian tubes are convoluted muscular canals that are very narrow at the portion where they enter the uterus, becoming wider toward the distal fimbriated ends. Each tube is divided into four portions starting from the insertion into the uterus: the interstitial portion, the isthmus, the ampulla, and the infundibulum. The narrowest portion is the isthmus; the widest portion is the ampulla. The infundibulum is fringelike, opens into the abdominal cavity, and is near the ovary. With the exception of the interstitial portion, the length of the entire tube is included in the upper portion of the broad ligament.

The cilia (small hairlike projections) within the tube aid in directing foreign bodies from the abdominal cavity into the uterus, a one-way process. The tubes are movable, and the musculature within the canals undergoes rhythmic contractions, which aid in moving the ovum along the tubes. The tubes are composed of elastic tissue and are richly supplied with blood vessels and lymphatics.

The ovaries are two almond-shaped organs responsible for developing and producing ova. They are attached to the posterior wall of the broad ligament. Their average size is from 2.5 to 5 cm. in length, 1.5 to 3 cm. in breadth, and 0.6 to 1.5 cm. in thickness. The ovarian ligament extends from the lateral and posterior portions of the uterus. The ovary is in close proximity to the fimbriated end of the tube, making it feasible for the ovum to be picked up at the time of ovulation. The ovary has two portions, an inner medulla, made up of connective tissue and blood vessels, and an outer portion, the cortex, in which are found the primordial cells.

MAMMARY GLANDS (BREASTS)

In the female the breasts are located on each side of the anterior chest wall extending from the second to the sixth or seventh rib. The breasts vary in size and shape depending upon individual differences and age.

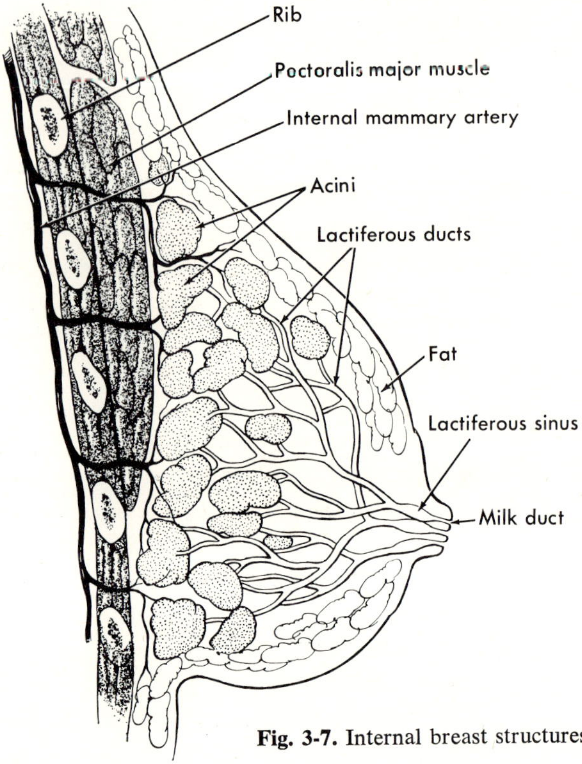

Fig. 3-7. Internal breast structures.

Fig. 3-8. External breast structures.

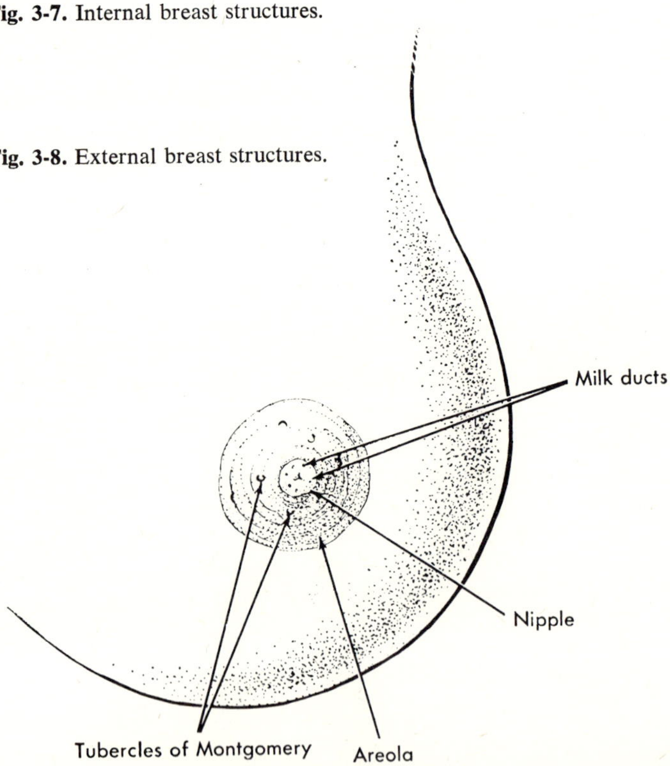

Each lobe contains several lobules composed of acini close to a vast blood and lymph supply. The acini (Fig. 3-7) in each lobe empty into lactiferous sinuses, which eventually terminate into openings called milk ducts in the nipples.

Breast tissue consists chiefly of glandular connective tissue and adipose tissue. The outer surface (Fig. 3-8) of the breast is composed of a delicate epidermis. The nipple is composed of erectile fibromuscular tissue. Completely circling the nipple is an area about 1.5 to 2.5 cm. in diameter known as the areola. The wrinkled, puckered areas of the areola are composed of sebaceous glands known as the tubercles of Montgomery. These glands secrete a lubricating substance that protects the nipple during lactation.

The blood supply to the breasts is derived from the thoracic branches of the axillary, intercostal, and internal thoracic arteries. Branches of these three main arteries supply the areola, the nipple, and the secreting parts of the gland. The mammary veins follow the same course as the arteries.

The lymphatic vessels of the breast originate in the interlobular spaces and in the walls of the lactiferous ducts. Lymphatic vessels in the center of the breast pass through an intricate plexus beneath the areola and drain laterally into the axillary nodes. The vessels draining the medial portion of the breast extend through the thoracic wall to the sternal nodes and through the pectoralis major muscle to the subclavian nodes.

Nerve supply is derived from the anterior and lateral cutaneous branches of the fourth, fifth, and sixth thoracic nerves, and from the supraclavicular nerves that supply the portion above the fourth rib.

Although the breasts are a distance from the pelvic female organs of reproduction, there is a functional relationship. The breasts are considered accessory organs of reproduction and develop in the female at the time of puberty. Their function is to supply the newborn with nourishment during the first few months of life at the termination of pregnancy.

The physiology of lactation will be discussed later in Chapter 15.

SELECTED REFERENCES

Eastman, N. J., and Hellman, L. M.: Williams obstetrics, ed. 13, New York, 1966, Appleton-Century & Appleton-Century-Crofts.

Kimber, D. C., and Gray, C. E.: In Leavell, L. C., editor: Anatomy and physiology, ed. 14, New York, 1961, The Macmillan Co.

Montagu, A.: The reproductive development of the female, New York, 1957, Julian Press, Inc.

Netter, F.: The reproductive system, Summit, N. J., 1964, Ciba Pharmaceutical Co.

Questions for study

1. Describe the anatomic structure and function of the external and internal organs in the male reproductive system.
2. Describe the anatomic structure and function of the external and internal organs in the female reproductive system.
3. What are the main sources of blood and nerve supply to the uterus?
4. Describe the muscles in the perineum.
5. Describe the anatomic structure and function of the breasts in the female.

CHAPTER 4

THE PELVIS

The pelvis is significant since it protects the female internal organs of reproduction. Safely within it lie the uterus, fallopian tubes, ovaries, and adjacent structures such as the ligaments supporting the uterus and blood vessels and nerve fibers that traverse the organs. It is through the bony pelvis and birth canal that the baby must pass in the birth process.

ANATOMY OF THE BONY PELVIS

The pelvis (Fig. 4-1) resembles a basin and is partly ligamentous and partly bony. It is supported by the movable vertebrae and rests upon the lower limbs. The pelvis is composed of four bones: two innominate bones, the sacrum, and the coccyx. Each innominate bone is composed of the ilium, the ischium, and the pubis.

The male pelvis is heavy and conical in appearance, is less flared at the iliac portion, and has strong muscular attachments. In comparison, the female pelvis is lighter in weight, less concave, markedly flared at the iliac portion, and is pliable and movable.

The bones of the female pelvis are joined by a fibrous cartilaginous tissue that becomes elastic and pliable during pregnancy because of the ovarian hormone relaxin. The joints are the following: the sacroiliac, joining the sacrum and iliac bones; the sacrococcygeal, joining the sacrum and the coccyx; and the symphysis pubis, joining the ischial bones anteriorly.

Division of the pelvis

The female pelvis is divided into the false pelvis and the true pelvis. The false pelvis (Fig. 4-2, *A*) lies above the linea terminalis and is bounded posteriorly by the lumbar vertebrae, anteriorly by the abdominal wall, and laterally by the iliac fossae. It serves no significant purpose in obstetrics, although as the baby grows the enlarged uterus rises into the false pelvis.

The true pelvis (Fig. 4-2, *B*) is that portion of the bony pelvis through which

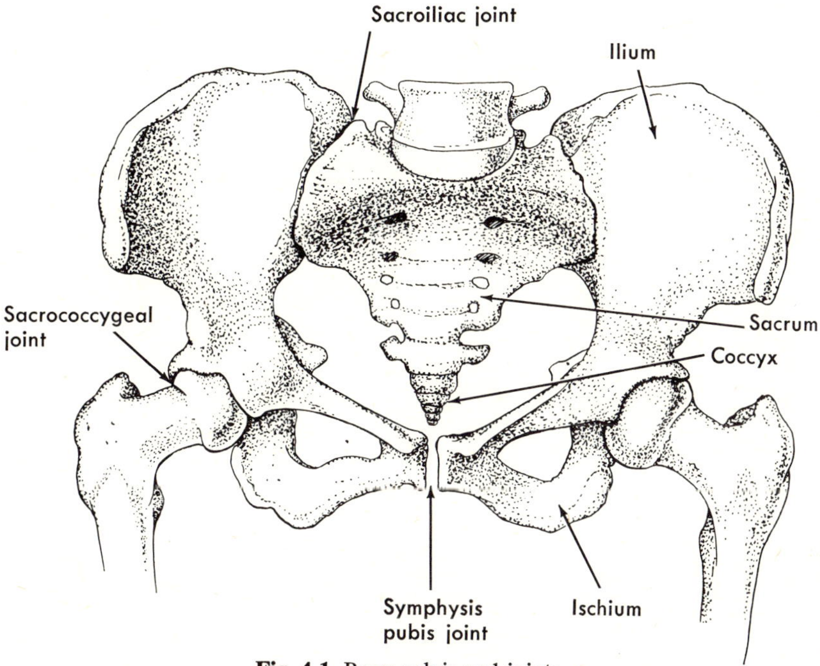

Fig. 4-1. Bony pelvis and joints.

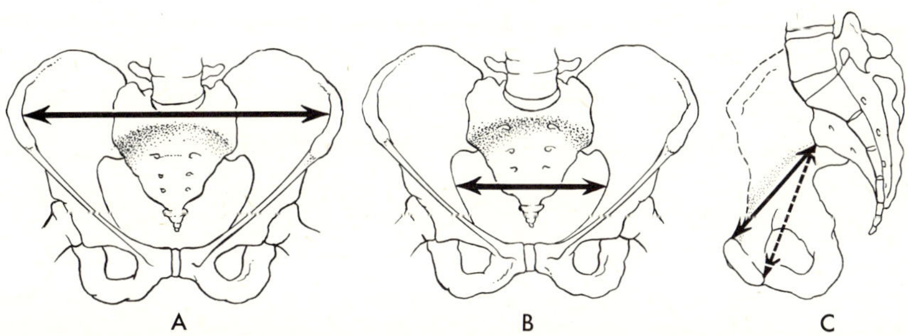

Fig. 4-2. Pelvis. **A,** False. **B,** True. **C,** Lateral view, false (above solid arrow) and true (below solid arrow).

the baby passes. It is bordered posteriorly by the anterior surface of the sacrum, laterally by the inner surface of the ischial bones and the sacrosciatic notches and ligaments, and anteriorly by the pubic bones and ascending rami of the ischial bones. The true pelvis is of great obstetric importance. It supports the muscles of the pelvic floor and gives form and direction to the birth canal.

Planes and diameters of the pelvis

The size and shape of the female pelvis adapt to its childbearing function (Fig. 4-3). The true pelvis has two planes of greater dimensions known as the inlet

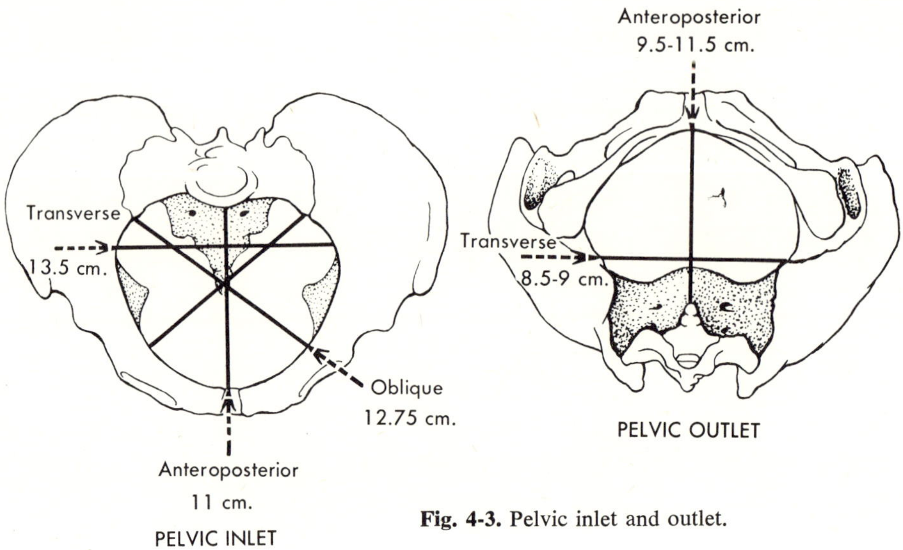

Fig. 4-3. Pelvic inlet and outlet.

(superior strait) and the outlet (inferior strait). The plane of least pelvic dimensions is the midpelvis.

The inlet (superior strait) is the upper boundary of the true pelvis. It is somewhat heart-shaped, being bordered posteriorly by the promontory of the sacrum, laterally by the linea terminalis, and anteriorly by the upper portion of the symphysis pubis. Four diameters traverse the inlet: the transverse, the anteroposterior, and the two oblique diameters. The anteroposterior diameter extends from the promontory of the sacrum to the upper margin of the symphysis pubis, known as the conjugata vera or the true conjugate. Normally the true conjugate measures 11 cm. or more and is an important obstetric diameter. The transverse diameter is at right angles to the conjugata vera, extending between the linea terminalis on either side. It normally measures 13.5 cm. Each of the oblique diameters extends from one of the sacroiliac joints to the iliopectineal eminence on the opposite side of the pelvis. The oblique diameters are designated as right and left, using the sacroiliac joints as starting points. These diameters normally measure 12.75 cm.

The outlet (inferior strait) is that portion of the true pelvis bounded anteriorly by the symphysis pubis and the pubic arch, posteriorly by the coccyx and the sacrosciatic ligaments, and laterally by the ischial tuberosities. Three diameters traverse the outlet: the anteroposterior, the transverse, and the posterior sagittal. The outlet resembles a triangle—the base is the distance between the tuberosities being completed by the pubic arch. The anteroposterior diameter extending from the lower margin of the symphysis pubis to the tip of the sacrum measures 9.5 to 11.5 cm. This variation in measurement depends upon the movability of the coccyx. The transverse diameter is the distance between the inner edges of the ischial tuberosities, which measures 11 cm. The posterior sagittal diameter extends from the tip

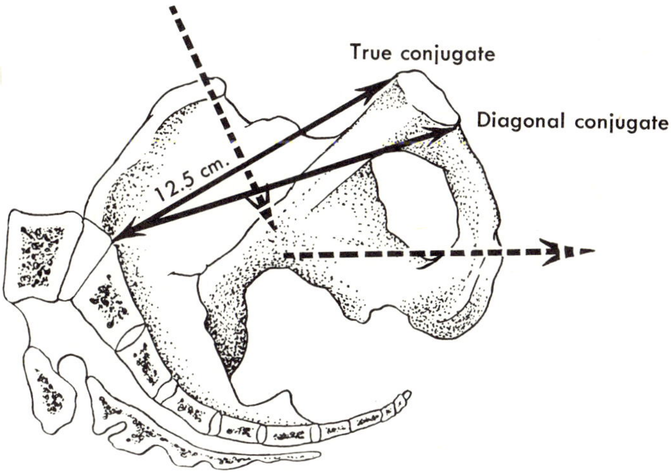

Fig. 4-4. Inclination of the pelvis.

of the sacrum to the right-angled intersection, with a line between the ischial tuberosities, and measures 7.5 cm.

The midpelvis has the plane of least dimensions. The anteroposterior diameter extends from the lower margin of the symphysis pubis to the sacrum, measuring 11.5 cm. The transverse diameter extends between the ischial spines and measures 10.5 cm.

It is apparent that at the inlet the larger diameter is the transverse and the smaller is the anteroposterior. At the outlet the reverse is true—the anteroposterior diameter is larger, and the transverse diameter is smaller.

Entrance into the true pelvis at the inlet finds the inclination is downward and curved backward, and midway it becomes downward and outward, stovepipe fashion (Fig. 4-4).

Classification of the pelves

The pelves of all women differ—no two are alike. The varying differences in pelves are a result of heredity, disease, injury, development, and nutrition. The pelves in most women do not ossify completely until approximately 20 to 25 years of age.

Not only does the size of the pelvis have significance, but also the shape or relationship of certain dimensions of the pelvis to each other is of equal importance. Caldwell and Moloy devised a classification that considers the type of posterior and anterior segments at the inlet. There are four types—the gynecoid, the anthropoid, the android, and the platypelloid (Fig. 4-5). The gynecoid or typical female pelvis is round and somewhat heart-shaped, the anthropoid or ape-like pelvis is oval-shaped, the android or masculine type pelvis is triangular at the inlet and narrowed at the midplane and outlet, and the platypelloid or flat pelvis has

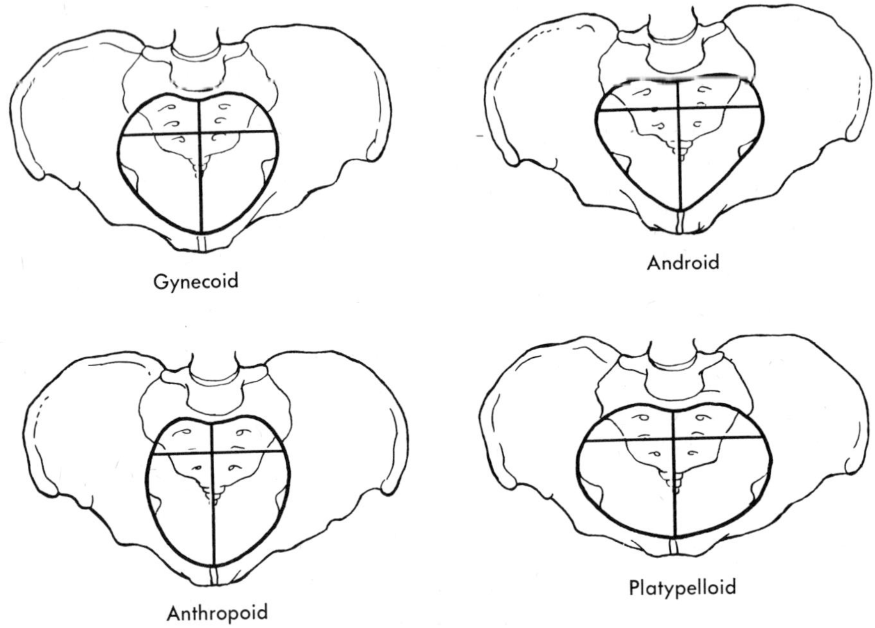

Fig. 4-5. Caldwell-Moloy classification of pelves.

a widening at the outlet. In many women there is a combination of these basic types.

Pelvic measurements

To assure a safe delivery a pelvic examination is an integral part of the physical examination of every pregnant women. Measurement is accomplished by external means, internal vaginal examination, or roentgenologic methods. External measurements provide only a limited amount of information concerning the size and shape of the true pelvis. The internal vaginal examination gives a true picture of the inner bony pelvis. Roentgenologic examination measures the size of the bony pelvis as well as the size of the baby and is more accurate.

External measurements. External measurements are done with a pelvimeter and provide a limited amount of information. Measurements commonly made are the intercristal diameter (the distance between the two lateral edges of the iliac crests), which averages 28 cm., the interspinous diameter (the distance between the external aspects of the superoiliac spines), which averages 25 cm., the intertrochanteric diameter (the distance between the external aspects of the trochanters of the femurs), which averages 31 cm., and the external conjugate (the distance between the anterior aspect of the symphysis pubis to the depression below the spines of the fifth lumbar vertebrae), which averages 18 to 20 cm.

The most important external measurement is that of the distance between the ischial tuberosities or the biischial diameter. This outlet measurement of the pelvis

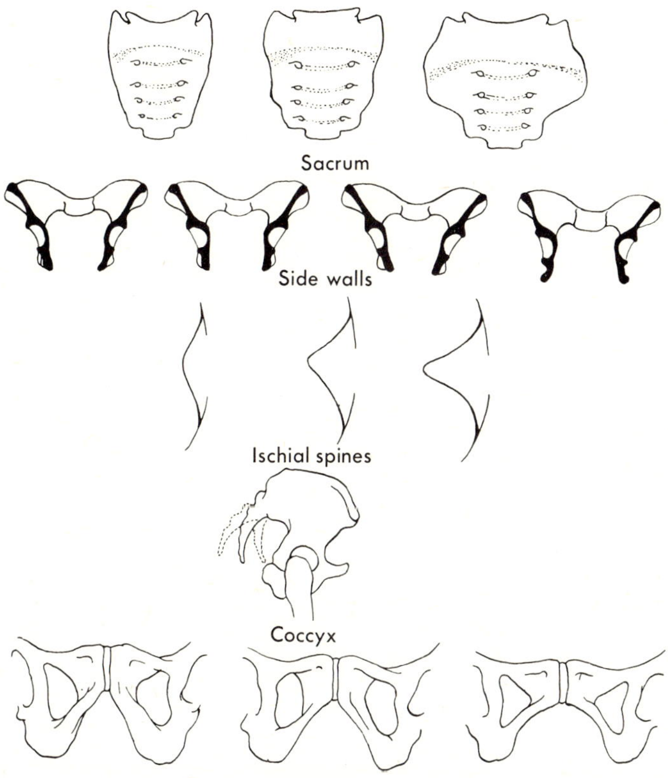

Fig. 4-6. Internal pelvic structures.

is made with a Thoms retractor with the mother in lithotomy position. Normally the distance between the tuberosities measures 8 cm. or more.

Internal measurements. Pelvic examination is done to determine the diameters of the inlet and to determine the shape and structures within the true pelvis (Fig. 4-6). With the mother in lithotomy position and her legs supported in stirrups, the evaluation is made. The fingers are introduced into the vagina, and by palpation the parts of the pelvis discussed in the following paragraphs are evaluated.

Sacrum. The width, length, and inclination of the sacrum are particularly significant. A sacrum that is narrow makes the entire true pelvis smaller; a sacrum that is long makes the pelvis deeper; a sacrum that is not concave makes the entire posterior diameter smaller. A normal sacrum is somewhat concave and is of average width and length.

Side walls. The inner portions of the ischium and the ilium form the side walls. Normally these are parallel, rounded, and concave. When the side walls converge, the pelvis becomes narrowed.

Ischial spines. The ischial spines are small protuberances midway in the true pelvis. This portion is the narrowest through which the baby passes. Normally the spines are rounded and blunt. At times they are prominent and sharp, shortening the diameter considerably.

Coccyx. Normally the coccyx is somewhat movable because of the coccygeal joint. At times the coccyx is immovable because of injury, trauma, or anatomic defect, which may constrict the diameter at the outlet.

Pubic arch. The pubic arch is that portion of the true pelvis extending from one ischial tuberosity to the other. Normally the pubic arch is moderate; however, should it be narrow the diameter of the triangle at the outlet is made smaller.

Diagonal conjugate. The diagonal conjugate (D.C.) is the distance between the promontory of the sacrum and the undersurface of the symphysis pubis. Normally this measurement is approximately 12.5 cm., 1.5 to 2 cm. longer than the true conjugate, since the width of the symphysis is included. This measurement is done by the physician, directing the fingers of the examining hand inward and upward so that the middle finger reaches the promontory of the sacrum. The point at which the examining hand meets the symphysis is marked by using the tip of the finger of the other hand, and measurement is made with a measuring device or a pelvimeter when the hand is withdrawn.

Roentgen-ray pelvimetry. Roentgen-ray pelvimetry is done to determine the transverse diameter of the outlet and to outline the bony pelvis more fully. It is indicated to determine the size of the baby's head when there is a history of a previous difficult delivery, or during a long labor without progress. The effects of irradiation on the mother and the baby need to be considered, particularly since the effect on the gonads of the baby cannot be predicted. The damage to the baby may be seen immediately or in later life—childhood leukemia sometimes develops. An increase in congenital malformations may appear in generations to follow. Potential hazards from roentgen-ray examinations are reduced when ultra-fast films, lightning screens, shielding, and high milliamperage are used. The Genetics Committee of the National Academy of Sciences has set specific dosage standards to be used—however, the Committee also states that even recommended dosage cannot be considered completely harmless. Roentgen-ray pelvimetry is therefore used only when there are obstetric complications.

ANATOMY OF THE BABY'S HEAD

Since 95% of all babies are born head first, a study of the fetal skull is important to understand the process by which it passes through the pelvis and birth canal.

The baby's head is composed of the bony skull and the face. The bony portion of the skull (Fig. 4-7) consists of the two frontal, the two parietal, the two temporal, the occipital, and the winged portions of the sphenoid bones. These bones are joined by membranous spaces called sutures. The frontal suture lies between the two frontal bones, the sagittal suture lies between the two parietal bones, the coronal suture lies between the frontal and parietal bones, and the

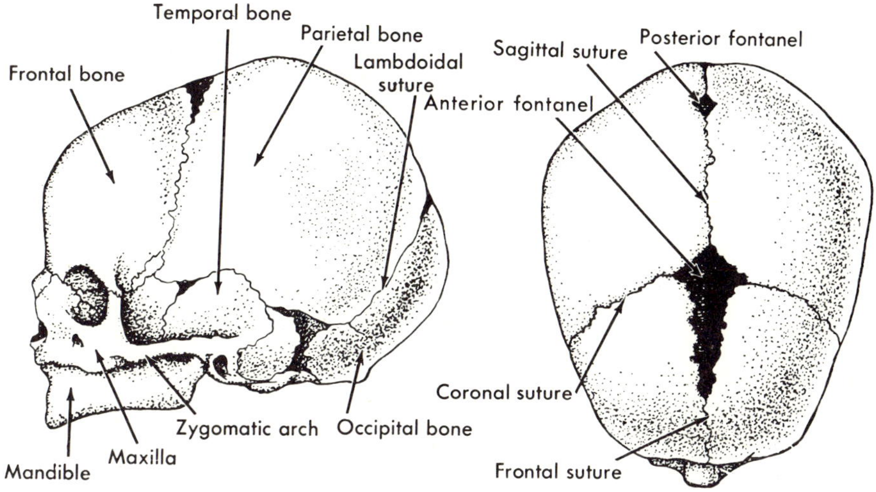

Fig. 4-7. Bones, sutures, and fontanels of the fetal skull.

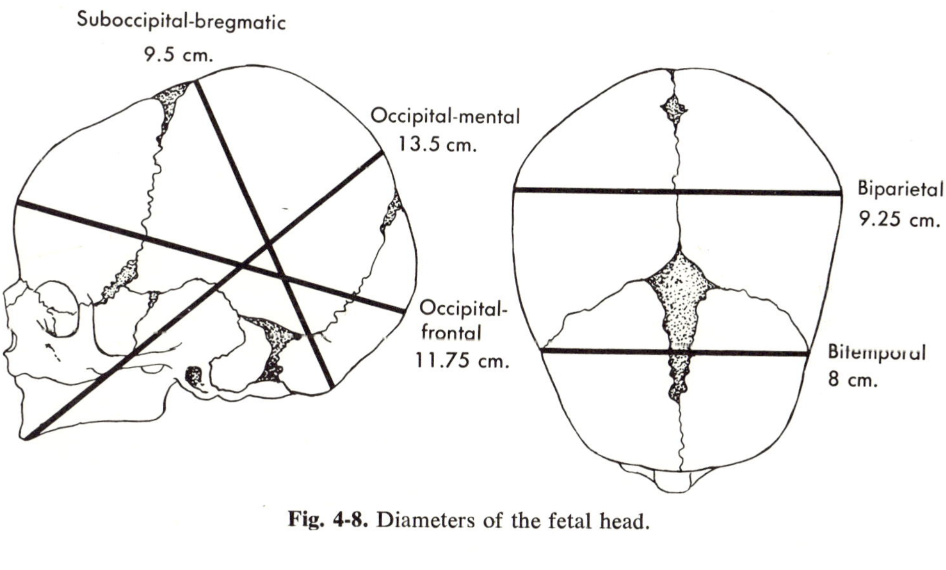

Fig. 4-8. Diameters of the fetal head.

lambdoid suture lies between the parietal and occipital bones. The areas where several sutures meet are wider and distinguishable; they are known as fontanels. The two most important fontanels in obstetrics that are also significant in normal growth and development of the child are the following: the anterior fontanel, which is diamond in shape (known as the soft spot), where frontal and sagittal sutures meet, and the posterior fontanel, which is triangular in shape, where sagittal and lambdoid sutures meet. These sutures are significant because they allow for overriding of bones in the baby's skull to facilitate delivery through the pelvis and the birth canal, and later to allow for proper brain growth before closure.

Of obstetric significance are various diameters and circumferences of the baby's skull. The occipital-frontal diameter (Fig. 4-8) measures 11.75 cm. It follows a straight line from the root of the nose to the most prominent portion of the occipital bone. The biparietal diameter measures 9.25 cm., which is the greatest transverse diameter from one parietal bone to the other. The bitemporal diameter measures 8 cm., which is the greatest distance between the two temporal bones. The occipital-mental diameter measures 13.5 cm. from the chin to the most prominent portion of the occiput. The suboccipital-bregmatic diameter measures 9.5 cm.—it follows a line from the middle of the anterior fontanel to the bony prominence of the occiput. For delivery purposes, it is well to remember that the greatest diameter of the infant's head is the occipital-mental and the smallest is the suboccipital-bregmatic.

SELECTED REFERENCES

See reference list following Chapter 13.

Questions for study

1. With a model of the pelvis, identify its bony structures and parts.
2. Identify the true pelvis, false pelvis, inlet, and outlet.
3. Which diameters of the pelvis are smallest and largest at the inlet? At the outlet?
4. Describe the inclination of the pelvis in relation to the birth process.
5. With a model of the pelvis, identify the significant structures in the true pelvis in determining adequacy for birth of the baby.
6. With a model of the baby, identify the bone sutures of the fontanels and head. Which diameter of the baby's head is smallest? Largest?

CHAPTER 5

PUBERTY

Puberty is a period during which the child incapable of reproduction is transformed into an adult capable of reproduction. During this transition there is a change in the gross morphology of the individual, in his reproductive organs, and in his psyche. Although there is a wide range as to the precise age of the onset of puberty, progression, once begun, occurs in an orderly pattern. Puberty begins when secondary sex characteristics begin to develop and ends when the individual is capable of reproduction.

PHYSICAL AND PHYSIOLOGIC CHANGES

In the male, puberty is less dramatic than in the female, beginning later and ending earlier. Any age between 10 and 14 years is within normal range for the onset of puberty. The first signs are an increase in the size of the scrotum and testes and a noticeable reddening of the scrotal skin.

Following the changes in the scrotum and testes there appears a sparse growth of hair at the base of the penis; this hair is longer and more deeply pigmented than the body hair. These changes continue for about a year. The penis begins to increase in length, the pubic hair becomes darker and coarser and covers a wider area of the pubes, the larynx enlarges, and a dramatic growth spurt begins.

A year later the pubic hair is similar to that of the adult, axillary and facial hair appears, and there is increased activity of the sweat glands. The penis continues to become larger in circumference and length, the glans penis becomes prominent, and a first ejaculation may occur. Once ejaculation occurs in the male, the fertile period has begun and puberty ends.

Along with these alterations, changes in the breasts, voice pattern, and musculoskeletal system are apparent. Marked changes occur in breast pigmentation, and an increase in the diameter of the areola occurs. There is a noted deepening of the voice, which is related to structural changes in the larynx. By the age of 16, the physique is masculine.

In the female, puberty occurs a year earlier than in the male. Unlike the male, the female undergoes changes that are dramatic and that occur suddenly between the ages of 9 and 13 years. The first signs of puberty in the female are development of the breasts and the appearance of hair on the labia majora. The growth spurt begins with these changes and reaches a peak at the end of the first year. The adolescent female may surpass the male in size because of this growth pattern.

There is a continuing growth of breast tissue for approximately 2½ years, with continuing deposits of adipose tissue in the mons veneris, buttocks, hips, breasts, and shoulders. Pubic hair then spreads from the labia majora to the mons veneris and the abdominal wall; hair also begins to grow in the axilla. The deposits of fatty tissue increase the size of the external genitalia.

The internal reproductive organs undergo many dramatic changes. The vagina increases in size and in vascularity. The epithelium of the vagina thickens to become stratified squamous epithelium. The vaginal pH, which is neutral or slightly alkaline in the child, becomes markedly acid with a pH of 2 to 3. The thickened vaginal epithelium begins to form glycogen, and there is a reappearance of Döderlein's bacillus. The bacillus oxidizes the glycogen to form lactic acid, which is responsible for the lowered pH. Glycogen and the Döderlein's bacillus are present in the adult vagina but are absent during childhood.

The uterus enlarges rapidly; the uterine tubes grow in length and diameter and become straightened. The ovaries, which were ribbonlike, become ovoid and function as endocrine glands.

Puberty in the female is heralded by the first menstrual flow or menarche. Although the menarche is considered the beginning of the fertile reproductive years, many of the first menstrual cycles are anovulatory and therefore infertile.

PSYCHOLOGIC CHANGES

Because of the many physical and physiologic changes, both sexes experience changes they do not quite understand. The changes in the reproductive organs make possible heterosexual interest, the degree of interest depending largely on the degree of change. Girls mature earlier than boys, and adolescents of the same ages become disinterested in each other during this time. The girls seek out older boys since the boys they once knew are not as mature. There is a strong tendency toward detachment of parental influence, and emancipation takes on quite a struggle. The adolescent becomes slow, daydreams, and needs other adults rather than his parents. He is clumsy as his rapidly changing body gets in his way. He strives for independence and yet needs some dependence in order to feel secure. He needs to belong, to be a member of his own peer group; through this process he gradually becomes an adult.

MENSTRUATION

Menstrual cycle

At birth the connective tissue of each ovary contains approximately 100,000 primordial follicles. Through a process of atresia the number at puberty ranges between 30,000 and 40,000.

At the time of puberty, a rhythmic, cyclic pattern occurs, influencing changes in the ovaries and uterus in preparation for the reproductive process. There are four phases of the menstrual cycle: follicular (proliferative), ovulatory, luteal (progestational), and menstrual. The pituitary controls the hormonal function of the menstrual cycle by producing three gonadotropins: follicle-stimulating hormone (FSH), luteinizing hormone (LH), and luteotropic or lactogenic hormone (LTH). These hormones stimulate the ovaries to produce estrogen and progesterone.

Follicular phase. Under the influence of FSH a follicular fluid containing estrogen accumulates in the center of the follicle, and the ovum becomes known as the graafian follicle. As maturation progresses, the ovum increases in size, the nucleus moves from the center of the cell to the periphery, and a rise in estrogen levels in the bloodstream releases LH, which causes rupture and extrusion of the follicle. This process is known as ovulation. The follicular or proliferative phase is conditioned by estrogen and extends from the end of menstruation to ovulation, the latter occurring near the middle of the cycle. During this phase the endometrium thickens as estrogen levels rise.

Ovulatory phase. No marked changes occur in the endometrium during the ovulatory process. There is, however, a distinct rise in basal body temperature, which remains high until the onset of the menstrual period. The rise in body temperature is attributed to the high titers of progesterone following ovulation.

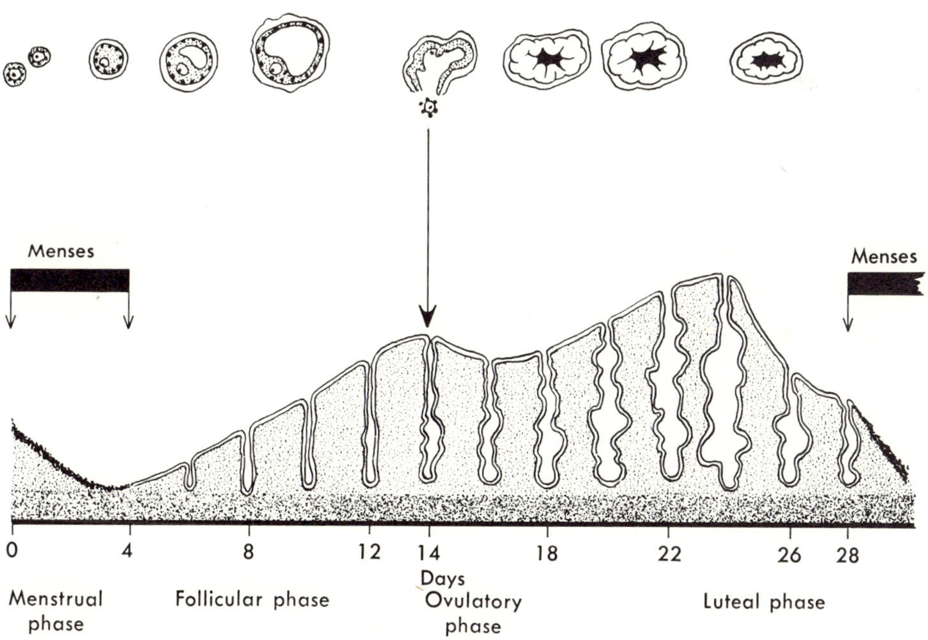

Fig. 5-1. Menstrual cycle.

Luteal (progestational) phase. Following ovulation the cavity of the ruptured graafian follicle becomes filled with a tissue known as the corpus luteum. During this phase the luteinizing hormone secretes estrogen and progesterone for a period of 8 days. The stroma of the endometrium becomes highly vascularized and edematous, the mucosa thickens, and the glands develop corkscrew and serrate features. The progestational endometrium is optimum for implantation of a fertilized ovum.

Menstrual phase. If the ovum is not fertilized by a sperm, there is a reduction in progesterone causing endometrial vascular stasis, vasoconstriction, and finally endometrial shedding with menstrual bleeding.

Clinical course of menstruation

The first menstrual period at puberty is called the menarche. The bleeding may be irregular and unpredictable at the onset. Eventually the cycle becomes rhythmic, continuing until the menopause. A typical cycle lasts anywhere from 26 to 35 days; however, individuals differ. The bleeding varies from 3 to 7 days and is usually no more than 2 to 4 ounces in amount. Menstrual blood contains mucus and destroyed cellular tissue from the endometrium that does not coagulate. When exposed to air it has a fleshy odor and can become offensive.

At the time of ovulation women experience engorgement, tingling in the breasts, an increase in vaginal secretions, spotting, and an increase in weight due to sodium and water retention. It has been found that a slight lowering with a decided sudden rise in basal body temperature is significant in determining periods of greatest fertility (Fig. 5-2).

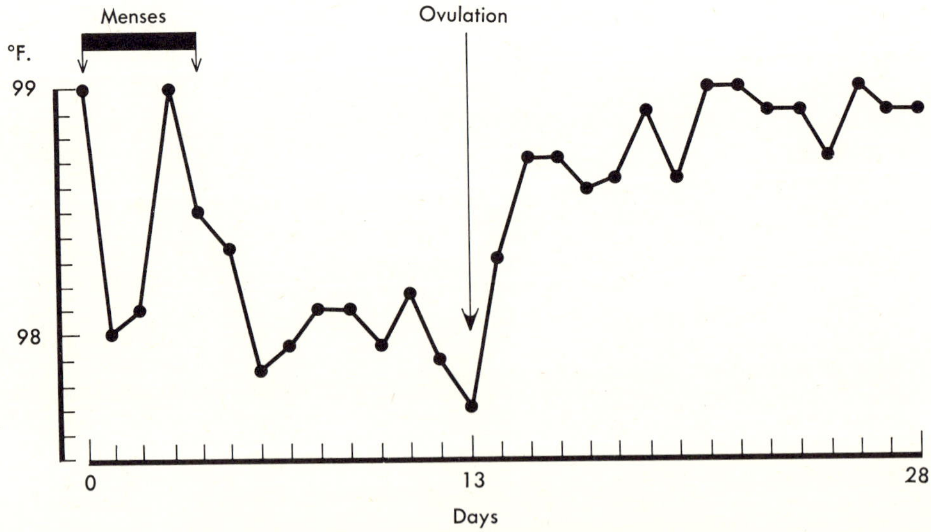

Fig. 5-2. Basal body temperature during menstrual cycle.

Premenstrual symptoms vary with individual women. Physical and mental disturbances a few days before menstruation and during the days of actual blood flow may be accompanied by headache, backache, breast fullness, abdominal discomforts such as distention and cramping, irritability, tension, drowsiness, and mental sluggishness. These symptoms may not occur in some women and in others occur in varying degrees. Most women will experience a feeling of general well-being immediately following the menstrual period.

Menstrual hygiene

At the time of puberty the knowledge of bodily functions is of primary importance in developing healthy attitudes toward normal body changes for the adolescent. Discussions with parents at home or at school are helpful in developing such attitudes. Schools have found that inviting parents to discussion classes on menstruation often clarifies erroneous misconceptions regarding personal hygiene.

Personal hygiene during menstruation is no different from daily hygiene at any other time. Frequent bathing and changing of perineal pads provide comfort and eliminate unpleasant odors. The perineal pad or tampon may be used to absorb the menstrual flow. The tampon (manufactured in various sizes) is inserted into the vaginal canal and unfolds following insertion. A string is attached to its distal end to facilitate removal. Perhaps the tampon may be difficult for the beginning young adolescent to use, and the perineal pad may serve the purpose until there is adjustment to the bodily change. The perineal pad is exposed, however, and the problem of unpleasant odor needs to be considered. This problem is not present with the use of the tampon.

Normal activity and exercise in moderation are continued during menstruation. An understanding of the discomforts will alleviate the fear and worry that something is wrong. Warm baths, good nutrition, and adequate rest will help relieve the discomforts. Heat to the abdomen and back and the knee-chest position will alleviate cramping. Symptoms that are exaggerated and prolonged or irregular menstrual periods should be reported to a physician.

SELECTED REFERENCES

Grollman, A.: Clinical endocrinology and its physiologic basis, Philadelphia, 1964, J. B. Lippincott Co.

Josselyn, I. M.: The adolescent and his world, New York, 1962, Family Service Association of America.

Lamers, W. M., Jr.: Understanding the teenager, Obstet. Gynec., vol. 33, no. 1, January, 1969.

Maddox, G.: Teenage diets, Child and Family, p. 58, Winter, 1963.

Montagu, A.: The reproductive development of the female, New York, 1957, Julian Press, Inc.

Newton, N.: Feminine hygiene, Amer. J. Nurs. **64:**100, December, 1964.

Parker, E.: The seven ages of woman, Baltimore, 1960, The Johns Hopkins Press.

Tampax, Inc.: Educational materials on menstruation, New York, Tampax, Inc.

Turner, D. C.: General endocrinology, Philadelphia, 1966, W. B. Saunders Co.

White, J. M.: Menstrual education in elementary school, Child and Family, Fall, 1962.

Questions for study

1. Define puberty.
2. Describe the function of the pituitary

gland in relation to the development of the gonads in the male and female.
3. What are the physical, physiologic, and psychologic changes occurring in the male and female at puberty? Why do these changes occur?
4. Define the physiology of the ovarian cycle. Which hormone is responsible for the follicular phase? The luteal phase?
5. Define ovulation. When does ovulation occur? How is the time of ovulation determined?
6. Contact school nurses in your community. Discuss the program in health education related to menstrual hygiene.
7. Research other facilities of health education offered to the adolescent in your community.

UNIT II MATERNITY CYCLE

CHAPTER 6

GROWTH AND DEVELOPMENT OF THE BABY

At the time of ovulation most ova find their way to the fimbriated end of the fallopian tube, and a few disintegrate into the peritoneal cavity. It is believed that migration of the ovum toward the fimbriated ends is produced by a current that attracts the ovum into the fallopian tube. The muscular action and movements of the tube also encourage entrance. It is within the tube that the ovum reaches further maturity or disintegrates, as most ova do. However, following sexual union should the mature ovum meet a mature sperm and union occur, fertilization (conception, impregnation) or new life begins.

OVUM AND SPERM

The ovum is a large round cell visible to the naked eye. It contains a nucleus with chromatin material and a large amount of cytoplasm and yolk granules. The ovum is surrounded by a thick outer membrane, the zona pellucida, and a thin inner lining, the vitelline membrane, which surrounds the cytoplasm. The surface extending beyond the zona pellucida contains follicular cells that adhere to the ovary proper when the follicle ruptures. The surrounding follicular cells are known as the corona radiata.

The spermatozoon is a slender, elongated structure resembling a tadpole. It has a flat, oval head, tapered body, and a long motile tail. The spermatozoon is one of the smallest body cells and is visible in the seminal fluid by microscopic examination. The head is the largest portion; it contains the nucleus and chromatin material.

At the time of ejaculation in the male, over 3 billion spermatozoa may be deposited in the female during copulation. Within 6 to 24 hours a large number find their way into the uterus and fallopian tubes.

Maturation of ovum and sperm

Since the chromosomes play a major role in maturation of the sex cells, heredity, and sex determination, a short study is essential. All human cells contain

23 paired chromosomes (total 46) in their cell nuclei. Of the 23 paired chromosomes, 22 pairs are homologous autosomes (nonsex chromosomes) and one pair are sex chromosomes. The sex chromosomes are designated as XX in the female cell and as XY in the male cell.

At the time of cell division, each chromosome is arranged as two identical arms above and below, joined at the center. The armlike structures are called chromatids, and the area at the center of union is called a centromere. The chromatids differ in length and size, and the position of the centromere may differ in chromosomes. On the basis of length, size, and position of the centromere, the following classification into seven groups has been made:

Group A Chromosomes 1, 2, 3
Group B Chromosomes 4, 5
Group C Chromosomes 6, 7, 8, 9, 10, 11, 12, and X
Group D Chromosomes 13, 14, 15
Group E Chromosomes 16, 17, 18
Group F Chromosomes 19, 20
Group G Chromosomes 21, 22, and Y

Although the preceding classification has been established, research is still being done with chromosomes that cannot yet be categorized.

OOGENESIS AND SPERMATOGENESIS

Most organisms exhibit two kinds of cell division—either mitosis or meiosis or both. Mitosis occurs in somatic cells in which the entire chromosome divides longitudinally, yielding two daughter cells with an identical number of chromosomes.

In germ cells two successive divisions occur. During maturation the first meiotic division occurs in which there is a reduction and division of maternal and paternal chromosome pairs. The second meiotic division is of a mitotic nature (longitudinal), and each daughter cell still has half the chromosomes following division. Through this division only one of the four cells in the female is functional; in the male all four spermatids become functional.

Each mature gamete following meiosis contains 22 autosomes and one sex chromosome, a total of 23. It is because of this chromosomal numerical difference that the mature ovum and sperm are attracted to each other. It is evident that half of the chromosomes of the male and half of the chromosomes of the female are transmitted to the new individual.

Since the new individual receives chromosomes from different germ cells, heredity potentials and sex determination are transmitted through chromosomes. The male sperm possesses the XY paired chromosome, and the female ovum possesses the XX paired chromosome. The uniting of the X chromosome from the male with the X chromosome from the female potentiates a female child, while the uniting of a Y chromosome from the male and an X chromosome from the female potentiates a male child. It is apparent that the father determines the sex of the new baby.

Ovulation, fertilization, and implantation

An understanding of the ovarian cycle indicates that the 12-hour to 24-hour period in which ovulation occurs is the most fertile for the female. When the mature sperm of the male are deposited during sexual union into the vagina of the female and a mature ovum is present, the environment is optimum for fertilization. Added factors for reception of the sperm are the following: (1) the increased secretions within the uterus and lubrication of the cervical and vaginal canal; (2) the increased contractility of the musculature of the fallopian tube, which propels the ovum along; and (3) the intense attraction the germ cells have for each other because of the maturation process.

Once the mature sperm penetrates the outer covering of the mature ovum, the cells unite (zygote), and new life begins—a process known as fertilization, conception, or impregnation. Penetration of the zona pellucida (ovarian outer covering) is facilitated by an enzyme present in the sperm known as hyaluronidase. The fertilized zygote immediately seals itself off so that no other sperm may enter. Fertilization usually occurs in the distal end of the fallopian tube (Fig. 6-1). Rapid division by cleavage commences, and in 1 week there are more than a hundred cells, yet there is no increase in the size of the developing cell cluster. The baby embryo at this time is no larger than the period at the end of this sentence.

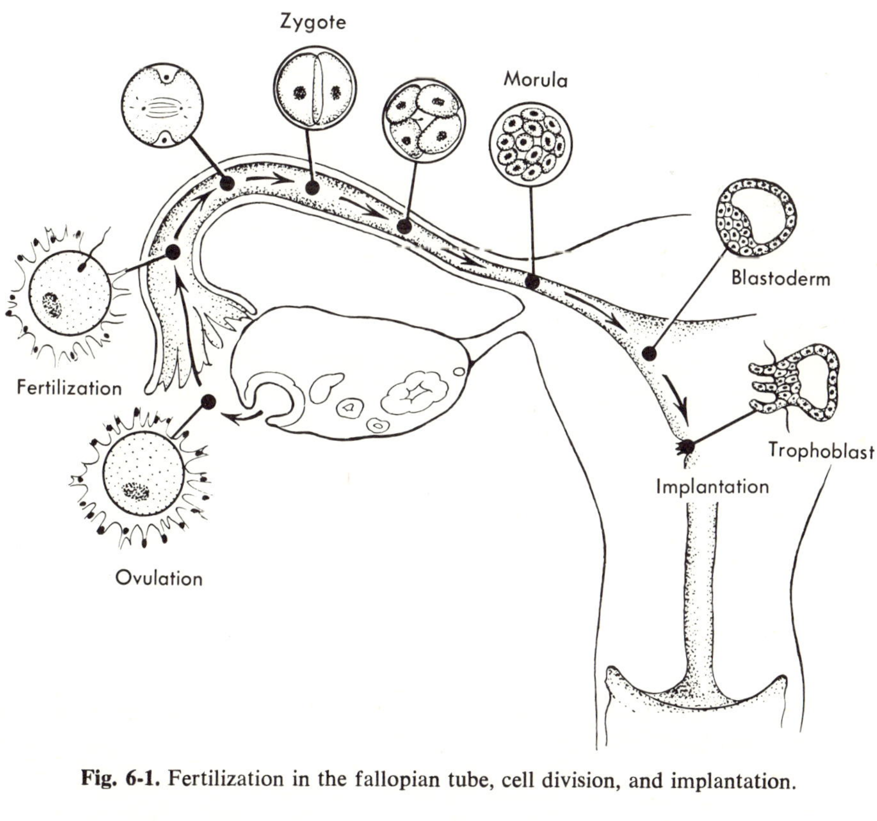

Fig. 6-1. Fertilization in the fallopian tube, cell division, and implantation.

The developing embryo is propelled by the ciliary current and the muscular contractions within the tube. The mucosa of the uterine tube is unique, and its histologic structure varies in each segment. The cells are ciliary and secretory and undergo cyclic hormonal changes. At the time of ovulation the secretory cells bulge out into the lumen of the tube and are believed to be of nutritional value to the conceptus and the migrating spermatozoa. The ciliated cells facilitate movement of the fertilized ovum toward the uterus.

By the fourth day the cell cluster (morula) moves down into the upper portion of the uterus, which, because of hormonal action of progesterones and estrogen, has become succulent and thickened for the reception of the embryo. The cells within the cluster have now arranged themselves so that a central fluid cavity (yolk sac), rich in sugars and salts, provides the necessary nutriments for proper development and survival. By the sixth or seventh day the zona pellucida is shed, and the trophoblastic shell of the blastocyte finds the endometrium in the fundus of the uterus a perfect environment and nestles within it, sinking deeper and deeper until it is enclosed within the rich endometrial lining. This process is called implantation or nidation.

The mulberry cell cluster then begins to sift out and rearrange its cells, separating the larger cell layers that will produce the embryo, the smaller cell layers that will become the placenta, and the outer cell layers that will house the growing baby. As the layers become differentiated, the embryo, now in a blastocytic state, has three distinct layers: the ectoderm, the mesoderm, and the endoderm. From the ectoderm (outer cell layer) will develop structures such as the nervous system, the spinal cord, the nerves, and special senses; from the mesoderm (middle cell layers) the supportive bony structures and circulatory, urinary, and reproductive systems develop; and from the endoderm (inner cell layers) the digestive and respiratory systems, which will provide for life, food, and oxygen, develop.

Once implantation occurs, there is further penetration of the maternal tissues since the growing embryo could not survive on nutriments from its own yolk sac. During this process a delicate network of projections called villi finds access to the succulent maternal tissue lying in close proximity. Penetration of the chorionic villi into the maternal surface is called the trophoblastic stage. It is from this delicate network that the placenta grows and develops, becoming the most important vehicle for exchange of nutriments and waste products between mother and baby.

GROWTH AND DEVELOPMENT OF THE BABY

By a process of invagination or turning inward of the various layers, the embryo begins to take form (Fig. 6-2). At 14 days the heart begins to beat, the brain looks like an early spinal cord bordered by vertebrae, and there are apparent muscle segments. At 26 days there are discernible tiny buds for arms, and at 28 days, only 2 days later, there are buds for the legs. From the very beginning growth and development occur in upper parts of the body first and then in lower parts (cephalocaudal development). At the end of 28 days the head, trunk, arms, and amniotic sac are well differentiated in the embryo. At 1 month the embryo has definite form, measures ¼ to ½ inch in length, is no larger than a pea, and is most fragile. The month-old embryo has a long way to go as refinement and growth continue in the ensuing months.

Amniotic fluid

During the first month the embryo receives most of its nourishment through a yolk sac. At 1 month rudimentary roots begin to form, and there develops a primitive umbilical cord through which nutriments and wastes are channeled between mother and baby, a meshwork that will eventually become the placenta. In the next 4 weeks the embryo becomes surrounded by amniotic fluid enclosed in a membrane having two linings, the amnion and the chorion. The amnion is closest to the developing embryo, the chorion is the outermost covering. The source of amniotic fluid is one of much dispute, and there are many speculations such as the following: (1) it is transudation from the mother's blood; (2) it is derived from fetal urine; (3) it is secreted by the amniotic epithelium; or (4) it may be produced by both mother and fetus.

Amniotic fluid is alkaline in reaction, consisting of 98% water and 2% solids. The solids are made up of the following: (1) organic materials such as protein, nonprotein nitrogen, uric acid, sugar, calcium, and phosphorus; and (2) inorganic substances such as fructose, lactic acid, carotene, adrenalin, citric acid, and the enzymes erepsin, pepsin, lipase, and rennin.

The main purpose of amniotic fluid is to provide an optimum medium for undisturbed intrauterine development. Amniotic fluid is in a dynamic equilibrium with the fluids in the maternal and fetal compartments. The amount of amniotic fluid increases rapidly with the growth of the baby, averaging 50 ml. at 12 weeks, 400 ml. at 20 weeks, and nearly 1,000 ml. at term. During the last few weeks of pregnancy the volume decreases somewhat but varies with individuals. An exchange of close to 6 gallons occurs in a 24-hour period.

The fluid provides an extracorporeal circulation for the fetus, which may be of great physiologic significance for fetal development. If this circulatory system is interrupted or impeded (as in fetal malformation), the equilibrium is disturbed, resulting in hydramnios or oligohydramnios.

Throughout pregnancy the amniotic fluid performs several important mechanical functions. It acts as a protective cushion, equalizes pressures, and prevents the adherence of the amnion so that the baby may change position.

Studies of amniotic fluid reveal fetal maturity, sex-linked diseases, Rh immunization, determination of sex prior to birth, and electrolyte qualities in relation to toxemia.

Growth between seventh and twenty-fourth weeks

By *7 weeks* the baby has a discernible face, eyes, ears, nose, lips, tongue, and teeth buds in the gums. The arm buds have fingers, and the slower growing legs

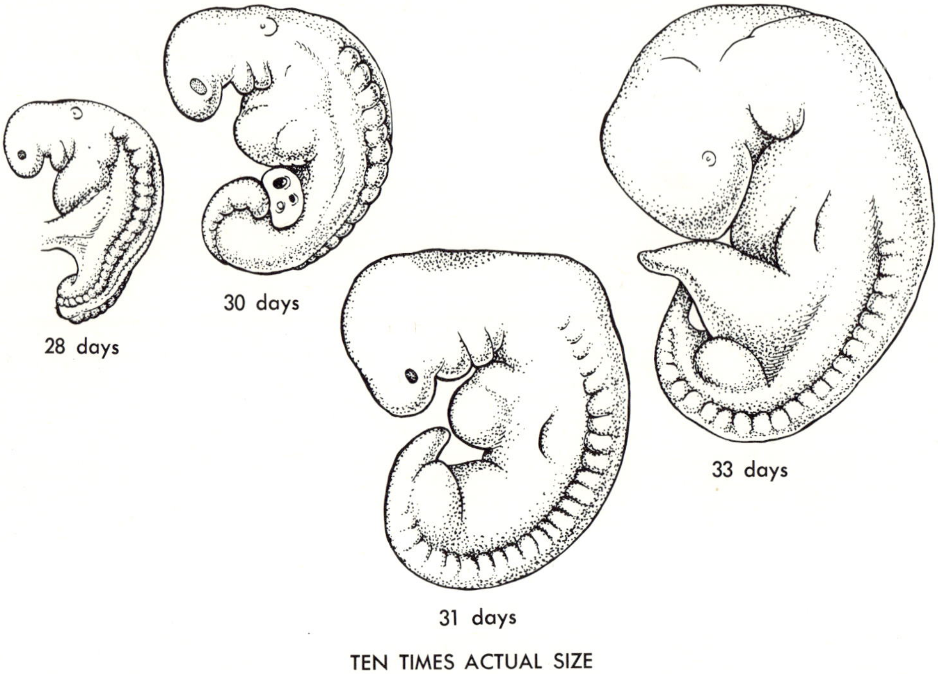

A

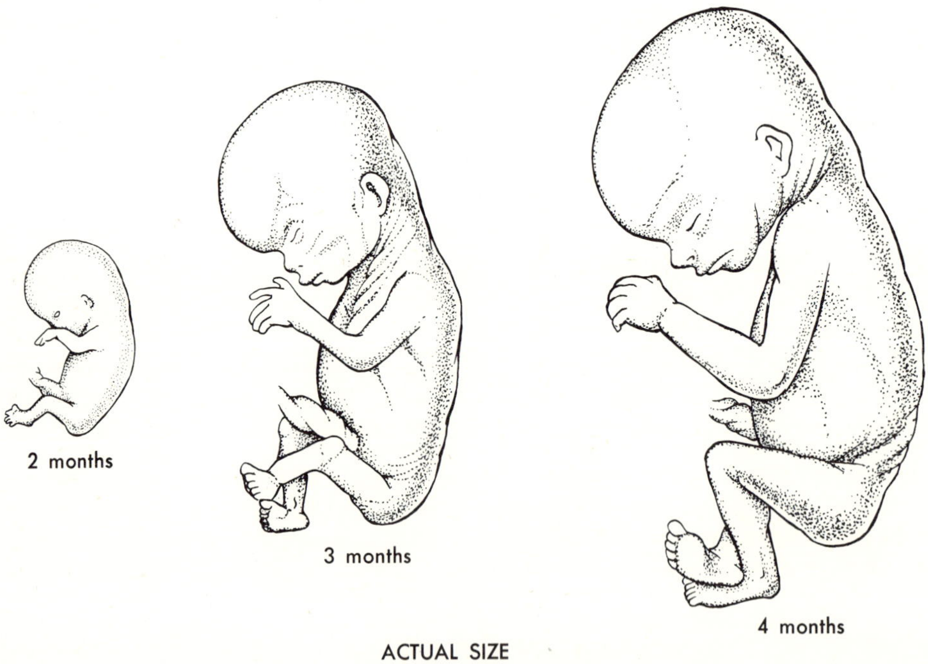

Fig. 6-2. A and **B,** Growth and development of baby.

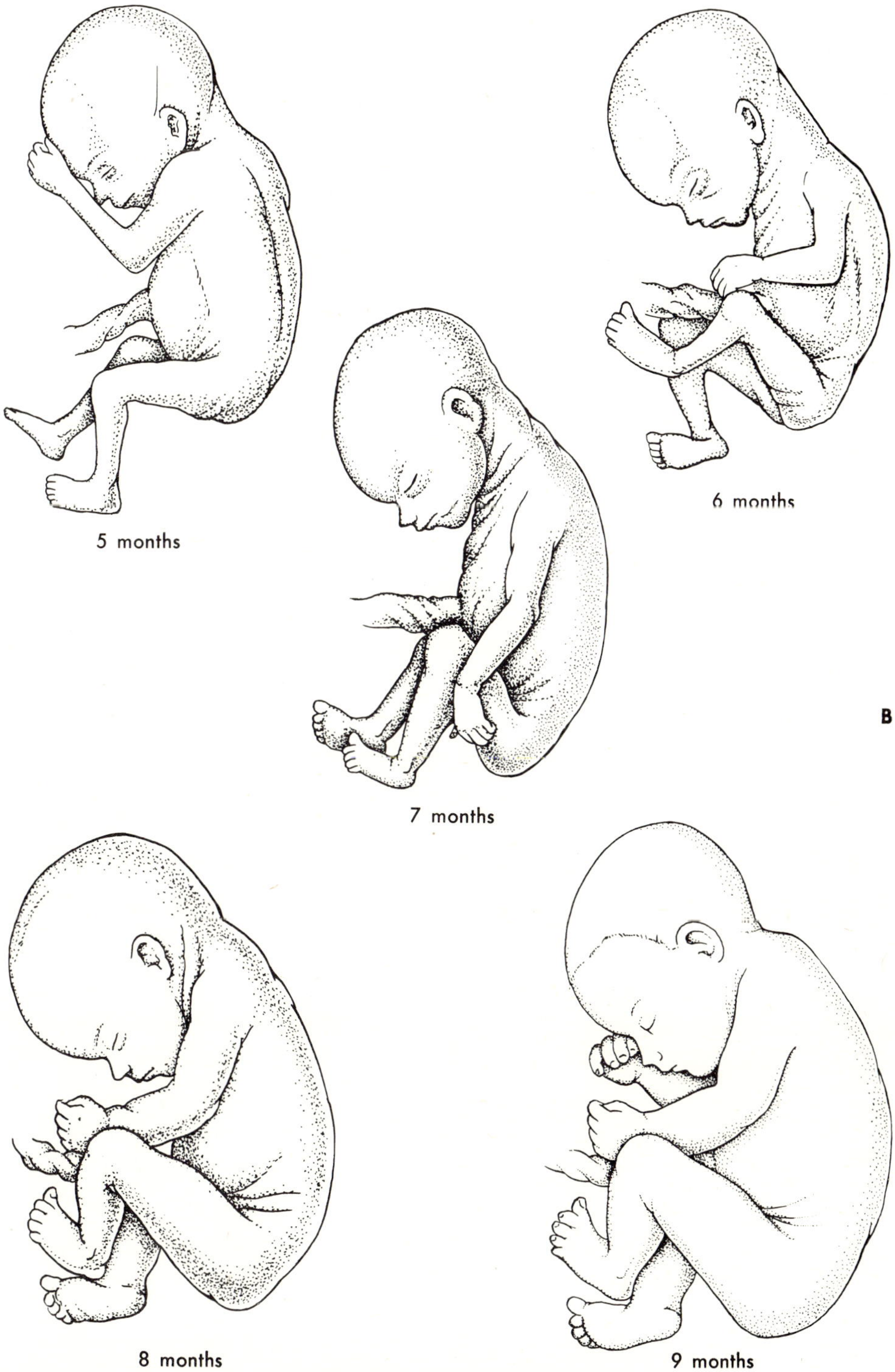

Fig. 6-2, cont'd. For legend see opposite page.

have knees, ankles, and toes. The head is quite large in comparison to the body, and the baby measures an inch in length and weighs 1/30 of an ounce. The embryo develops with precision, and embryologists can now tell an embryo's exact age in prenatal days by looking at it. For instance, at 30 days the arm buds are rounded knobs; at 31 days the arm buds are subdivided into hand, arm, and shoulder; and at 33 days there are definite finger outlines. The embryo grows 1 mm. daily—the growth is not in even progression throughout the body, however, since different sections grow more on some days than on others.

By 46 to 48 days the first bone cells replace the cartilage, appearing initially in the upper arms. It is after this period when first bone cells appear that we begin to call the embryo a fetus (from the Latin for young or offspring). By the end of the second month the embryo resembles a baby.

At *12 weeks* the baby weighs 1 ounce and becomes active. He moves parts of his body, opens his mouth, and can even swallow and breathe at this time. Although his lungs are not functioning, in his ability to exercise them he practices inhaling and exhaling. If amniotic fluid is ingested, it is believed to aid proper formation of the air sacs in the lungs. There is no damage since the baby does not depend on his lungs for oxygen; he receives his supply via the umbilical vein and the placenta.

At 16 weeks he increases his weight six times. He now weighs 6 ounces and measures 8 to 10 inches in length. He is more vigorous, and his movements will now be felt by the mother. This "feeling of life" by the mother is referred to as *quickening,* occurring at approximately 18 to 20 weeks in most women.

At *20 to 24 weeks* the baby (still enclosed in a translucent amniotic sac) is 1 foot long and weighs 1 pound. There is hair growth on his head, eyebrows, and eyelashes, yet the eyelids are still closed. The mammary glands develop, and the skeletal system hardens. Fetal heart rate can now be heard with a stethoscope, and fetal parts can be palpated easily through the abdominal wall. Periodic quiet and active episodes are experienced by the mother as the baby sleeps and wakens. At 24 weeks he begins to gain weight, and there are apparent fat deposits.

At the end of 24 weeks the baby weighs 1¼ pounds. His eyelids now open, and he can maintain regular breathing for 24 hours if born prematurely, yet he still has a slim chance for survival outside the uterus. At this time the amniotic fluid increases to 1 quart, being constantly replenished and freshened every hour. There is a daily total exchange of 6 gallons, and yet how this occurs is still not known. The fluid acts as a protector against external blows, ensures maintenance of the baby's body temperature, and makes it easier for him to exercise in a weightless environment. The skin is protected from this liquid environment by a cheesy white coating called vernix caseosa.

In the last trimester, from *28 to 40 weeks,* the baby gains a considerable amount of weight. In the seventh month there is a weight gain of 1½ pounds, and in the last 6 weeks an additional 4 pounds are gained. During this time he begins to store proteins that he will need after birth. As he grows steadily, the uterus becomes a cramped environment. The placenta, which was once a most efficient organ, begins to deteriorate, and the baby's increasing needs outweigh his ability to survive in utero.

Haase's rule is used to determine weeks of gestation by measuring the length of the fetus. Taking the square root of the length of the fetus in centimeters for the first 5 months and multiplying its length by 5 thereafter will provide an approximate gestational age. For example:

1 month	$1 \times 1 = 2$ cm.	6 months	$6 \times 5 = 30$ cm.
2 months	$2 \times 2 = 4$ cm.	7 months	$7 \times 5 = 35$ cm.
3 months	$3 \times 3 = 9$ cm.	8 months	$8 \times 5 = 40$ cm.
4 months	$4 \times 4 = 16$ cm.	9 months	$9 \times 5 = 45$ cm.
5 months	$5 \times 5 = 25$ cm.	10 months	$10 \times 5 = 50$ cm.

Placenta

It is during the fourth month that the placenta, a temporary organ, plays a vital part in supplying food, oxygen, and water to the growing baby. The placenta, now adherent to the maternal surface, is no more than 3 inches in diameter and weighs 4 ounces. At birth, in comparison, the placenta is 8 inches in diameter, weighing 1 to 1½ pounds. The placenta has three functions: kidney, lung, and endocrine gland. As a lung the placenta exchanges carbon dioxide for oxygen, which is carried to the baby by the mother's bloodstream. The baby's blood traverses the placenta through the cord and never leaves its closed vessels; therefore there is no mixing of blood. The exchange occurs through the porous walls of the closed blood vessels. In the same way, nutriments such as iron are utilized, and wastes are excreted by way of the mother's kidneys.

The placenta, well formed by 12 weeks, takes on the function of producing female sex steroids, estrogen, progesterone, and the protein hormone chorionic gonadotropin. The placenta contains all three major estrogens, a larger amount of estriol, and lesser amounts of estrone and estradiol-17B. Estriol levels increase as pregnancy advances to term. An estriol level of 4 mg. or less during the last trimester indicates fetal death, and levels of 4 to 12 mg. indicate fetal distress. Progesterone quantities of 1 to 2 mg. have been known to be extracted from the placenta, together with a number of adrenal substances such as hydrocortisone, cortisone, tetrahydrocortisone, aldosterone, and 11-hydrocorticosterone. High levels of progesterone and gonadotropin are essential for maintaining a quiescent uterus and for further development of the mammary glands for lactation.

The baby, attached to the placenta via the umbilical cord, has his own blood system pumped by his own heart. The umbilical cord, the life line to the baby, is composed of one large vein to transport nutriments and oxygen and two arteries by which wastes are returned to be eliminated by the mother. The cord is protected by a slippery, shiny, jellylike substance called Wharton's jelly. Although the cord is approximately 18 to 20 inches in length, it rarely becomes tangled or knotted, since the blood force within it keeps it distended and straightened.

Mother and baby have separate blood systems, and the exchange occurs through diffusion at the placental site. It is known that substances entering the mother's bloodstream can reach the baby within a short time. It is apparent that the placenta is an efficient organ and system for exchange. The quality and quantity of transmittable material through the placenta are dependent on the permeability of its membrane and on the size of the organisms. Certain drugs, bacteria, and gases are known to traverse the placenta quite rapidly, affecting the baby as well as the mother. It is worthy to note that in late pregnancy sodium is transferred 70 times faster than during the first trimester.

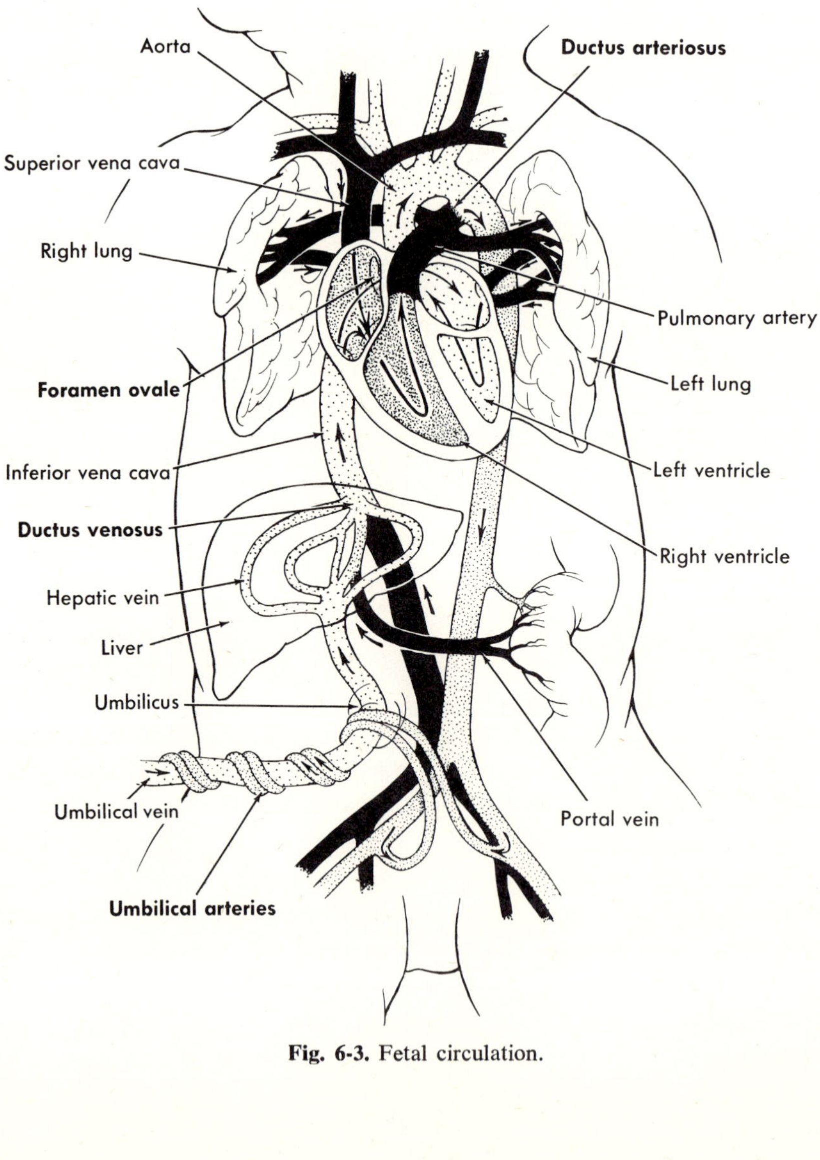

Fig. 6-3. Fetal circulation.

Fetal circulation

Structures existing in fetal circulation (Fig. 6-3) that disappear following birth are the following: (1) placenta and umbilical cord (one umbilical vein and two umbilical arteries); (2) foramen ovale, an opening between the right and left atrium of the heart; (3) ductus arteriosus connecting the vessel between the pulmonary artery and the aorta; and (4) ductus venosus connecting the vessel between the umbilical vein and the ascending vena cava.

Since the lungs do not function in fetal circulation, nutriments are brought to the fetus through the placenta and umbilical vein. The umbilical vein penetrates the abdominal wall of the fetus, dividing into two branches. A smaller branch unites with the portal vein and circulates blood through the liver, gaining access to the inferior vena cava through the hepatic vein. The larger branch, the ductus venosus, empties directly into the inferior vena cava and enters the right atrium, mixing with the return flow from the superior vena cava. Since the blood entering the right atrium has more oxygen saturation, it is forced into the left atrium and aorta, supplying the head and trunk with nourishment. The blood returning from the right atrium goes directly into the right ventricle and through the ductus arteriosus into the lungs and lower portion of the body, returning to the placenta via the umbilical arteries to be reoxygenated. It is evident then that the blood circulating through the fetus is mixed blood; however, the oxygen content in the inferior vena cava is higher than in the aorta. A small portion of the blood is sent to the lungs for nourishment purposes rather than for aeration. Changes that occur in fetal circulation at birth are discussed in Chapter 13.

SELECTED REFERENCES

Abramovich, D. R.: The volume of amniotic fluid in early pregnancy, J. Obstet. Gynaec. Brit. Comm. **75**:728, 1968.

Anderson, A. B.: Estimation of duration of gestation by amniotic fluid cytology, J. Obstet. Gynaec. Brit. Comm. **75**:300, 1968.

Arey, L. B.: Developmental anatomy, ed. 1, Philadelphia, 1962, W. B. Saunders Co.

Balinsky, B. I.: An introduction to embryology, Philadelphia, 1960, W. B. Saunders Co.

Bonner, D. M.: Heredity, Englewood Cliffs, N. J., 1961, Prentice-Hall, Inc.

Eastman, N. J., and Hellman, L. M.: Williams obstetrics, ed. 13, New York, 1966, Appleton-Century & Appleton-Century-Crofts.

Flanagan, H. L.: The first nine months of life, New York, 1962, Simon and Schuster, Inc.

Fujimoto, W. Y., and others: Biochemical diagnosis of an X-linked disease in utero, Lancet **2**:511, 1968.

Gordon, H.: Cytology of amniotic fluid—a new text for fetal maturity, Obstet. Gynec. **30**:652, 1967.

Karchmer, S., and others: Study of electrolytes of amniotic fluid in pregnancy toxemia, Obstet. Gynec. **24**:71, July, 1968.

Martin, P. C.: Human development, New York, 1960, The Ronald Press Co.

Moya, F., and Thorndike, V.: Passage of drugs across the placenta, Amer. J. Obstet. Gynec. **84**:1778, 1962.

Mungula, H., and others: Determination of fetal sex by amniotic fluid cytology, Obstet. Gynec. **21**:765, September-October, 1966.

Pitkin, R. M.: Fetal contribution to amniotic fluid, Amer. J. Obstet. Gynec., March, 1968.

Plentl, A.: Formation and circulation of amniotic fluid, Year Book of Obstetrics and Gynecology, Chicago, 1965-1966, Year Book Medical Publishers, Inc.

Reid, D. E.: A textbook of obstetrics, Philadelphia, 1962, W. B. Saunders Co.

Stewart, A. G., and others: Amniotic fluid bilirubin levels and the Rh-isoimmunized mother, Amer. J. Obstet. Gynec. **97**:338, 1967.

Vincent, E. L.: Human psychological development, New York, 1961, The Ronald Press Co.

Waddington, C. H.: Principles of embryology, New York, 1956, The Macmillan Co.

Yerushalmy, J.: Mother's cigarette smoking and survival of infant, Amer. J. Obstet. Gynec. **88**:505, 1964.

Questions for study

1. Define gamete, zygote, maturation, ovulation, fertilization, and implantation.
2. Describe oogenesis and spermatogenesis.
3. Of what importance are the chromosomes in fertilization?
4. Describe mitosis and meiosis when cell division occurs.
5. Where does fertilization occur? Describe the three stages in early embryonic development.
6. Prior to implantation, how does the embryo derive nourishment for survival?
7. Describe the three primary germinal layers, and the systems derived from each.
8. Describe significant changes in growth and development of the baby in utero at 4 weeks, 8 weeks, 12 weeks, 16 weeks, 20 weeks, 24 weeks, 36 weeks, and 40 weeks.
9. Describe the structure and function of the umbilical cord and placenta during intrauterine life.
10. Draw a fetal heart. Label structures that differ from adult circulation. Trace the blood flow when it enters the fetus through the umbilical vein and its return by the hypogastric arteries to the mother's circulation.

CHAPTER 7

PHYSIOLOGIC CHANGES DURING PREGNANCY

Although pregnancy is a normal physiologic process, all the body systems are affected when a woman is pregnant. The changes in the body systems are directly related to the progressive growth and development of the baby in utero. The physical, physiologic, and psychologic needs of the mother evolve with due respect to these changes.

FIRST TRIMESTER CHANGES

Endocrine and reproductive system

The endocrine and reproductive systems play leading roles during pregnancy. In the first trimester (conception through 12 weeks) symptoms of fatigue, amenorrhea, breast changes, and leukorrhea are commonly experienced by the mother. Changes in the size, shape, and consistency of the uterus are noted by the doctor.

Fatigue. Excessive fatigue may be an early symptom, yet it is seldom related to a possible pregnancy. Fatigue results from a change in metabolism whereby sodium and water are retained and relaxation of smooth muscle occurs.

Amenorrhea. Cessation of menstruation may be an early sign of pregnancy, but there are other causes of amenorrhea. Pregnancy may occur in a girl prior to puberty, the amenorrhea may be occurring during lactation, the amenorrhea may be caused by tuberculosis, stress, or other factor, or it may occur following curettage or following the menopause. The ovary may continue to function during gestation; thus menstruation may continue, concealing pregnancy. However, pregnancy is suspected in the woman who menstruates normally and whose flow suddenly ceases. Once pregnancy is confirmed, any bleeding that occurs should be reported and checked immediately.

Leukorrhea. Increased vaginal secretions are common during pregnancy since there is activity of the glandular tissue in the lower uterine segment. Added secretions lubricate the cervix and vaginal canal, markedly increasing the acidity, which acts as protection from bacterial invasion.

Vagina. A bluish, dusky hue to the vestibule and anterior wall of the vagina is known as Chadwick's sign. It appears about the eighth to twelfth week of gestation and becomes more pronounced as pregnancy advances. It is presumably caused by local venous congestion. It is, however, a presumptive sign, since it may be present with pelvic tumors, obesity, and heart disease.

Tissue changes usually noted are thickening of the mucosa, hypertrophy of the muscle cells, and a loosening of connective tissue. The vaginal secretions are markedly acid (pH of 3.5 to 6) because of the presence of lactic acid (derived from glycogen) within the vaginal epithelium. Increased acidity during pregnancy prevents the invasion of pathogenic organisms. Increased vascularity extends beyond the genitalia to the pelvic tissue.

Cervix. Softening of the cervix occurs in the sixth week because of congestive hyperemia of the pelvis. This is known as Goodell's sign; it is a presumptive sign of pregnancy, since it is often an early sign of pelvic infection.

Other changes include increased vascularity, edema, and hyperplasia of the cervical glands. The glands undergo marked proliferation so that the mucosa comprises half the entire cervix. The glands in proximity to the external os proliferate beyond the stratified mucosa, giving the cervix a velvety appearance. In 20% of women the hyperactivity of basal cells, which is produced by an increase in estrogens, can produce histologic findings similar to those seen in carcinoma in situ; however, normally these regress with the termination of pregnancy. As pregnancy advances, changes in the cervix resembling erosions are common as gland proliferation of endocervical glands occurs because of estrogenic stimulation.

Uterus. Softening or compressibility of the lower uterine segment is known as Hegar's sign. This is determined by the physician by means of bimanual examination; he places one hand on the abdomen behind the uterus and two fingers in the anterior fornix. Softening appears at 6 weeks in the multigravida and at 8 weeks in the primigravida, and it is definitely discernible by the tenth week. Of all the signs it is the most highly presumptive. The uterus also increases in size, becomes soft and spongy in consistency, and is markedly anteflexed over the bladder.

Breasts. The increased secretion of estrogen and progesterone during pregnancy prepares the breasts for lactation. The higher titer of estrogen has an inhibitory effect upon the pituitary gland, suppressing lactation. Following delivery of the baby, lactation is established as the estrogen titer drops, releasing the pituitary mammogenic hormone prolactin.

As early as the fourth week of pregnancy the mother experiences tingling, tenseness, or soreness of the breasts. During the second month an increased blood supply to the glandular tissue, with hypertrophy of the mammary alveoli, produces breast enlargement. The nipples become deeply pigmented and enlarged, and a yellowish fluid known as colostrum may be expressed by gentle massage. The areola becomes broader in diameter and deeply pigmented, and the tubercles of Montgomery become prominent. Should the breasts become excessively enlarged, striae may appear because of skin stretching. The former belief of an existing nervous connection between the uterus and the breasts has been disproved since lactation can be established following the severance of nerve supply to the breast.

Basal body temperature. The basal body temperature (taken upon awakening) can be a great help in the early diagnosis of pregnancy. A level of 98.8 to 99.8° F. for a period of more than 16 days after ovulation is highly suggestive of pregnancy. This method, however, can be used only by women who have kept records of their basal body temperatures prior to pregnancy.

Digestive system

Nausea and vomiting. The combination of nausea and vomiting, commonly known as "morning sickness," is a symptom of early pregnancy. It occurs as early as 2 weeks after the first missed menstrual period and may last through 8 weeks of pregnancy. The reduction of free hydrochloric acid decreases gastric motility, resulting in heartburn and flatulence. Heartburn occurs when free hydrochloric acid is regurgitated by reverse peristalsis into the esophagus. Ingestion of a carbohydrate such as dry toast or crackers increases gastric secretions and motility, thereby alleviating discomfort. Aluminum antacids such as Amphojel, Maalox, and Gelusil are commonly ordered. Should excessive nausea and vomiting continue, adequate nutritional needs of the mother and baby are to be considered. Usually excessive nausea and vomiting is pathologic and is known as hyperemesis gravidarum.

SECOND AND THIRD TRIMESTER CHANGES

Quickening

At about 16 to 18 weeks the mother begins to experience a fluttering feeling in the abdomen, caused by the movements of the fetus. For the primigravida it may go unnoticed for a week, but for the multigravida, who knows the sensation, it may be noticed earlier. In some mothers the fluttering may be felt as late as the sixth or seventh month; however, it is rare that it is never experienced. Quickening or the "feeling of life" is often used to estimate date of confinement—22 weeks are counted ahead for the primigravida, 24 weeks for the multigravida. Quickening is a presumptive sign, since intestinal peristalsis may give the impression of fetal movements. As the baby grows, active fetal movements may be felt by placing the hand on the abdomen.

Uterus

Marked changes occur in the uterus during pregnancy; the changes affect its size, weight, anatomic position, musculature, and circulation.

Size and weight. Enlargement of the uterus in early pregnancy is caused partially by hypertrophy of the muscle cells or by the formation of new cells; in the second and third trimesters, enlargement is essential to accommodate the growing baby, the placenta, and the amniotic fluid. In the prepregnant state the uterus is an almost solid muscular organ measuring 6.5 cm. in length and weighing 1 ounce. At the end of pregnancy the uterus measures 32 cm. in length and weighs approximately 2 pounds, 2 ounces.

Early in pregnancy the uterine walls are thick and at term become thinner; this thinning is apparent as fetal movements occur and palpation of the baby is possible. Enlargement of the uterus is not symmetric—it is most marked in the fundal portion. From its original piriform shape the uterus changes and becomes globular; it is almost spherical by the third month. After the third month the uterus increases more rapidly in length than in width, and it takes on an oval form until the end of pregnancy.

The pregnant uterus, with its upper portion free in the abdominal cavity and its lower portion anchored at the cervix, can easily change position. In a standing position the uterus rests mainly upon the anterior abdominal wall. In a prone position the weight of the uterus falls backward, resting upon the vertebral column. The growing uterus has a tendency to rotate slightly to the right since the rectum occupies the left portion of the pelvis.

Musculature. The muscle fibers become two to seven times wider and seven to eleven times longer as pregnancy progresses. With the resulting increase in width and length, there is an increase in mesenchymal tissue between the muscle bands. The amount of elastic tissue forms a strong network of muscle bundles, giving added strength to the tissue walls. At the same time there is an increase in the size of blood vessels (especially the veins) at the placental site, forming placental sinuses. Marked hypertrophy of the lymphatic and nerve supplies to the uterus is also apparent.

The muscle fibers of the pregnant uterus are arranged in three ways: (1) a hoodlike layer arches over the uterus and extends into the various ligaments; (2) an internal layer contains sphincterlike fibers around the orifices of the tubes and the internal os; and (3) a dense portion of muscle fibers perforated by many blood vessels—the muscle fibers of the middle layer are so interlaced that they resemble the figure eight.

Interlacing of fibers allows for effective constriction of blood vessels following delivery; this constriction prevents hemorrhage. The muscles of the pregnant uterus have an increased capacity to contract, and painless, irregular contractions occur from the first trimester to the end of pregnancy. These contractions (called Braxton Hicks) are sporadic, unrhythmic, and not felt by the palpating hand at first, but during the last month of pregnancy they become rhythmic and simulate labor contractions.

Abdominal walls

As the baby grows and develops, the abdomen becomes enlarged and the skin becomes taut; reddish streaks known as striae gravidarum develop. These streaks are caused by the hyperactivity of the adrenal cortex. At times the abdominal wall may be unable to withstand the tension as enlargement occurs, with a resulting separation of the recti muscles, known as a diastasis recti abdominis. The separation may resemble a hernial protrusion.

In the first trimester the abdominal wall is not noticeably enlarged. At the end of the third trimester, the uterus rises out of the pelvis upward toward the xiphoid of the sternum. On vaginal examination there is a softening of the body of the uterus known as Hegar's sign. At 6 months the height of the fundus of the pregnant uterus is at the umbilical level. At 8 months the fundus may be felt between the umbilical level and the xiphoid, and at 9 months the fundus reaches the xiphoid. At 40 weeks, once lightening (engagement of the baby's head into the true pelvis) occurs, the height of the fundus can be felt just below the xiphoid. Enlargement of the abdominal wall may be less pronounced in primigravidas than in multigravidas, since the former have better muscle tone.

Circulatory system

Blood volume. The hypervolemia present during pregnancy first appears at about 6 weeks of gestation. The levels rise rapidly until 24 weeks, and then rise more slowly until term is reached. The rise in blood volume varies among women and sometimes shows a 50% increase above the nonpregnant state. The increased blood volume is essential to meet the demands of the enlarging uterus and helps protect the mother and the fetus with return blood flow and loss during delivery. The blood volume increases more slowly in the last trimester and is believed to reach a plateau a few weeks prior to term. Since hemoglobin particles are more widely dispersed, there is a resulting physiologic anemia.

Determination of a hemoglobin level below 10 gm./100 ml. is usually followed by oral administration of ferrous sulfate. Ascorbic acid is given to enhance the absorption of iron. If the patient is told that iron is better assimilated if taken with meals or following meals and that it tends to constipate and produce tarry stools, many unnecessary anxieties will be avoided. Increasing fluid and fruit intake may alleviate the constipation.

Cardiac output. Oxygen consumption during pregnancy increases and in the last month is 20% higher than that of the nonpregnant state. The need for added oxygen is met by an increase in cardiac output; this increase begins at the end of the second month and reaches its peak at the seventh and eighth months. At 36 weeks cardiac output falls abruptly, and it returns to the nonpregnant levels at 40 weeks. The fall in cardiac output during the last month is related to gradual closing down of placental circulation. A 30% increase in cardiac output occurs immediately following delivery as the contracting uterus empties blood into the circulation. By the end of the second postpartal week the level returns to normal.

Heart rate. The heart rate increases ten beats per minute in the latter half of pregnancy, accounting for 14,000 extra beats in 24 hours.

As the uterus enlarges with advancing pregnancy, the diaphragm rises, lifting the heart and rotating it to the left. This gives a false impression of cardiac enlargement. Postural hypotension is an occasional occurrence since there is compression of the inferior vena cava against the spinal column, resulting in syncope, low blood pressure, and tachycardia.

Intermittent uterine contractions. As early as the tenth week of pregnancy the mother may experience intermittent contractions and relaxation of the uterus, known as Braxton Hicks contractions. These continue throughout pregnancy, and in the latter weeks are known as false labor contractions. They do not cause any dilatation of the cervix.

Auscultatory signs. Between 18 and 20 weeks gestation, fetal heart tones may be heard with a stethoscope; these tones resemble the tick-tock of a watch—there is a tick, a short pause, then a tock and a long pause. Fetal heart rates vary from 120 to 160 and may go as high as 190 with fetal activity or palpation of fetal parts. Uterine contractions or pressure on the fetal skull slow the rate. At times the sound of blood rushing through the umbilical arteries may be heard. This is commonly known as a fetal or funic souffle.

Integumentary system

Diaphoresis. Diaphoresis is not uncommon during pregnancy since the baby's wastes are excreted through the mother's kidneys and skin. Daily bathing brings added comfort for the mother.

Skin changes. Skin changes include darkening of the genitalia, areola of the breast, linea nigra (line separating the abdominal rectus muscles midline from the umbilicus to the symphysis), and occasional pigmentation of the face known as chloasma. Under the influence of estrogens, melanin is produced in the basal cells, causing chloasma. Should it not disappear following pregnancy, large doses of vitamin C are helpful.

Striae are spindle-shaped streaks occurring on the abdomen, hips, and breasts after the fifth month. They are associated with hyperfunction of the adrenal cortex (absorption of adrenocortical hormone by the fatty tissue).

Herpes gestationis are erythematous spots, urticaria, papules, and vesicles associated with pruritus, burning, and pain. The areas usually involved are the extensor side of the extremities, and scapular and sacral regions.

During pregnancy nail and hair growth is accelerated as secretions of growth hormones (ACTH) are increased. Erythema of the palmar surfaces of the hands is also common.

Respiratory system

Dyspnea. Dyspnea is not uncommon from 36 to 38 weeks gestation. As the baby grows, the fundus rises, with resulting pressure on the diaphragm and lungs. When lightening occurs (settling of the presenting part in the true pelvis before labor commences), dyspnea usually subsides. Dyspnea at this time is not to be confused with true dyspnea related to circulatory problems.

Vital capacity. Although there is crowding of the lungs because of fetal growth, the lungs increase in width and more air is inspired, with a resulting increased vital capacity.

Excretory system

Frequency of urination. Frequency of urination is present in early and late pregnancy—in early pregnancy the increased vascularity of the enlarging uterus and in late pregnancy the engaging fetal head decrease bladder volume. Educating the mother so that she understands this to be a normal phenomenon alleviates fear and anxiety.

Dilatation of the renal pelvis, ureter, and bladder is caused by hormonal influence. Dilatation is seen early in pregnancy. The degree of dilatation is independent of presentation, position, and attitude of the child. Slight dilatation occurs when women are receiving gonadal hormones. The frequency of ureteral peristalsis decreases during pregnancy. Any dilatation persisting 4 months following pregnancy is indicative of permanent structural damage.

Lowered specific gravity. Lowered specific gravity accounts for the finding of sugar in the urine in the last trimester. However, possible diabetes should always be ruled out with fasting blood sugar and glucose tolerance tests.

Gonadotropic hormones. Gonadotropic hormones may be found in the urine of pregnant women, which is significant for diagnostic purposes.

Kidney infections. Kidney infections during pregnancy are enhanced because of a physiologic dilatation of the right ureter and relaxation of the smooth muscles. Stasis of urine in the kidney is an ideal environment for bacterial growth. Tenderness or pain in the lumbar region or elevation of the basal temperature should be reported and treated immediately. Bed rest and chemotherapy usually alleviate the signs and symptoms. Proper positioning in bed (lying on the affected side) splints the area against pain and promotes urinary drainage. Forcing fluids promotes hydration when there is an elevation in basal body temperature.

Edema of the extremities

In the last trimester blood stasis is occasionally present in the extremities because of relaxation of the smooth muscles in the blood vessel walls. In mothers who already have varicosities this stasis can present problems. Ace bandages applied properly from below the toes to the knee before arising can improve circulation (Fig. 7-1). For some women well-fitted elastic stockings serve the same purpose if there is minimal leg edema. Simple elastic straps suspended from the shoulders with attached garters should be recommended in place of round constricting leg garters. Women who work at desk jobs need an opportunity for occasional short walks in order to improve circulation and prevent stasis.

Leg cramps. Leg cramps during pregnancy occur with pressure of the enlarging uterus on the peripheral vascular system, resulting in sluggish drainage and buildup of waste metabolites in the muscles. Leg cramps result from insufficient calcium or occur when huge quantities of phosphorus are ingested. Decreasing

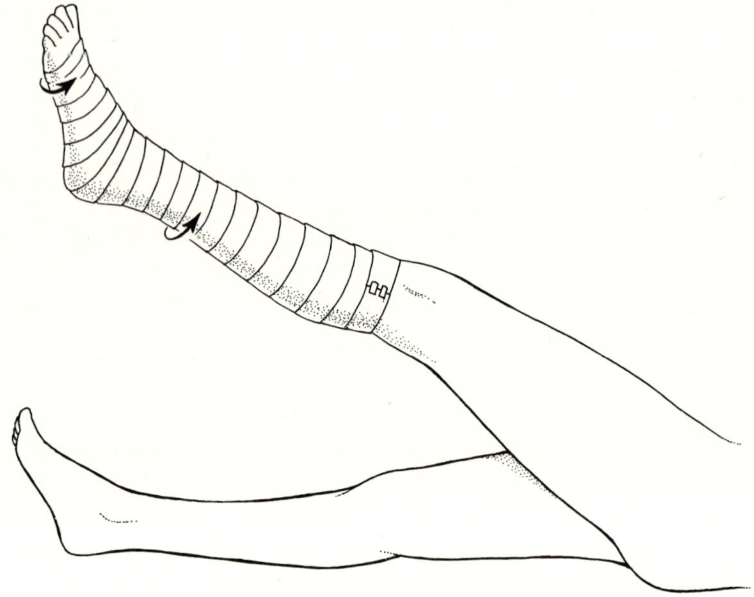

Fig. 7-1. Ace bandage to the leg.

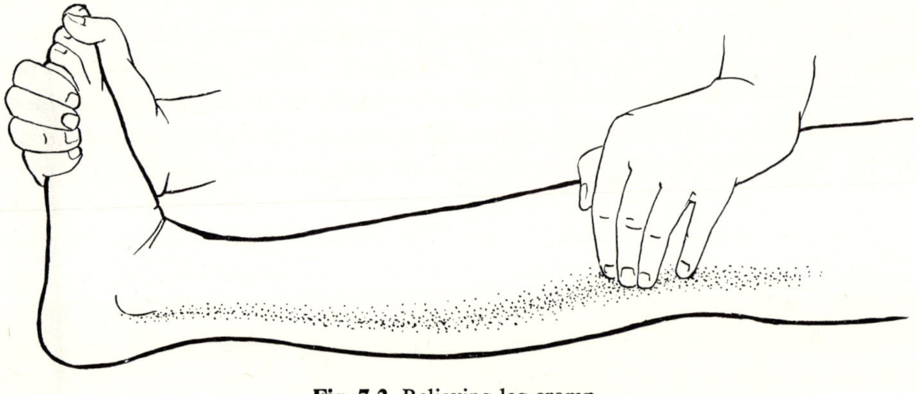

Fig. 7-2. Relieving leg cramp.

the intake of foods high in phosphorus and adding aluminum hydroxide gel to the diet help to remove phosphorus from the intestinal tract.

Cramps are common during labor because of hyperventilation. Immediate relief is attained by firm pressure over the knee in order to straighten the leg and by exerting a force with flexion of the toes, thus relaxing the calf muscle (Fig. 7-2).

DIAGNOSTIC TESTS FOR PREGNANCY

In 1927 Aschheim and Zondek demonstrated that urine of pregnant women contained a gonad-stimulating substance later identified as chorionic gonadotropin. This introduced the first valid pregnancy test. The Aschheim-Zondek test originally required 5 mice and a 96-hour waiting period for results. In 1930 Friedman reported a test done on a rabbit that required a shorter waiting period (48 hours) for results. Following these several tests, the use of toads, frogs, and immature rats was developed with a reduced time interval. All these tests were based on the ability of chorionic gonadotropin in pregnant urine to produce hemorrhagic changes in the ovary of the mice or rabbit, the extrusion of ova in the female toad, the ejection of sperm from the testes of the male frog or toad, and the development of ovarian hyperemia in the immature rat. The latest rat ovarian test was modified by Kupperman so that a 2- to 6-hour reading is possible.

Chorionic gonadotropic hormone (produced by the chorionic villi) is present in the blood and urine of pregnant women by the tenth day of pregnancy. The concentration reaches a peak between the sixtieth and seventieth days of pregnancy and is at its lowest level by approximately the one hundred twentieth day.

A hormone-induced withdrawal bleeding test is currently being used as a presumptive test in the diagnosis of early pregnancy. The test is accomplished by giving an oral hormone containing progesterone and estrogen for 2 or 3 days. The effect of the medication takes place within 15 days following the administration of the last dose. Physiologically the increase in these hormones will develop the secretory endometrium, and upon withdrawal of the drug menstruation will occur. However, if the woman is pregnant, the corpus luteum and the placenta will produce sufficient hormones to keep the baby implanted, and there will be no effective change following withdrawal. Therefore bleeding would indicate that pregnancy has not occurred, and absence of bleeding would indicate a positive pregnancy. This test is done immediately following the first missed menstrual period, whereas the animal tests can be used only after the first month of pregnancy since the hormone concentration is increased at that time.

Advances since 1960 in immunology have made it possible to detect the hormone by observing hemagglutination inhibition, complement fixation, and precipitation reactions. A common hemagglutination inhibition test is the Pregnosticon. In February, 1965, a simple slide test was introduced; this test, done with Gravindex,* can be easily accomplished as an office procedure. A drop of antiserum is mixed thoroughly with a drop of urine for 30 seconds. An additional 2 drops of antigen indicator are then added and mixed thoroughly by rocking the slide gently for not more than 2 minutes. Visible agglutination indicates a negative reaction for pregnancy. Absence of agglutination indicates a positive test for pregnancy. This test has been proved 90% accurate.

An ultrasonic diagnostic unit can diagnose a pregnancy in the first 6 weeks, before most urine tests give positive results. It is used to diagnose low implantation of the placenta, hydatidiform mole, tubal pregnancy, ovarian tumors, and fibroids. It can be used safely with no effect on the mother or the fetus.

---

*Ortho Pharmaceutical Corp., Raritan, N. J.

METABOLIC CHANGES DURING PREGNANCY

Weight

Alterations in weight are attributed to the growing baby, the uterus, the placenta, the amniotic fluid, and water retention. The normal weight gain during pregnancy is 18 to 24 pounds. Twelve pounds are gained in the last trimester. The average weight gain constitutes 7½ pounds for the baby, 1 to 1½ pounds for the placenta, 1½ pounds for the amniotic fluid, 3 pounds for the increased weight of the reproductive organs (the breasts), 3 pounds for the uterus, and 2 to 3 pounds for the storage of tissue proteins outside the uterus and for water retention in the mother's blood. Sudden weight gain deviating from these proportions may be the first sign of beginning toxemia.

Skeletal system

Increased hormonal action (relaxin, ovarian hormone) causes softening of all the pelvic ligaments and joints. This allows for pliability and facilitates passage of the baby through the pelvis at the time of delivery. Excessive mobility of the joints may cause a wide separation of the symphysis pubis, with a resulting waddling gait; this produces great discomfort. A low, firm elastic band support over the symphysis gives some relief.

Nervous system

Changes in the nervous system depend upon the woman's prepregnant state. If there was a tendency before pregnancy for a woman to be depressive or manic, these symptoms can become aggravated. If, on the other hand, the woman was quiet, happy, and tranquil, she can have the same reaction. There are, however, emotional changes such as fear and apprehensions that will be discussed later. Some of the differences in attitudes result from the great hormonal changes that affect mood swings or from awareness and apprehension over altered physiology.

SELECTED REFERENCES

Barnes, C. G.: Medical disorders in obstetric practice, ed. 2, Oxford, England, 1965, Blackwell Scientific Publications.

Donald, I., and Abdulla, U.: Ultrasonics in obstetrics and gynecology, Brit. J. Radiol. **40**:604, 1967.

Eastman, N. J., and Hellman, L. M.: Williams obstetrics, ed. 13, New York, 1966, Appleton-Century-Crofts.

Lund, C. J., and Donovan, J. C.: Blood volume during pregnancy: significance of plasma and red cell volume, Amer. J. Obstet. Gynec. **98**:393, 1967.

Questions for study

1. Describe the physiologic changes occurring in the body systems during pregnancy.
2. In retrospect of the changes occurring in the body systems during pregnancy, what are the needs of mothers during the antepartal period?
3. Read the following and bring to class to discuss:

Mr. and Mrs. Oliver, a Negro couple, aged 34 and 32, respectively, are expecting their third baby. They are both high school graduates and of the lower socioeconomic status. The other children are Mary, aged 2, and John, aged 4. Mrs. Oliver arrives at the prenatal clinic for her first visit. She gives a history of having missed two menstrual periods; she feels tired and complains of nausea and vomiting and frequency of urination:

a. On the basis of the preceding symptoms, is Mrs. Oliver pregnant?
b. Relate the preceding symptoms to the physical, physiologic, and emotional changes occurring during pregnancy. In light of these changes, how would you plan to help this mother?
c. What measures would be taken to ensure a healthy outcome for Mrs. Oliver during this pregnancy?
d. What are the changes in the family constellation with the anticipated arrival of a new baby?
e. Considering the cultural and socioeconomic background, what would you include in health teaching for this family?

CHAPTER 8

PRENATAL CARE

THE FIRST PRENATAL VISIT

At the first prenatal visit, a family history is usually recorded by the doctor. Such a history includes medical, surgical, gynecologic, and obstetric data. Interviewing involves tactful use of the appropriate terminology so that the mother understands and can give accurate and substantial data. This information is important in planning and providing optimum supervision. Medical data include family and personal histories of diabetes, heart disease, tuberculosis, kidney ailments, and venereal diseases, which give clues to hereditary and communicable diseases; for example, diabetes is hereditary, tuberculosis is communicable, and each has specific implications for pregnancy.

A complete gynecologic history includes information regarding age of first menarche, regularity of menstrual cycle, and length of and pain during menstrual periods. Gynecologic surgery and previous obstetric data are significant. The mother with a history of toxemia, cephalopelvic disproportion, or difficult labor can then be more closely supervised during the present pregnancy.

Childhood diseases are significant since the mother who has never had measles would be a candidate for the vaccine should she be exposed. German measles during the first trimester of pregnancy may be harmful to the growing fetus. Teaching the importance of taking only those drugs prescribed by the physician assures safe care of mother and baby.

Physical examination

The physician performs a complete physical examination, which includes examination of the thyroid, teeth, lungs, heart, abdomen, and pelvis. Diagnostic measures include attention to weight, blood pressure, and urinalysis.

Thyroid. Palpation of the thyroid often reveals a slight enlargement, which is temporary during pregnancy. Disturbance in thyroid function may result in fluctuation in hormonal levels and may be a contributing factor in interruption of pregnancy prior to term.

Teeth. Dental examination and good oral hygiene contribute to adequate nutrition. Dental caries may interefere with food assimilation, affecting the health of mother and baby.

Lungs. Auscultation for adequate lung aeration assures sufficient oxygen intake, which ultimately keeps the infant well supplied. A chest radiograph (with adequate shielding of the abdomen) is performed to rule out tuberculosis and cardiac complications. Immunization for poliomyelitis is highly recommended.

Heart. Careful examination by auscultation for impaired cardiac function is performed on the initial visit. Elevations in blood pressure readings are a warning sign of impending toxemia.

Abdomen. Abdominal palpation is regularly included in the physical examination after the first trimester. Measurement of the height of the fundus with a pelvimeter determines gestational weeks and proper fetal growth. As pregnancy progresses, fetal parts can be palpated, and fetal movements and fetal attitude may be determined. At 18 to 20 weeks the fetal heart tones may be heard (by means of a stethoscope) through the abdominal wall.

Pelvis. At the first visit it is the pelvic examination that is of most concern to women. They know of its importance, yet they often think of it as associated with embarrassment and discomfort. The nurse can alleviate some of the anxiety by explaining the procedure, instructing the mother to keep her back flat on the examining table and to take slow, deep breaths so that she may be better able to relax.

With the mother in lithotomy position, her legs and abdomen are draped to expose the pudenda. The physician will put on a glove and observe the external genitalia for anomalies, growths, or varicosities. A vaginal speculum lubricated with warm water is inserted to examine the vaginal mucosa and cervix. Smears of the cervix and vaginal canal are taken for cancer cells, monilia, or trichomonal organisms. A thick, white leukorrhea may be indicative of monilial invasion; a cheesy leukorrhea is usually characteristic of trichomonal infection. These are not uncommon during pregnancy since the vaginal pH is somewhat altered. (For treatment, refer to Chapter 25.) A Papanicolaou smear of Class 1 or 2 is indicative of normal cell growth. Class 3, 4, or 5 is suggestive or positive evidence of carcinoma of the cervix. The cervix is inspected for erosions and is immediately treated with silver nitrate application. Because of increased vascularity, the cervix and vaginal canal take on a purplish hue.

Following speculum examination, the physician lubricates his gloved fingers and proceeds with a bimanual examination of the uterus and surrounding structures, together with a complete pelvic estimation. The pubic arch, sacrum, side walls, ischial spines, coccyx, and conjugate diagonal measurements are checked. (See Pelvic Measurements in Chapter 4.) Following pelvic examination the mother is offered tissues to remove the excess lubricant. The nurse should be in attendance to support, instruct, and assist during the pelvic examination. After two missed periods, a tentative diagnosis of pregnancy may be made on the basis of a pelvic examination. By the end of the third month (12 weeks), a positive diagnosis is made.

All of these examinations are included in the first prenatal visit. Regular monthly return visits are scheduled until the twenty-eighth week of pregnancy, followed by return visits every 2 weeks until 36 weeks, and then weekly visits to term. Should the health of the mother warrant more frequent visits, these are arranged and discussed with her. Revisits include urinalysis, weight measurement, blood pressure readings, abdominal examination for growth of the baby, and auscultation of fetal heart tones. On revisits mothers are more often ready to discuss their needs and concerns.

Diagnostic measures. On the first visit the mother is weighed and is asked what her normal weight is. Normal weight gain during pregnancy is approximately 20 pounds. Half the baby's weight is gained in the last 8 weeks of pregnancy. Any marked decrease or increase in weight warrants the attention of the physician. A high-protein, low-sodium, low-calorie diet is ordered when weight gain is excessive.

Microscopic examination of urine is done on the first visit. On subsequent visits sugar, acetone, and albumin determinations are performed to rule out toxemia and diabetes. When findings are abnormal, follow-up with blood work or midstream urinalysis is indicated.

Blood is drawn on the first visit for complete blood count, typing, Rh, and V.D.R.L. Hemoglobins of 10 Gm. or lower are treated by supplementing iron to the diet. Typing and Rh are essential should bleeding occur during the maternity cycle. Mothers with Rh-negative factors are supervised carefully, and blood titers are frequently taken in the last trimester. Should the titers increase, amniocentesis or further treatment may be instituted. (Refer to discussion on Rh incompatibility.) A positive V.D.R.L. is followed by dark-field microscopic examinations. Treatment is begun immediately with large doses of penicillin to prevent damage to the growing fetus.

Estimation of delivery date

Duration of pregnancy is approximately 280 days (40 lunar weeks, 10 lunar months) or 276 days (36 calendar weeks, 9 calendar months). Estimated date of delivery (E.D.D.) can be arrived at by counting back 3 months from the first day of the last menstrual period and adding 7 days; this is known as Nägele's rule. It is normal for a baby to arrive 2 or 3 weeks prior to the estimated date; however, it is rare for a pregnancy to go more than 3 weeks past term. Placental insufficiency is a hazard in such a pregnancy.

Should the last menstrual date not be known, the date quickening occurs, the height of the fundus, the size of the baby on x-ray examination, or changes in effacement and dilatation of the cervix may be used to determine an expected date of delivery.

THE NURSE'S ROLE DURING THE MATERNITY CYCLE

Optimum health care of the mother during the maternity cycle is essential for growth and development of the baby in utero. Health care incorporates medical and nursing supervision of the family; community health agencies are consulted when necessary. Agencies involved in family health care are the following: public health agencies, the welfare department, the social case worker, clergy, heart and diabetic associations, homemaker service, educational facilities, maternity shelters for unwed mothers, agencies that include services to the unwed father, adoption agencies, family counseling for marriage and family planning, and other allied medical services.

The nurse, who is sometimes the first contact the mother makes in seeking medical supervision, has every opportunity to evaluate needs at each visit and plans for the most effective nursing care, promoting optimum well-being of mother and baby. The nurse becomes for the mother an essential part of the complete care she anticipates. The nurse is one who is interested, kind, warm, understanding, a good listener, and a helper—the fact that she is a woman herself is never to be forgotten.

For the nurse, working with families during the childbearing period is more often a normal course, yet identifying and meeting the needs of expectant parents bring with them many psychologic as well as physical and physiologic considerations. The advent of pregnancy is not always a happy, wanted one, not always an expected one; at times, although parenthood is expected and welcomed, parents react rather peculiarly to the sudden realization that the responsibilities of parenthood will shortly be theirs. The nurse, being aware that a crisis does exist at this time of change in family constellation, is prepared by being perceptive and nonjudgmental and by giving support through anticipatory guidance. Her objectives in light of these factors would necessarily include the ability to listen carefully, interpret behavior, and communicate effectively. The nurse identifies needs, plans accordingly, and evaluates her plan to measure its effectiveness. She also needs to develop skills for teaching. Her knowledge of the social sciences prepares her to consider cultural influences in her plan of family care. As she helps each new family, she is fostering their knowledge of community health facilities.

PREPARATION FOR CHILDBEARING

It is true that childbearing is a "natural" process that has been going on for centuries with little knowledge on the part of women. We also know, however, that it is only the woman who can help in the delivery of her baby, and she is the sole participant. In our society young girls are beginning to question bodily functions and want to know and participate so that they might derive satisfaction in the maturing process of motherhood.

It is also understandable that progress in the education of youngsters includes the biologic sciences, since interest in this area is optimum. Improved health programs in schools and mass educational media such as literature, television, and radio make our young people aware of the importance of education in preparation for childbearing.

Community agencies

The health professions and related fields are involved in supplying adequate educational facilities in preparation for childbearing. The American Red Cross, nurses in hospitals, public health nurses, adult education departments, church groups, family life agencies, and private agencies in most communities offer these services. The content offered parents varies with the agency providing the services. Some agencies charge fees for services offered, while others do not. All agencies require permission from the physician supervising the care. A team, such as an obstetrician, a pediatrician, a nutritionist, a nurse, a nurse midwife, a physiotherapist, a psychiatrist, a social worker, and parents themselves, may be involved in the teaching.

Programs for parents

Preparation for childbearing includes instruction in which expectant parents are taught simple anatomy and physiology and the psychology of pregnancy, labor, and delivery. Such education helps parents understand the changes that are occurring during pregnancy, alleviating many fears and anxieties. Exercises are taught to the mother to prepare muscles that will be used during labor and delivery, so that she may participate as she brings forth her newborn infant. The father is included in the classes since he supports and helps his wife during pregnancy, and in some settings he can be with her during labor and delivery.

Classes offered to parents vary in the method used in teaching. The person conducting the classes usually decides on the method, taking into consideration the educational level of the group and using the method with which she (the instructor) is most comfortable.

Lecture methods. The lecture method is a structural approach in which all meetings are prearranged by the instructor. The material is presented by the instructor, and the lecture is followed by questions from the group. These sessions usually include discussion of (1) the importance of medical supervision and the hygiene of pregnancy, (2) the anatomy and physiology of the reproductive system, (3) the growth and development of the baby, (4) the physiology of pregnancy, (5) labor and delivery, and (6) baby care and infant feeding. A tour of the obstetric unit is also sometimes arranged by the instructor to acquaint the parents with the personnel and the hospital.

Discussion method. The discussion method is an unstructured approach in which the instructor acts as a group leader and the parents discuss whatever is of paramount interest to them. The instructor conducting these sessions needs to be quite flexible and also needs to have a broad understanding of the content area, including group dynamics and behavior.

Regardless of which method is used, the members of the group have similar interests, goals, feelings, and experiences. These similarities are helpful as expectant parents prepare for the roles of mother and father.

Tools used in teaching. Tools used in teaching include visual aids and pamphlets.

Visual aids. Posters, models, and films are helpful when chosen carefully. The more senses one gets the learner to use, the greater the amount of learning that takes place. It is relatively useless to discuss the uterus without simultaneously showing a picture of it. Models of the pelvis and the baby reveal and clarify the process by which the baby gets through the pelvis. Films chosen carefully to meet the needs of the group may be a useful tool in stimulating further discussion.

Pamphlets. The United States Department of Health, Education, and Welfare publishes excellent pamphlets to reinforce or supplement materials already used. Assigned readings will serve for an interesting discussion at a future group meeting. Many agencies have a collection of books given as donations from satisfied parents. Other excellent sources for materials related to maternal child health* are insurance companies, formula distributors, pharmaceutical firms, and so on. Many of the lay magazines have numerous articles related to childbearing and child rearing that are often clarified during group discussions.

TEACHING DURING PREGNANCY

In teaching the mother, the nurse should keep in mind the physiologic and psychologic changes that occur as pregnancy advances. For example, Caplan's works indicate that most women are angry when they first learn of pregnancy. They become passive and are greatly concerned with their own health. Nurses, to capitalize on this knowledge, should expend their energies in focusing on the mother's health; such concern would be greatly appreciated. It is during the first 3 months of pregnancy that the nurse might focus her instructions on the expression of feelings about becoming pregnant, the reasons for the nausea and vomiting, the alterations in mood and why they occur, and so on. Nurses should remember that the mother's general health is of primary importance during this time; the baby at this point is of relatively little concern to the mother.

As pregnancy advances, however, the second trimester brings a change in body contour and a feeling of the baby's movements; the mother begins to accept that a life is truly growing within her, and she experiences a general feeling of well-being. She begins to focus her attention on the baby; she begins to fantasize and dream of what the baby will be like. She likes to explore and discuss the baby's growth and the sensations she may be experiencing, and she enjoys getting things ready for the baby. Discussions centered about her dreams and fantasies might be helpful in giving clues to early mother-infant relationships. Caplan's studies show that not only do dreams and fantasies predict relationships, but the content of these dreams is most significant. The mother who dreams of her baby

*Maternity Center Association, 440 East 92nd St., New York, N. Y. International Childbirth Education Association, Seattle, Wash.

being of school age may be fearful of the responsibility of a tiny newborn. The mother who never fantasizes may be denying the fact that she is pregnant. What the mother says about her infant may also be significant. Some mothers immediately talk to their baby in utero, and others may never relate to the life growing within. Instructions during the second trimester might well focus on fetal growth and development, exploration of what the baby will be like, and preparation for the new family member.

The third trimester heralds exaggerated growth of the uterus, lesser agility, discomforts of pressure, and probably the longest waiting period of the entire pregnancy. The mother now focuses on the impending labor and delivery process and is most amenable to preparation in this area. Preparation for labor and delivery, then, is best taught during the last trimester. Discussions of what labor will be like will foster expressions of fears and anxieties in most women. Some of the fears and anxieties are a result of previous experiences; others result from what has been heard in relation to childbearing, from cultural influences, or simply from limited knowledge of the childbearing process. It has been proved that with knowledge there is less fear, and with less fear there is less anxiety. It is evident that preparation is a component of, and has a direct relationship to, performance. Therefore the preparation of parents is most important for satisfactory childbearing.

EXERCISES IN PREPARATION FOR CHILDBEARING

Exercises should be included in a comprehensive program of parent education. The purposes of exercises are to promote comfort during pregnancy, to facilitate childbirth, and to aid in strengthening muscles during the puerperium.

There are two specific differences in the approach to exercises and breathing techniques used. One uses principles of relaxation (the Read method), and the other uses conditioning (the Lamaze method).

The Read method

Relaxation position. In the relaxation position the woman lies on her side; a pillow is placed under her head (Fig. 8-1). All body parts including both arms and legs must be supported by the mattress. The abdomen rests on a small pillow or folded towel for additional support. A small pillow under the left leg (when the woman is lying on her right side) may give added back and abdominal comfort. To promote relaxation, muscle groups must be trained to tighten and then relax; this training should start with the face, hands, and toes.

The relaxation position may be assumed at any time during pregnancy and is most useful during the relaxation phase of labor. Along with complete breath and breath control, it will often induce sleep. After practicing the relaxation position, the woman brings back the circulation slowly by moving her hands and feet first. To rise from this position she should slowly push herself to a half-sitting position, kneel with buttocks up, and then rise to a standing position off the mattress.

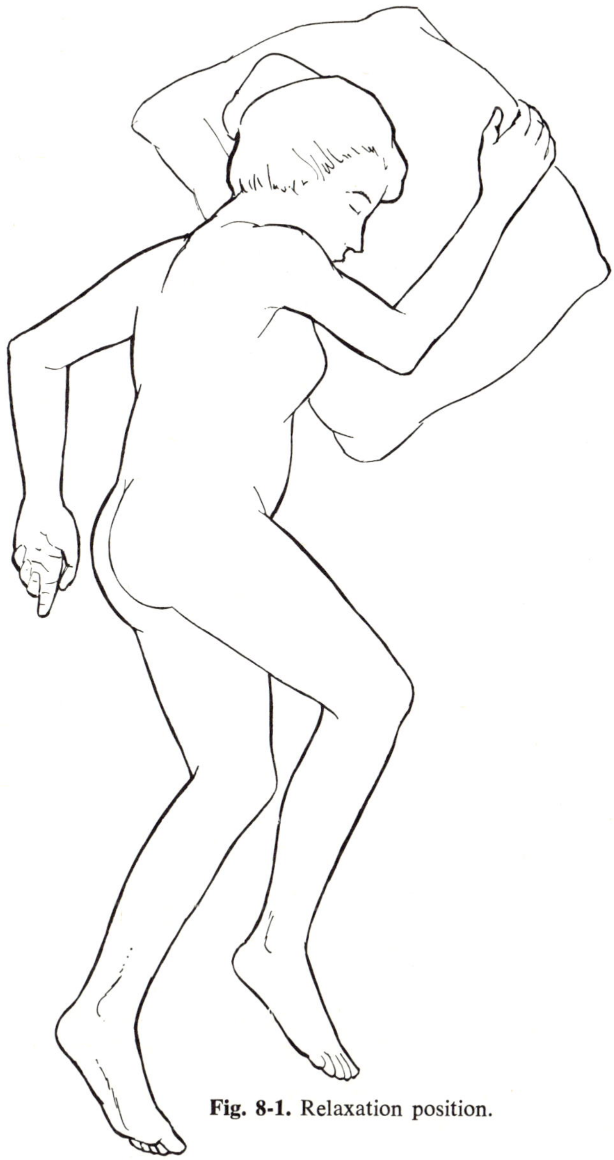

Fig. 8-1. Relaxation position.

Squatting and tailor sitting. Squatting and tailor sitting aid in stretching the perineal muscles and in increasing the circulation to that area (Fig. 8-2). These positions also make the pelvic bones more pliable. Loose, comfortable clothing should be worn; the feet are flat, the knees are bent, and the buttocks are slowly brought down as close to the heels as possible. From this position the buttocks are brought down to the floor, and the feet undersurfaces are brought together. In rising from this position, the buttocks are brought up first and then a standing position is resumed.

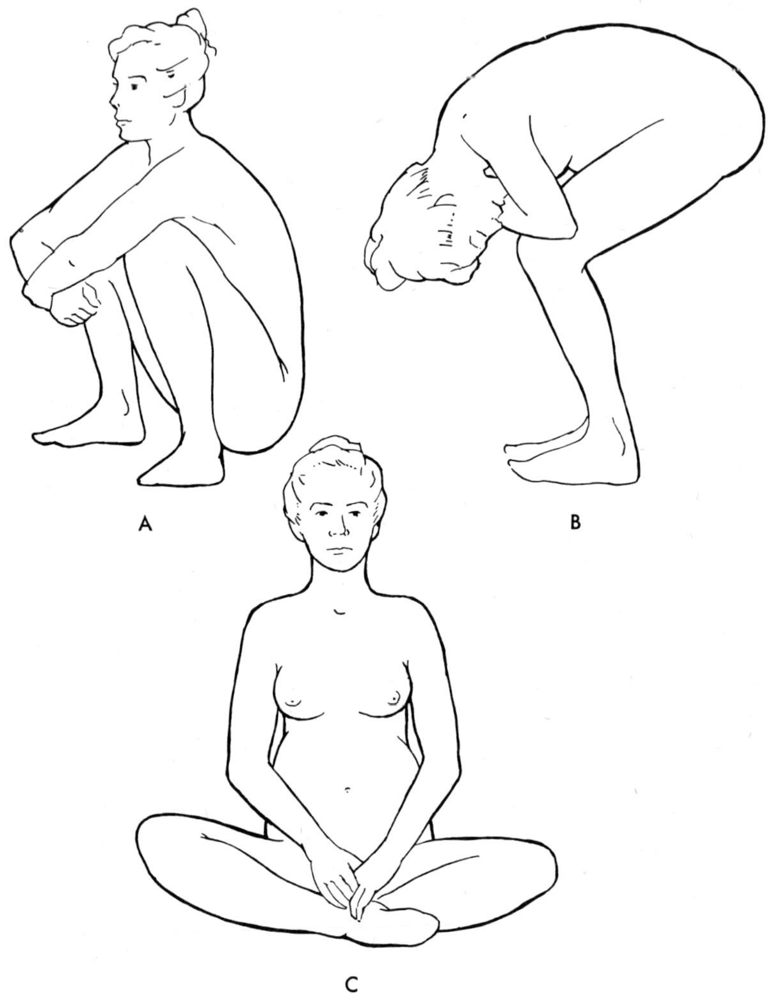

Fig. 8-2. A, Squatting. **B,** Rising. **C,** Tailor sitting.

Pelvic rocking. This exercise will help relieve abdominal pressure during pregnancy and low backache during pregnancy and early labor (Fig. 8-3). It can also be used following delivery to strengthen abdominal muscles. Pelvic rocking may be done in various positions: standing, sitting, lying down, or on all fours. In a standing position the feet are slightly separated, the back is arched, and the pelvis is tilted forward. In a supine position (with a pillow under the head) the small of the back is arched upward so that the abdomen rises and relaxes; this is repeated. In a kneeling position (with knees and hands on the floor), the back is arched and the abdomen is dropped forward.

Abdominal contractions. This exercise helps strengthen abdominal muscles during pregnancy and during the postpartum period. It may be done in a stand-

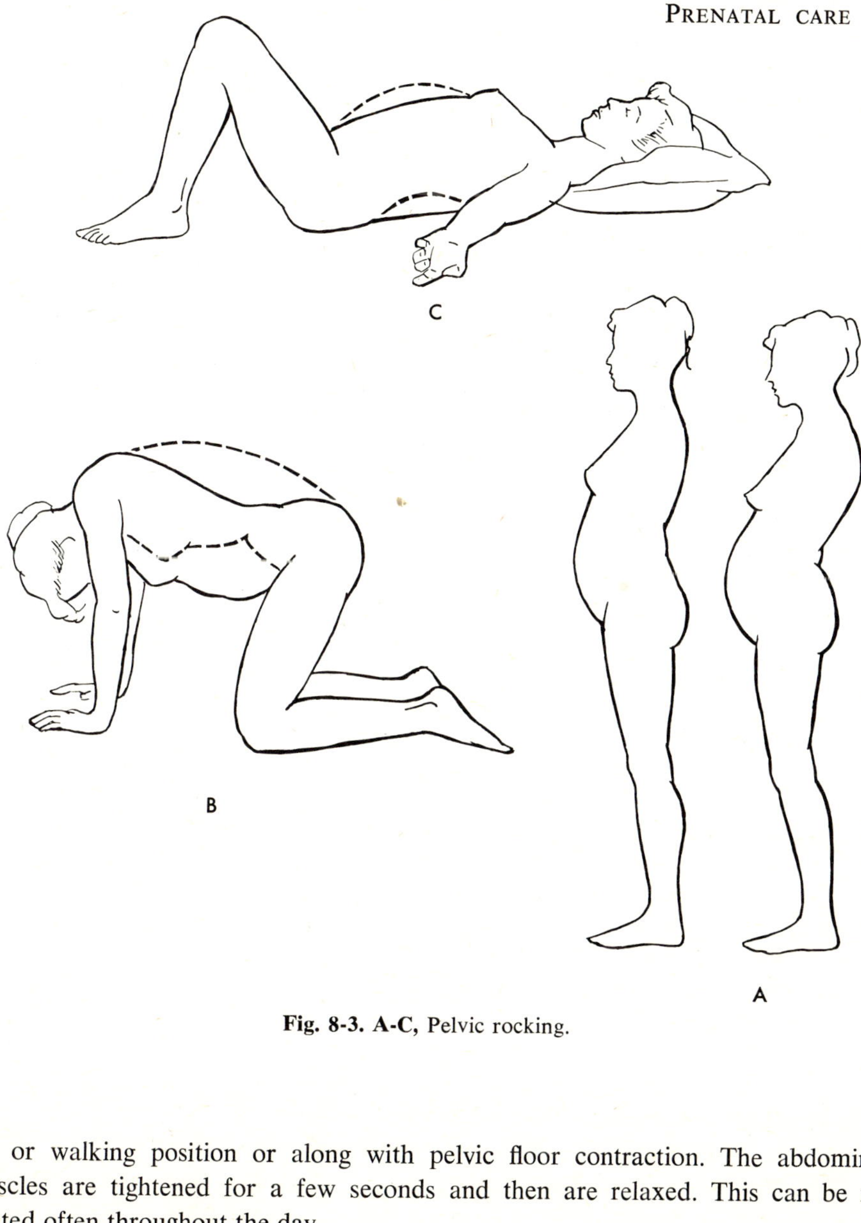

Fig. 8-3. A-C, Pelvic rocking.

ing or walking position or along with pelvic floor contraction. The abdominal muscles are tightened for a few seconds and then are relaxed. This can be repeated often throughout the day.

Pelvic floor contractions. This exercise relieves congestion and discomfort in the pelvic region and also increases the ability to control muscles surrounding the vagina, rectum, and bladder. It is done during pregnancy in preparation for labor and for the postpartum period. In a standing, sitting, or reclining position the muscles around the vagina and rectum are tightened for a few seconds and are relaxed slowly.

Modified knee-chest position. This exercise (Fig. 8-4) helps relieve pelvic pressure and cramps in the thighs or buttocks, and is beneficial for discomfort from hemorrhoids. In a kneeling position with knees apart, the abdominal muscles

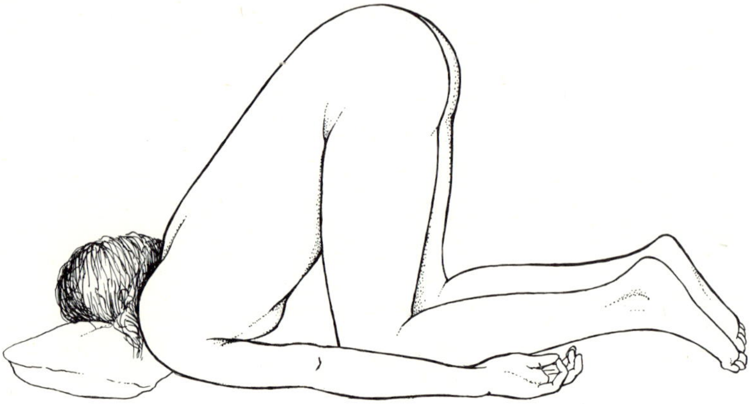

Fig. 8-4. Knee-chest position.

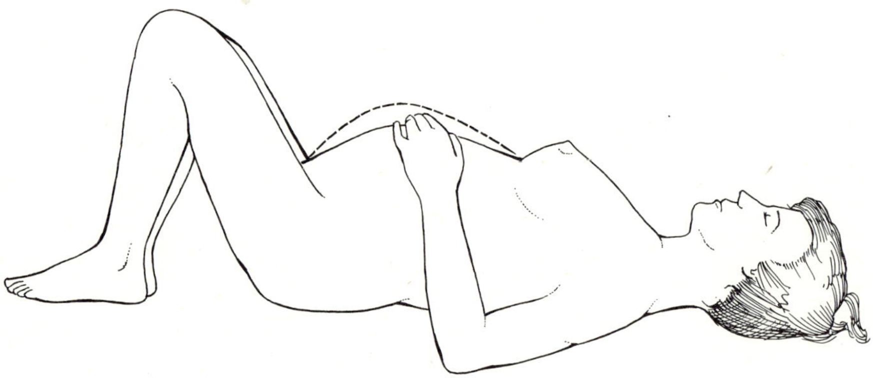

Fig. 8-5. Abdominal breathing.

are slightly tightened to relieve pressure of the baby on the abdominal wall. The arms are encircled about the head, the pelvis is higher than the rest of the body, and the back is straight. This position may be assumed for a minute or two.

Complete breath and breath control. This exercise (Fig. 8-5) is used to aid in relaxation and may be used throughout pregnancy and during the relaxation phase of labor. A deep breath is taken; on exhalation the air is forced out by blowing or hissing as the whole body becomes limp. The breathing is continued quietly, slowly, and rhythmically until complete relaxation is achieved. During early labor the entire breath exercise is practiced by starting with a deep breath, breathing slowly and rhythmically during the contraction, and ending with a deep breath.

Modified complete breath. This exercise is used as contractions become more forceful and increase in strength and length. The initial deep breath is taken; as the contraction nears its peak, four or five short, shallow breaths (throat breaths) are taken. At times dizziness and light-headedness may be experienced; a few

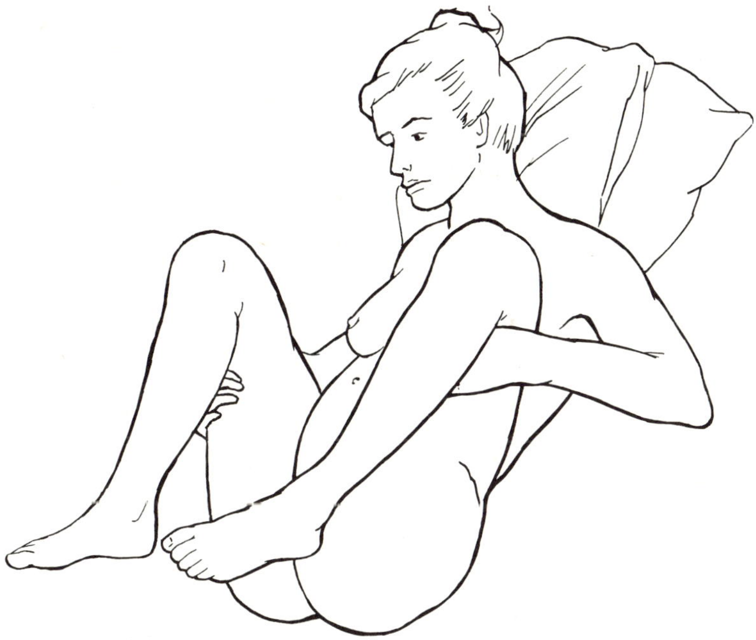

Fig. 8-6. Balloon breathing, pushing position.

quick, deep breaths will relieve these symptoms. The breath pattern again ends with one complete breath.

During transition there is often a tendency to hold the breath and a strong desire to push. During transition the modified complete breath can be done with one change. During the light breathing, puffing during exhalation on the third or fourth breath will decrease the urge to push.

Panting. This type of breathing is useful when the baby's head is crowning during delivery—it prevents rapid delivery through the birth canal. Panting is done by taking quick, shallow breaths with the mouth open.

Pushing position with pushing breath. This exercise is done during the second stage of labor as the mother actively helps in the delivery of the baby (Fig. 8-6). In a semi-Fowler's position, the knees are bent, and the legs are separated. The mother may hold the undersides of her thighs with her feet elevated from the mattress. An initial deep breath is taken, with a blow out on exhalation. With the next deep, quick breath, the breath is held and effort is made to fix the diaphragm on the abdominal wall for effective downward pressure in the uterus as pushing follows. During the actual pushing the head is raised, and the chin is bent on the chest while the mouth remains closed. Following this, a short catch breath and another push can be maintained if the contraction is still felt; complete relaxation should follow. During pregnancy the position and initial breath are practiced; however, pushing is contraindicated.

Lamaze method*

Neuromuscular control exercises:

Object: To learn muscular control of muscle groups.

Position: Lie on your back with one pillow under your head. If desired, place one pillow under knees. Rest arms on floor a little distance from your body.

1. Contract right arm. Release. Contract left arm. Release.
2. Contract right leg. Release. Contract left leg. Release.
3. Contract right arm and right leg. Release. Contract left arm and left leg. Release.
4. Contract right arm and left leg. Release. Contract left arm and right leg. Release.

Pay particular attention to contracting strongly where indicated while absolutely relaxing the rest of the body. Practice daily, husband giving commands and checking relaxation.

Body building exercises:

All exercises must be practiced every day on a hard surface (not in bed) without pillows. Repeat Exercises 1 through 5 three to five times:

1. Sit cross-legged for pelvic stretch, stretching of thigh muscles, and training of pelvic floor muscles.
2. Sit on floor. Pull feet as near body as comfortable. Press knees gently toward floor.
3. Lie down, arms at side, inhale through nose, raise right leg slowly, point toes. Exhale through lips, flex foot, lower right leg slowly. (Repeat with left leg.)
4. Lie down, spread out arms, inhale through nose, raise right leg, point toes. Exhale through lips, flex foot, lower leg as far as possible to right side. Inhale through nose, point toes, raise leg sideways, exhale through lips, flex foot, lower leg forward down. (Repeat with left leg.)
5. To rise from lying position: bend knees, turn from back to side, push up with the help of both arms.
6. Pelvic rocking: lie on back with legs bent, feet firmly on ground. Press back and shoulders firmly against floor, contracting abdominal muscles at the same time. Release. With breathing: flatten back while *exhaling,* release back while *inhaling*. (Repeat 10 times.)

First stage of labor:

Breathing exercises:

1. Preliminary labor: Slow rhythmic chest breathing, inhalation through nose, exhalation through lips. Preceded by deep inhalation-exhalation; followed by deep inhalation-exhalation. To be practiced with massage for abdomen or back. (Practice for one minute three times daily. Use 6-9 breaths for one minute.)

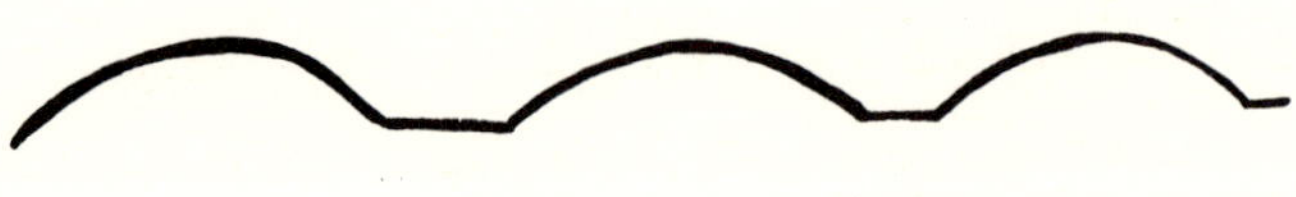

*From the American Society for Psycho-prophylaxis in Obstetrics, Inc., New York, N. Y.

2. Accelerated or active labor: Panting with acceleration as contraction builds up, deceleration as contraction subsides. Preceded and followed by deep inhalation-exhalation. (Practice for one minute three times a day.) Keep 4/4 rhythm at plateau of contraction:

Accelerated
Decelerated
Panting

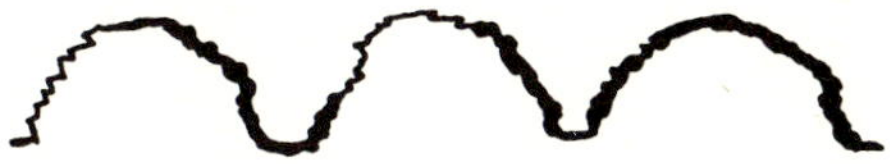

3. Transition: 4—6—8 fast shallow breaths, blow. Repeat. Preceded and followed by deep inhalation-exhalation. (Practice for 60-90 seconds, three times daily.)

Practice blowing only to avoid pushing when permission to push has not yet been given.

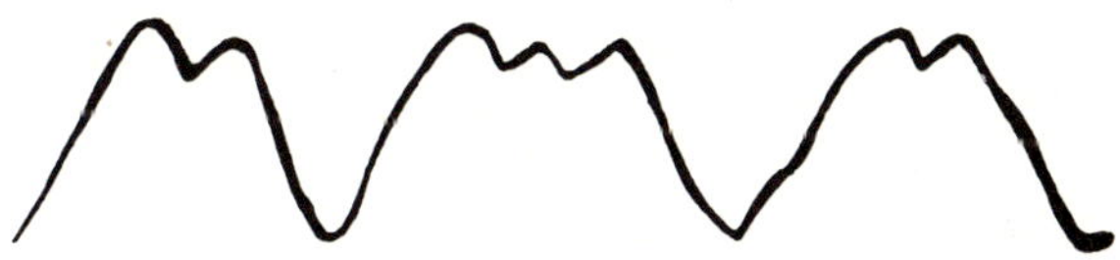

Second stage of labor:

Expulsion exercises:

1. Pelvic floor contraction-release: contract sphincter, vagina, and urethra, hold to a count of six, then release. (Practice as often as possible.)
2. Assume 45 degree angle position as for pushing in the labor room: inhale-exhale, inhale-exhale, inhale, hold breath, hold legs, under the knees, bring knees as close to shoulders as possible, elbows out, bend head forward, lean on diaphragm, push through vagina, exhale, relax head. Inhale, hold breath, bend head forward, lean on diaphragm, push, etc. Release when contraction is over. Take two or three deep breaths. (Practice pushing once a day for a few seconds.) When asked in delivery room not to push, use transition breathing or blow if urged to push is very strong.

NURSING CARE DURING THE PRENATAL PERIOD

Since there are physical and physiologic changes in all the body systems during pregnancy, care of the pregnant mother is planned accordingly. However, the emotional changes during pregnancy need also be considered since they greatly influence the general well-being of the mother and her relationships with family members.

EMOTIONAL ASPECTS OF PREGNANCY

Pregnancy at times may occur without readiness—family plans centered about financial stability are threatened, causing much anxiety. Young married parents or parents having a subsequent pregnancy may have planned savings for larger living quarters, or perhaps a much-needed summer vacation for family togetherness, or for the higher education of other family members. The awareness of a possible pregnancy leaves parents with distorted feelings, and they begin to question, "Why weren't we more careful?" "How could this have happened with all our planning?" "Just when we thought we could get away from washing diapers and getting up nights, we have to start all over again," "What will the older children think after all these years, and how will this affect them?" "I don't mind the pregnancy part, but thinking about another difficult labor and delivery makes me want to scream," "What will the neighbors think since we have so many children already?"

These are merely a few of the underlying realities that leave married people with many mixed feelings. All these reactions are to be expected by the nurse since she has great perception and understanding of human beings. The nurse should be ready to act as a sounding board—she knows that only in this way can parents ventilate, relieving their anxieties, and eventually with support there is acceptance. At times talking through does not solve problems and relieve anxiety, and the nurse may need the help of other paramedical personnel; then referral is pursued. Helping parents with emotional upheavals often involves education in preparation for what is happening, which helps in making the experience joyous rather than burdensome. The nurse helps the husband understand the changes occurring in his wife, that is, why she behaves so differently, so that he too may be able to help her at this time. Group discussions, where a small group of parents meet to discuss common experiences such as childbearing and the responsibilities of parenthood, are an essential part of every prenatal program. All the medical and physical care given is sold short when preparation for childbearing is not included.

NUTRITION

Nutrition requirements

Progressive growth and development of the baby make many demands on the nutritional status of the mother during pregnancy. Adequate nutrition aids the mother in maintaining her own optimum health status as well as that of the growing baby during pregnancy and later for breast-feeding.

Although caloric requirements during pregnancy are only slightly increased, the protein, mineral, and vitamin requirements are greatly increased as pregnancy advances. Dietary habits are established early in life, and food habits the pregnant mother already has need evaluation before any teaching is done. Dietary habits are essentially evaluated on the first prenatal visit, and planning with the mother through discussions should continue throughout pregnancy.

Protein. The protein needs are increased from 1 gm. to 1.5 gm. per kilogram of body weight. The added protein allows for storage of nitrogen, which is essentially supplied to the uterus, meeting the baby's need for growth and also supplying the mammary tissue in preparation for lactation. The greater portion of proteins ingested should be of animal origin (such as meat, milk, eggs, cheese, poultry, fish) since these contain essential amino acids.

Table 1. Recommended daily dietary allowances for a moderately active woman during pregnancy and lactation*

Essential nutrients	*Nonpregnant woman (58 kg. 25 yr.)*	*Pregnancy (second and third trimesters)*	*Lactation (850 ml. daily)*
Calories†	2,100	2,300	3,100
Protein, gm.	58	78	98
Calcium, gm.	0.8	1.3	1.3
Iron, mg.	15	20	20
Vitamin A, I.U.	5,000	6,000	8,000
Thiamine, mg.	0.8	1.0	1.2
Riboflavin, mg.	1.3	1.6	1.9
Niacin equivalent,‡ mg.	14	17	21
Ascorbic acid, mg.	70	100	100
Vitamin D, I.U.		400	400

*Food and Nutrition Board National Research Council, revised, 1963.

†Niacin equivalents include dietary sources of the preformed vitamin and the precursor tryptophan.

‡Energy requirements will vary with size, age, and activity.

Diet during pregnancy

Whole milk: 1 qt. (1 ounce of cheddar cheese is equivalent to 8 ounces of milk).

Lean meat: 1 liberal or 2 small servings (4 oz.) of meat, fish, or fowl; liver is desirable at least once a week.

Egg: 1 each day.

Fruit: 2 or more servings (1-1½ cups, 200-300 gm.) each day; 1 serving should be citrus fruit or other good source of ascorbic acid.

Vegetables: 2 or more servings of cooked or raw vegetables (1-1½ cups, 200-300 Gm.) each day; these should include dark green leafy or deep yellow vegetables; in addition, a medium potato (150 gm.) should be eaten daily.

Bread and cereal: Whole-grain or enriched bread, at least 4 slices daily (½ cup of cereal is equivalent to 1 slice of bread).

Butter or margarine: 1 to 2 tablespoons.

Additional foods: Consisting of either more of the foods already listed or other foods of one's own choice adjusted to individual energy needs in relation to desired weight gain.

Vitamin D: Some form of vitamin D to supply 400 I.U.

A diet with adequate protein requirement will of necessity also include ascorbic acid, vitamin A, and vitamin D. Deficiency in protein deprives the mother of adequate calcium, phosphorus, iron, and vitamin B.

Studies show that deficiency in proteins is responsible for nutritional edema, anemia, poor uterine muscle tone, abortion, prematurity and deformities, lowered resistance to infections, and failure to lactate. It has also been found that protein deficiency can be related to toxemia of pregnancy. The Food and Nutrition Board of the National Research Council recommends adding 20 gm. protein to the diet daily in the latter half of pregnancy (Table 1). Amino acids also facilitate calcium absorption if a calcium deficiency exists.

Calcium, phosphorus, and vitamin D. Since vitamin D is essential for the synthesis of calcium and phosphorus, their values must be considered at the same time. The fetus retains 65% and 64% phosphorus and calcium, respectively, in the last 2 months of pregnancy. Again, if protein requirements are adequate, so are phosphorus values.

Iron. The growing fetus stores iron in his tissues and circulating hemoglobin for use during the first months of life. The daily diet should contain 20 mg. iron during pregnancy.

Oral preparations of 100 to 110 mg. of supplemental iron are given daily in the last trimester since iron absorption is increased during this time. Large milk intakes may interfere with iron absorption. Folic acid, 5 mg. daily, is often prescribed for mothers of lower socioeconomic status. Severe anemia in which the hemoglobin is 8 Gm. per 100 ml. or less is common with amylophagia. Amylophagia is the ingestion of large quantities of starch to the exclusion of other dietary substances; it is a form of pica.

Iodine. Added demands upon metabolism by the thyroid make iodine a necessary constituent in the diet. The use of iodized salt is sufficient to maintain the proper amount of iodine in the diet.

Vitamins. Demand for all vitamins is increased during pregnancy, as shown by recommendation of the National Research Council. Studies suggest that vitamin E is necessary for normal development of the fetus and for the completion of pregnancy. Vitamin K, 5 mg., may be given to the mother at the time of labor or to the infant at the time of birth (2.5 mg.). Since vitamin K is not produced until the infant ingests nourishment, this practice stabilizes prothrombin level.

Caloric intake. Although the basal metabolic rate increases from 6% to 14% during pregnancy, the increase in caloric requirement is not needed until the latter half of pregnancy. The Food and Nutrition Board of the National Research Council recommends an additional 300 calories during the latter half of pregnancy, since the metabolic rate increases and the appetite is stimulated. If overweight is a problem, the diet can be restricted in calories—however, all the essential nutriments should be included for adequate nutrition of the mother and the baby.

Milk can be taken between meals if desired. During the latter half of pregnancy when 300 added calories are required, 1 ounce of meat and 1 pint of milk will fulfill the requirements for essential proteins, calcium, and vitamin C. If whole milk cannot be tolerated, skim milk or buttermilk can be used. Other alternatives to milk are soups, custards, puddings, and ice cream if weight is under control. Cheese can be another substitute for milk and can be taken when salt is not restricted. The fluid requirement will aid in promoting intestinal peristalsis and in controlling constipation common during pregnancy.

Education in nutrition

Dietary planning begins with the first prenatal visit. A printed diet list is not sufficient in dietary health teaching. A more effective approach would be to dis-

Table 2. Cultural food habits

	Food habits	*Food likes*	*Food deficiencies*
Mexican	Tomatoes and corn Rice, beans Use mostly white flour Lard in large amounts Beef, pork, and veal cooked with vegetables or in soup Eggs, fried or boiled Fish on Fridays Sugar used abundantly	Dried beans Peppers Potatoes Bread	Milk Fresh citrus fruits Green leafy vegetables
Armenian Syrian, Greek, Turkish	Yogurt Very little butter Vegetables fried with meats, nuts, and beans and cooked in lamb broth Peppers, tomatoes, cabbage, and grape leaves Cucumbers, squash Few potatoes used Dried apricots and raisins Nuts substituted for meat Dried peas, beans, lentils Lamb used extensively Honey, sugar for sweetening Like fruit compotes Lamb fat and olive oil Olives in place of butter Turkish coffee, thick and sweetened	Cracked wheat and dark bread Vegetables Dried fruit	Milk Fresh fruits Butter
Polish	Milk and sour cream, especially in soups Cheese Butter on bread Dark rye bread Vegetables, cabbage and root vegetables cooked a long time, in soup or with hot milk Fruits, limited for economic reasons Prefer pork	Dark grain Vegetables Coffee Sweets	Milk Citrus fruits Beef and lamb Raw vegetables
Scandinavian Denmark, Finland, Norway, Sweden	Cream in coffee, gravies Sweet butter preferred Whole wheat, rye, and barley flour Vegetables, coleslaw, root, avocados Fruit, berries a favorite Meat, wild game, reindeer Fish, fresh, smoked, or salted	Dark bread, whole grains Milk, dairy products Dried fruit Fish	Less food between meals Fresh fruits, vegetables

Continued.

Table 2. Cultural food habits—cont'd

	Food habits	*Food likes*	*Food deficiencies*
	Hard-cooked eggs Sweets, cakes, cookies, pastries Pickled meat and fish Molasses and ginger used in breads and cakes		
Italian	Cereals, use of cornmeal substitute, farina Starches, macaroni with sauce and cheese Breads, white crusty breads, whole wheat Vegetables and fruits, potatoes, fried, vegetables, cooked too long, eggplant, a favorite Salads a favorite, but expense a factor Meat, eggs, use more for flavoring, highly seasoned Dried beans in soups and main dishes Eggs, fried with vegetables, peppers, spinach Sweets, fruits for dessert, spumoni ice cream Olive oil used for frying and cooking Salt pork used as a substitute, garlic and pepper for flavoring	Leafy vegetables Fruits	Milk, whole grains in breads and cereals American cheeses Inexpensive oils when finances are low Butter
Puerto Rican	Spices used in foods Plantains, called "Tostones," fried, baked, broiled, boiled Beans with onions, bacon, and garlic Peppers, part of everyday food Fish with sauces Breadfruit, like cantaloupe boiled, tastes like bread Corn, large sweet yams Avocados	Grapefruit, pineapple, oranges, limes	Meat and eggs not used since they are expensive in Puerto Rico Milk, expensive
Chinese	Eggs, meat, fish, cereals, vegetables, cheese Radish leaves, bean and bamboo sprouts Rice instead of bread Wheat, corn and millet seed		

Table 2. Cultural food habits—cont'd

	Food habits	*Food likes*	*Food deficiencies*
	Noodles Meat: lamb, goat, duck Milk: water buffalo or soybean Pigeon eggs		
Japanese	Rice, bean paste soup Raw or cooked fish Pickles Wheat noodles with broth Vegetables Salty crisp seaweed		

cuss what the mother is eating at each meal. Evaluation of her existing dietary habits might eliminate unnecessary teaching, starting with the principle of giving the mother credit for what she is already eating that is good nutrition. Perhaps it would be better to discuss the family menu since the mother cooks the food for the family, and alterations for herself might appear to be a chore. If, for instance, it is necessary to restrict her salt intake, the cooking of foods without salt and then adding it for the family would be feasible. Discussing the food budget at times might be necessary in suggesting less expensive cuts of meat. Cultural food patterns are also considered and need not be changed, but at times methods used in preparation need modification. It is always good psychology to allow at least one well-liked (cultural) food so that the rest of the diet can be assimilated. A good nutritionist is an essential member of the health team in planning dietary needs.

Food habits of nationality groups

Cultural food customs (Table 2) are as much a part of the culture of an individual as his habit of speech, mode of dress, or way of life. Helping the Puerto Rican, Italian, Scandinavian, Polish, Finnish, Mexican, and people of the Near East is made easier if the nurse is aware of their particular food habits. Emphasizing good nutrition that includes cultural food habits is a needed prerequisite in accepting other essential diet requirements.

Nutrition for the adolescent mother

The problem of hunger and malnutrition was the major discussion topic at the December, 1969, White House Conference at Washington, D. C. The incidence of malnutrition in teen-agers is unknown. It is, however, higher among the poor and among those who are under tensions at home or at school. "The girl teen-ager is the least well-fed member in our society" has often been said. Yet the food habits of teen-agers are aberrations in an attempt to express independence, freedom to choose, and a desire to be associated with their peer group.

Dietary surveys show that adolescents have less than two thirds of the recommended dietary allowances for calcium, iron, ascorbic acid, and vitamin A. Adolescent girls are more aware of being fat, and when caloric intakes are less than 2,000 calories per day, the recommended 20 mg. of iron is deficient. Anemic, underweight teen-agers are prone to infections, colds, and tuberculosis.

The nutritional state of the teen-ager prior to conception is more important than the quality of her diet during pregnancy. There is a higher incidence of toxemia, with resulting premature births and a higher infant mortality, among teenagers who have not had proper nutrition prior to pregnancy.

Health aspects of pregnancy in adolescents began to receive national concern because of the alarming infant mortality and morbidity rates in the United States during the early 1960's. Because of these startling statistics there has been a renewed interest in the role of maternal nutrition as it affects the outcome of pregnancy.

In 1966, Children's Bureau requested that the Food and Nutrition Board of the National Academy of Sciences, National Research Council, constitute a Committee on Maternal Nutrition with the purpose of synthesizing scientific information as it applies to nutrition in maternal and child health. In January, 1970, two conferences explored the subjects of the pregnant school-age girl and parenthood in adolescence. The results of these conferences follow.

> There must be a national affirmation that every woman has the right to high quality and high standard health care. This includes a food intake that will prepare her for and carry her through a healthy pregnancy and childbirth and permit her infant to flourish. It affirms that the right to adequate nutrition is an inseparable part of the basic right to health care and that women require and are entitled to sufficient amounts of nutritious food.
>
> The Panel believes that the increasing numbers of pregnancies among adolescent girls and the decreasing age at which girls become pregnant, jeopardize national health goals and comprise the status of the present generation as well as those to follow. The nutritional status of many adolescents in the United States is such as to contribute unfavorably to the outcome of pregnancy as reflected by maternal mortality, maternal morbidity, perinatal and infant mortality and morbidity.*

The preceding conclusions are important and of great concern since there is an increasing number of pregnancies at younger ages. During the period from 1957 to 1968, there was a steady decline in birth rate (live births per 1,000 population). However, in 1969 the total number of live births in the United States increased 2% as compared to 1968. The children born during World War II are now entering the childbearing age, and, with proper nutrition prior to pregnancy and adequate health care during pregnancy, this rise in live births will continue.

Another factor in the increasing number of adolescent mothers is that girls are reaching sexual maturity earlier; the average age for onset of menses is approximately 13 years. For instance, in 1965, there were 196,372 children born to girls 17 years of age, 29,000 were born to girls 15 years of age and under, and over 56,000 were born to girls 16 years of age. This same year's statistics

*Food and Nutrition News, National Live Stock and Meat Board, Chicago, Ill., May, 1970.

showed an increase of low birth weight infants, with higher infant mortality rates. These pregnancies were also complicated by toxemia, anemia, and difficulties during labor and delivery.

The Committee on "Nutrition and the Pregnant Adolescent" found that:

1. Pregnant and nonpregnant adolescents have bizarre dietary habits, and their intakes of iron, calcium, vitamin A, and ascorbic acid are inadequate.

2. Caloric requirements during adolescence parallel the growth curve, and each individual has a unique pattern of development.

3. Young adolescents tolerate caloric restrictions poorly.

4. Impact of pregnancy occurring during adolescent growth on the achievement of body growth remains to be determined.

5. Once pregnancy occurs it is too late to improve nutrition; the nutritional state of the pregnant adolescent prior to becoming pregnant is more important.

The National Research Council also found that:

> Society, because of its punitive attitudes toward early pregnancy, especially if out-of-wedlock, is prone to withhold the understanding and support that are so important to girls in this circumstance. A punitive attitude reflected in restrictive practices may force the young pregnant girl to discontinue her education, may make it difficult for her to obtain medical care, and even prevent her from getting married in many states. These social and psychological difficulties are superimposed on the emotional adaptations and problems characterizing adolescence.

Therefore the Panel at the White House Conference on Food, Nutrition, and Health made the following recommendations:

1. Steps to be taken to eliminate all local statutes which disqualify the pregnant adolescent from continuation of schooling and the receipt of appropriate health care, nutrition education, and nutrition.

2. Adequate support be made available to initiate and maintain special school programs in conjunction with comprehensive health and social programs, to ensure continuity of education and necessary health care for all girls who become pregnant.

3. Action be initiated to develop practices, regulations, and laws which will make available family planning information and services, upon request, to the adolescent, whether married or unmarried.

4. The Panel recognized that an essential step to reduce the incidence of pregnancy in young adolescent girls is the inclusion in the curricula of our schools instructions in health, nutrition, social and physiological aspects of human reproduction and the importance and means of achieving responsible parenthood.*

Nurse's role in teaching the adolescent nutrition. The adolescent has difficulty making a decision to change dietary habits. The nurse who learns to listen and to let the girl talk allows her to make the change. In planning with the adolescent, consideration of the social, economic, psychologic, and cultural factors is primary

---

*Pregnancy in school age girls, Food and Nutrition News, National Live Stock and Meat Board, Chicago, Ill., June, 1970.

in bringing about effective change. Change must be gradual, and current food habits must be explored and used as a "takeoff."

The meaning of food to the adolescent is different from its meaning to adults. Criticism of certain foods does not help, but rather lessening consumption of nonessential foods and gradual change to other foods are more successful.

Change is brought about more readily when there is a reward available. Stress on appearance of the skin, hair, and body contours may help the adolescent to acquire new food habits. Adolescents are known to skip meals because both parents are working, and they have no companion with whom to share a meal. Nutrition education for the adolescent should become a part of preschool, grade school, and high school education.

The nurse who recognizes the environmental, cultural, and economic aspects of adolescent motherhood and develops interest for nutrition will be successful in working with the teen-age mother.

PHYSICAL ASPECTS OF PRENATAL CARE

Care of the teeth

Good dentition, requiring regular visits to the dentist and adequate dental hygiene, should be maintained during pregnancy. Occasionally some women develop dental caries requiring immediate care. Massaging of the gums is good practice prior to morning and evening mouth hygiene.

Clothing

Wearing apparel during pregnancy should not only allow for comfort and easy laundering but should also be flattering. The enlarging breasts and abdomen change body posture, gait, and appearance, which may be greatly altered by clothing. Shoes should of necessity provide comfort and safety and be conducive to good posture and proper balance. Well-fitting brassieres should be worn to support the breast tissues, as the increased blood supply to the breasts prepares the tissues for their lactating function. Dresses that hang from the shoulder, are loose about the waist and abdomen, provide comfort, and are stylish, since the popularity of the "shift," are commonly worn. Playclothes for the summer are available for sunbathing and water wading when desired. Since increased diaphoresis is common during pregnancy, materials that are lightweight and washable are more practical. Wearing apparel that is attractive and comfortable minimizes many of the ambivalent feelings often associated with increasing size as pregnancy advances.

Bathing habits

Daily bathing is refreshing, stimulates circulation, and adds comfort as body wastes are increased. The selected method used for bathing should be safe and satisfying for the mother. Bathing the extremities becomes a chore during the last month of pregnancy, and perhaps the husband's cooperation can be encouraged at this time.

Care of the breasts

The increased blood supply to the breasts causes some enlargement; therefore adequate support is needed. The brassiere should have a large enough cup to support the breast tissue. The mother who does not plan to breast-feed her infant need concern herself only with providing proper support and with keeping the breasts clean.

Niles Newton discourages the use of soap for the mother planning to breast-feed; soap tends to dry the natural secretions of the tubercles of Montgomery in the areola. The added secretions around the nipple are not dirt particles, but rather are a common occurrence during pregnancy.

In cultures in which women's breasts remain exposed there is a definite toughening of nipple tissue, and there are rarely problems with tissue breakdown. Since women in our society must adhere to proper attire, other techniques are recommended. The mother may be taught to toughen the nipples by rubbing them briskly with a towel at bath time. Also, nipple rolling and breast massage are advantageous for the mother who is at ease in handling her breasts.

Directions for breast care in preparation for nursing*:

Breast massage

Wash hands well with soap and water; have lotion and towel available; sit in a comfortable chair. Then proceed as follows:

1. Lubricate hands with lotion.
2. Place one hand on top of other above one breast.
3. Draw hands apart with firm pressure.
4. Turn hands downward on each side of breast; press firmly and evenly.
5. Cup breast as hands sweep downward to areola and nipple, bringing breast forward and upward.
6. Allow breast to fall gently as fingers and thumbs slide off; do not touch areola or nipple.
7. Repeat (several times) for each breast.

Colostrum expression (Fig. 8-7)

1. Support breast with one hand.
2. With other hand, feel gently for lacteal sinuses around edge of areola.
3. Grasp breast with fingers below and with thumb above edge of areola.
4. Exert pressure inward; compress and release lacteal sinuses.
5. Look for beads of yellow-orange colostrum at nipple ducts; wipe away with towel.
6. Repeat pressure with finger and thumb around areola.
7. Continue until flow of colostrum ceases (usually in 1 or 2 minutes).
8. Repeat with other breast; do once daily.

Nipple rolling (Fig. 8-8)

1. Grasp nipple between thumb and forefinger.

---

*From Iorio, J.: When your patient wonders about breast feeding, RN **26**:44, November, 1963.

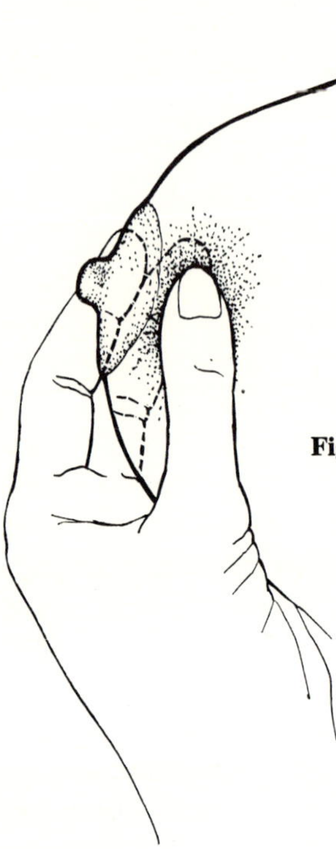

Fig. 8-7. Colostrum expression.

Fig. 8-8. Nipple rolling.

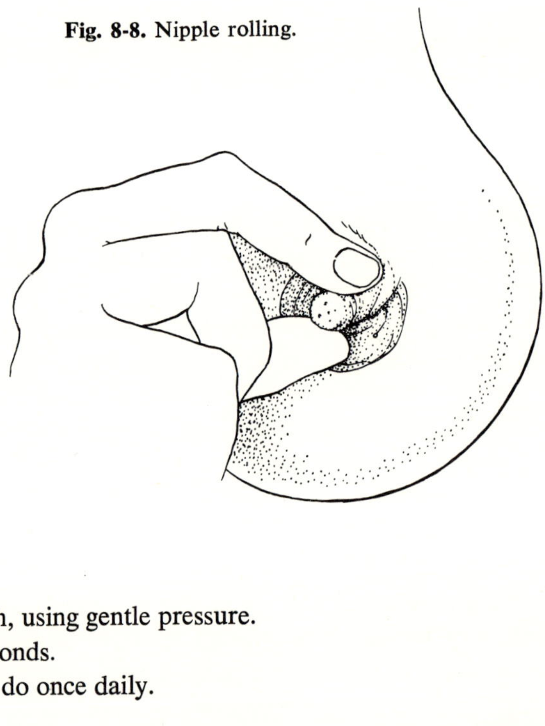

2. Roll nipple back and forth, using gentle pressure.
3. Continue for 15 to 30 seconds.
4. Repeat with other breast; do once daily.

Excretory system

Constipation resulting from bowel relaxation and impaired tone is a constant complaint of pregnant women. Addition to the diet of fresh fruit and vegetables, intake of adequate fluids to increase peristalsis, and engaging in adequate exercise will prove beneficial. When vitamins with an iron supplement are ordered, discussing the possibility of dark stools and constipation eliminates worry and concern.

Occasionally mild cathartics that have a lubricating effect or those increasing bulk are ordered by the physician. Mineral oil, milk of magnesia, Colace, or Senokot are common laxatives ordered. Harsh cathartics and enemas are seldom ordered during pregnancy.

Relaxation, rest, and social activity

During the first and last trimesters, mothers complain of fatigue. The increased secretions of the ovarian hormone relaxin in the first trimester, and the size and weight of the abdomen during the last trimester, result in fatigue. Rest, in either a comfortable sitting or lying down position, is essential when needed. As the baby gets larger, backache caused by pressure on the coccyx may be relieved by a side-lying position, which promotes relaxation, or by the pelvic-rocking exercise. When varicosities are present, stasis of blood causes leg edema and discomfort. Ace bandages or elastic stockings applied in the early morning and elevation of the extremities without pressure on the popliteal space provide comfort.

Some mothers are employed during pregnancy, and sitting can be just as tiring. Since blood volume is increased, occasional mild exercise is important to improve circulation and promote adequate oxygenation to the growing baby.

Relaxation and social contact are much needed during pregnancy. Engaging in strenuous exercise would depend upon previous habits. For some mothers strenuous exercise engaged in before pregnancy may be within normal range. However, heavy lifting, pushing, or pulling should be avoided.

The advisability of traveling during pregnancy depends upon the course of pregnancy and the general health of the mother. When fetal growth and development are occurring, the hazards of maternal infections are increased in crowded areas and with changes in environment. During the last month of pregnancy, the hazards of premature labor may also present problems. Traveling is not contraindicated, provided the safety of the mother and thc baby is ensured.

Douching

Douching is not a part of routine feminine hygiene during pregnancy. Should there be irritation and leukorrhea resulting from bacterial invasion, a cleansing douchc may bc ordered. For safety purposes douching is done in reclining position in a clean bath tub. The douche nozzle should be inserted 2 or 3 inches, and the level of the irrigating can should be no higher than 2 feet above hip level. Gentle rotation of the nozzle assures effective irrigation of the vaginal canal. Bulb type syringes are contraindicated since the force may cause air embolism.

Smoking

Studies reveal that smoking mothers have smaller babies than nonsmoking mothers, and the decrease in birth weight is closely related to the amount of smoking during pregnancy. Smoking should be limited during pregnancy.

Marital relations

Normally sexual intercourse during pregnancy is not contraindicated unless there is bleeding (indicating possible abortion) or unless ill health is present in either partner. Occasionally alterations in position during marital relations may be more comfortable as the uterus enlarges. Often there are fluctuations in sexual desires during pregnancy that are not understood by parents, and free discussion should be encouraged. Unless there is contraindication or discomfort, sexual union is not harmful. Physicians usually advise abstinence in the last month of pregnancy for comfort and safety.

PUBLIC HEALTH SUPERVISION OF THE FAMILY

Referral for added supervision by the public health nurse enhances prenatal care. Evaluation of the home in preparation for the new baby assures readiness and facilitates family equilibrium following delivery. The mother in her own home is more at ease and feels free to discuss many things she does not think of during a hurried clinic visit. Her first visit to the clinic, in which blood work is done and complete physical examination is followed by a pelvic examination, is hardly the time to verbalize added fears of oncoming labor and delivery. Preparation of clothes and crib for the new infant is discussed and handled with greater ease in the home. Planning visits at mealtime may prove beneficial if help is needed in diet planning. Involving the father may be accomplished by arranging a visit when he is at home. Continued public health supervision following delivery is essential since the postpartal hospital stay has been shortened. The responsibility of parenthood in our present-day society needs consideration in the total care of families.

SELECTED REFERENCES

Alvarez, H., and Caldeyro-Barcia, R.: Contractility of the human uterus recorded by new methods, Surg. Gynec. Obstet. **91:**1, 1950.

Apgar, V.: Drugs in pregnancy, Amer. J. Nurs. **65:**104, March, 1965.

Assali, N. S., Rauramo, L., and Peltonen, T.: Measurement of uterine blood flow and uterine metabolism. VIII. Uterine and fetal blood flow and oxygen consumption in early human pregnancy, Amer. J. Obstet. Gynec. **79:**86, 1960.

Beebe, J. E.: Bench conferences in a large obstetric clinic, Amer. J. Nurs. **68:**85, January, 1968.

Belkin, M., Suchman, E. A., Rosenblatt, D., and others: Mothers' utilization of the child health station and evaluation of child health conference, Amer. J. Public Health **54:**2023, 1964.

Biancardi, P.: Special delivery, RN **32:**52, August, 1969.

Boissoneau, R. A.: Satellite obstetric center services patients in their own neighborhood, Hospitals **42:**50, March 1, 1968.

Caplan, G.: Concepts of mental health and consultation, U. S. Department of Health, Education, and Welfare, Children's Bureau, 1959, Publication No. 373.

Chow, B. F.: Maternal nutrition and metabolism of the offspring: studies in rats and man, Amer. J. Public Health **58:**668, 1968.

Cooper, L. F., Barber, E. M., and Mitchell, H. S.: Nutrition in health and disease, Philadelphia, 1963, J. B. Lippincott Co.

Cunningham, J.: Abdominal decompression for pregnancy and labour; the Heyns method, Nurs. Times **63:**1285, 1967.

Davis, C., and Morrone, F.: An objective evaluation of a prepared childbirth program, Amer. J. Obstet. Gynec. **84:**1196, 1962.

Day, G. A.: Early discharge of maternity patients, Nurs. Outlook **11:**825, 1963.

Eastman, N. J., and Hellman, L. M.: Williams obstetrics, ed. 13, New York, 1966, Appleton-Century & Appleton-Century-Crofts.

Editorial: Human pregnancy nutrition, a clinical view, Obstet. Gynec. **30:**605, 1967.

Elliott, J. M.: Pica and pregnancy, Nurs. Clin. N. Amer. **3:**299, 1968.

Estey, G. P.: Natural childbirth—word from a mother, Amer. J. Nurs. **69:**143, July, 1969.

Friedman, W. L.: Prophylactic use of iron in pregnancy, Obstet. Gynec. **25:**495, 1965.

Goodrich, F. W.: The problem of anxiety in

obstetrics, Child and Family, p. 62, Winter, 1965.
Henry, J. B., Little, W. A., and Christian, C. D.: Modified immunologic test for pregnancy, Techn. Bull. Regist. Med. Techn. **34:**99, 1964; Amer. J. Clin. Path. **42:**109, 1964.
Hilliard, M. E.: The changing role of the maternity nurse, Nurs. Clin. N. Amer. **3:**277, June, 1968.
Hoff, F. L.: Natural childbirth—how any nurse can help, Amer. J. Nurs. **69:**145, July, 1969.
Hommel, F.: Natural childbirth—nurse in private practice as monitrices, Amer. J. Nurs. **69:**146, July, 1969.
Jacobson, B. D.: A simple and rapid immunologic test for pregnancy, based on agglutination-inhibition, Obstet. Gynec. **25:** 192, 1965.
Keane, V.: An evolving philosophy of maternity care, Bull. Amer. Coll. Nurse Midwifery **12:**40, May, 1967.
Kitzinger, S., and Litt, B.: A fresh look at antenatal exercises, Nurs. Mirror **129:**14, Sept. 5, 1969.
Kumabe, K. T.: A prenatal clinic in a rural area, Children **11:**214, 1964.
Lindner, E. M.: Childbirth practices in two primitive cultures: implications for modern maternity care, Bull. Amer. Coll. Nurse Midwifery **11:**130, 1966.
Litz, A. W.: Maternal care, Bull. Amer. Coll. Nurse Midwifery **13:**18, February, 1968.
Loughlin, B. W.: Pregnancy in a Navajo culture, Nurs. Outlook **13:**55, March, 1965.
Madore, E. C., and Deutsch, Y. B.: Talking with parents, Amer. J. Nurs. **62:**108, November, 1962.
McDonald, R. H.: Current programs for childbirth, Child and Family, p. 4, Winter, 1963.
Milio, N.: Values, social class and community health services, Nurs. Res. **16:**26, Winter, 1967.
Morris, E.: How does a nurse teach nutrition to patients? Amer. J. Nurs. **60:**67, January, 1960.
Natural childbirth—a most thrilling experience, RN **32:**40, April, 1969.
Newton, M., and Newton, N.: The normal course and management of lactation, Clin. Obstet. Gynec. **5:**44, March, 1962.
Nyirjesy, I., and others: Clinical significance of total weight gain in pregnancy, Obstet. Gynec., vol. 32, no. 3, September, 1968.
Perchard, S.: Hypnosis and the pregnant woman, Nurs. Mirror **124:**1, April 7, 1967.
Preparation for childbirth, Maternity Center Association, E. 92nd St., New York, N. Y., 1965.
Robinson, G., and Filkins, M.: Group teaching with outpatients, Amer. J. Nurs. **64:** 110, November, 1964.
Russell, J. K.: Pregnancy in the young teenager, Nurs. Mirror **126:**30, June 28, 1968.
Saunders, P.: A family oriented program for students in obstetrics, Canad. Nurse **64:** 32, January, 1968.
Shyne, A. W., Aline, F. L., and Kogan, L. S.: Evaluating public health service to the maternity patient and her family, Nurs. Outlook **11:**56, January, 1963.
Simpson, M. J.: The medium for the message in maternal child health nursing, Amer. J. Nurs. **67:**2343, November, 1967.
Stitt, P.: The family health clinic, Child and Family, p. 68, Winter, 1963.
Ten Berge, B. S.: Pregnancy chemistry management, Springfield, Ill., 1965, Charles C Thomas, Publisher.
Vellay, P.: Psycho-prophylaxis, Child and Family, p. 18, Winter, 1964.
Young, E. W.: Prepared childbirth: its impact on nursing, Canad. Nurse **64:**39, January, 1968.

Questions for study

1. What are the objectives of a prenatal program for parents?
2. What are the essential components of a first prenatal visit?
3. What are some of the methods used to diagnose early pregnancy?
4. Define the nurse's role during pregnancy.
5. Make a survey of agencies in your community offering services to parents in preparation for parenthood. Share and discuss the objectives of the services offered with your fellow classmates, evaluating the services in light of their contribution toward optimum health of families.
6. Visit maternity departments in your community to become familiar with market prices and style of clothes for mothers during pregnancy.
7. Study the exercises used in preparation for labor and delivery and practice them in preparation for helping mothers during clinical practice experience. Keep a record of their effectiveness so that your

experiences can be shared with those of your classmates.

8. How do the dietary requirements of the pregnant woman differ from those of the nonpregnant woman? For the lactating mother?
9. As you discuss diet with mothers during the prenatal period, keep a record of cultural differences, likes, and dislikes and the recommendations and alterations made in helping mothers. Sharing these at a clinical conference will be a valuable learning.
10. What common fears have mothers expressed during pregnancy? How did you handle them? Evaluate your plan of care.
11. What opportunities did you have for health teaching while caring for mothers during prenatal clinic visits? Keep a daily diary of principles used in teaching, with a self-evaluation.

CHAPTER 9

ATTITUDE, LIE, PRESENTATION, AND POSITION OF THE BABY IN UTERO

ATTITUDE AND LIE

Most babies in utero assume an attitude (relationship of fetal parts to each other) in which the baby accommodates itself to the uterine cavity. The baby's head is markedly flexed with his chin upon the chest, thighs are flexed over the abdomen, and arms are crossed over the chest. In this attitude most babies lie head down (cephalic presentation) (Fig. 9-1) since the head is the heaviest and largest portion of the baby and yet smaller than the buttocks with flexed extremities. However, there are times when the buttocks or feet are presenting at the inlet (a breech presentation) (Fig. 9-2). The baby accommodates body parts to the piriform contours of the uterus.

The term lie refers to the relation of the long axis of the baby in utero to that of the mother. In 99% of all pregnancies the longitudinal lie takes precedence over the transverse lie.

PRESENTATION

The presentation or presenting part refers to the portion of the baby that engages into the true pelvis. In a longitudinal lie the head or breech can present, and in a transverse lie the shoulder becomes the presenting part. When the head presents at the pelvic inlet we refer to a cephalic presentation (Fig. 9-3), when the buttocks or feet present we refer to a breech presentation, and when the shoulder presents we refer to a shoulder presentation.

Cephalic presentations are divided further with consideration to the degrees of flexion of the baby's head in relation to the body. The majority of cephalic presentations are vertex, in which the head is flexed sharply so that the baby's chin is in contact with his chest. In rare instances the neck can be extended sharply so that

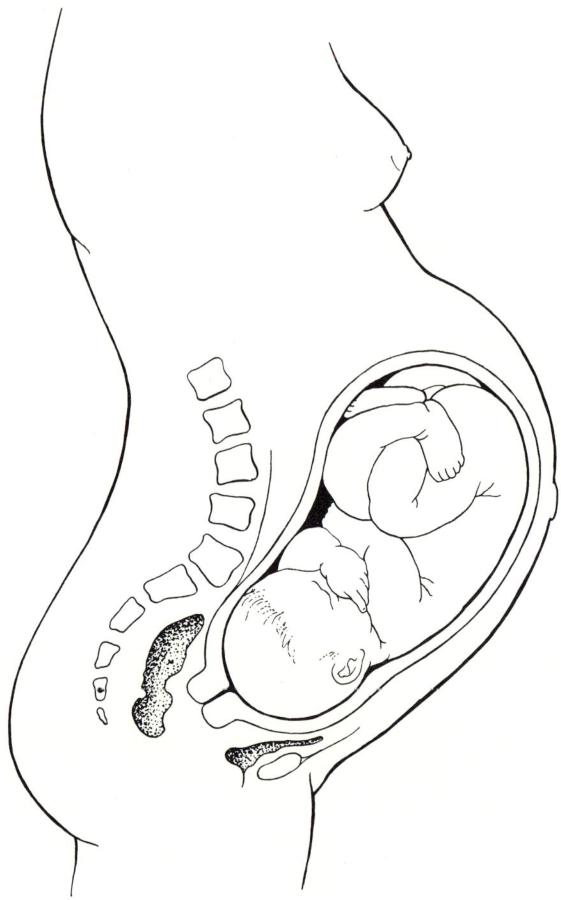

Fig. 9-1. Cephalic presentation.

the occiput and back are in close contact and the face engages at the inlet, known as face presentation. At other times the head can assume a position at points between these two extremes, such as when the large fontanel engages, known as sincipital presentation, or when the brow engages, known as brow presentation (Fig. 9-2, *D* and *E*). At times the latter two presentations become either a vertex or a face presentation as labor progresses, with flexion or extension, respectively.

There can be varying degrees of breech presentations. When the buttock presents itself into the true pelvis with the thighs flexed on the abdomen and the legs upon the thighs, this is called a full or complete breech presentation. Should the thighs be flexed with the legs extended over the anterior surface of the baby's body, this is called a frank breech presentation (Fig. 9-2, *A* and *B*). Occasionally one foot or both feet can present, known as a footling presentation, or one foot or knee can present, known as an incomplete foot or knee presentation.

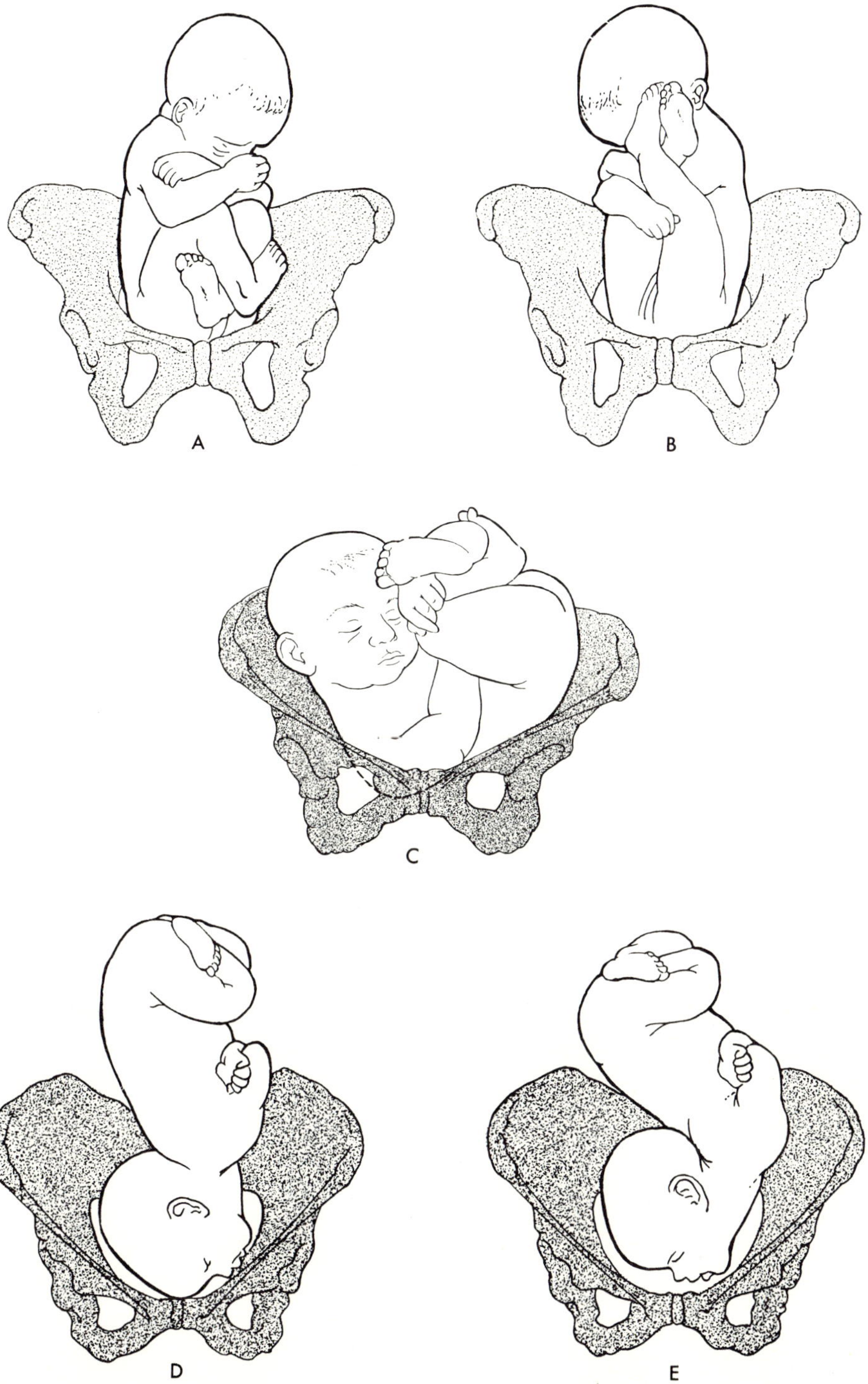

Fig. 9-2. A and **B,** Breech presentation. **C,** Shoulder presentation. **D,** Brow presentation. **E,** Face presentation.

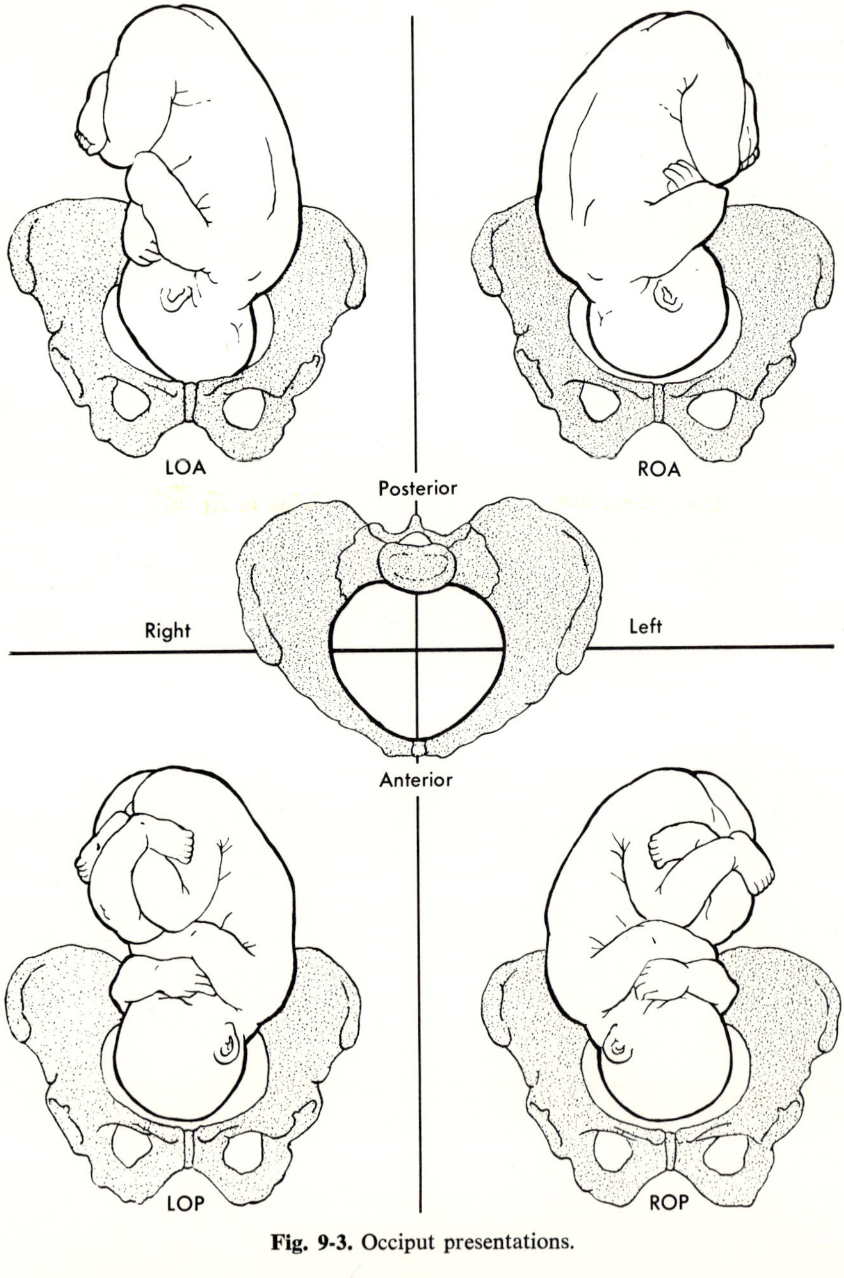

Fig. 9-3. Occiput presentations.

POSITION

Position refers to the relationship of the presenting part to the four quadrants of the mother. In order to determine position, a designated portion of the presenting part is chosen. With a cephalic presentation, the occiput, chin, or brow is used, depending upon the amount of head flexion. When the pelvic extremities are presenting the sacrum is used, and when a shoulder is presenting the scapula is used. The vertex is designated *O* for occiput in cephalic presentations (Fig. 9-3), *M* for mentum in chin presentations, *S* for sacrum in breech presentations, and *Sc* in shoulder presentations since the scapula is used. With each presentation the designated point is either anterior, posterior, transverse, right, or left in relation to the four quadrants of the mother's pelvis.

Table 3 contains a classification of the varieties of positions in cephalic and breech presentations.

Shoulder presentations are not included in Table 3 since they are known as transverse lies of the baby in utero. The frequency of vertex presentations is 95%, breech presentations, 3.5%, face and shoulder presentations, 0.5%. It has been found that two thirds of vertex presentations are in the L.O.A. position, and the remaining one third are in the R.O.A. position.

Determining presentation and position

Presentation and position can be determined by abdominal palpation, by vaginal or rectal examination, by auscultation of fetal heart tones, and in selected instances by roentgen-ray examination.

Table 3. Classification of positions in cephalic and breech presentations

Presenting part	*Position*	*Presentation*	*Variety*	*Abbreviations*
Vertex	Left	Occiput	Anterior	L.O.A.
	Left	Occiput	Transverse	L.O.T.
	Left	Occiput	Posterior	L.O.P.
	Right	Occiput	Anterior	R.O.A.
	Right	Occiput	Transverse	R.O.T.
	Right	Occiput	Posterior	R.O.P.
Face	Left	Mentum	Anterior	L.M.A.
	Left	Mentum	Transverse	L.M.T.
	Left	Mentum	Posterior	L.M.P.
	Right	Mentum	Anterior	R.M.A.
	Right	Mentum	Transverse	R.M.T.
	Right	Mentum	Posterior	R.M.P.
Breech presentation	Left	Sacrum	Anterior	L.S.A.
	Left	Sacrum	Transverse	L.S.T.
	Left	Sacrum	Posterior	L.S.P.
	Right	Sacrum	Anterior	R.S.A.
	Right	Sacrum	Transverse	R.S.T.
	Right	Sacrum	Posterior	R.S.P.

Abdominal palpation. Palpating the abdomen is commonly known as Leopold's maneuver. Four suggested maneuvers are carried out with the mother in a dorsal recumbent position and the abdomen exposed for palpation. The first maneuver explores with the fingertips to locate what is in the fundus. A hard, round object that is freely movable is the head of the baby, whereas a large, irregular-shaped body is the breech. The second maneuver explores with the palms of the hands what is felt on the right and left sides of the abdomen. A hard, firm surface is the back of the infant, and an irregular portion is the baby's extremities. The third maneuver is carried out by placing the thumb and finger of one hand just above the symphysis to grasp what portion of the baby is in the lower section of the abdomen. When the presenting part is not engaged in the true pelvis, the head or

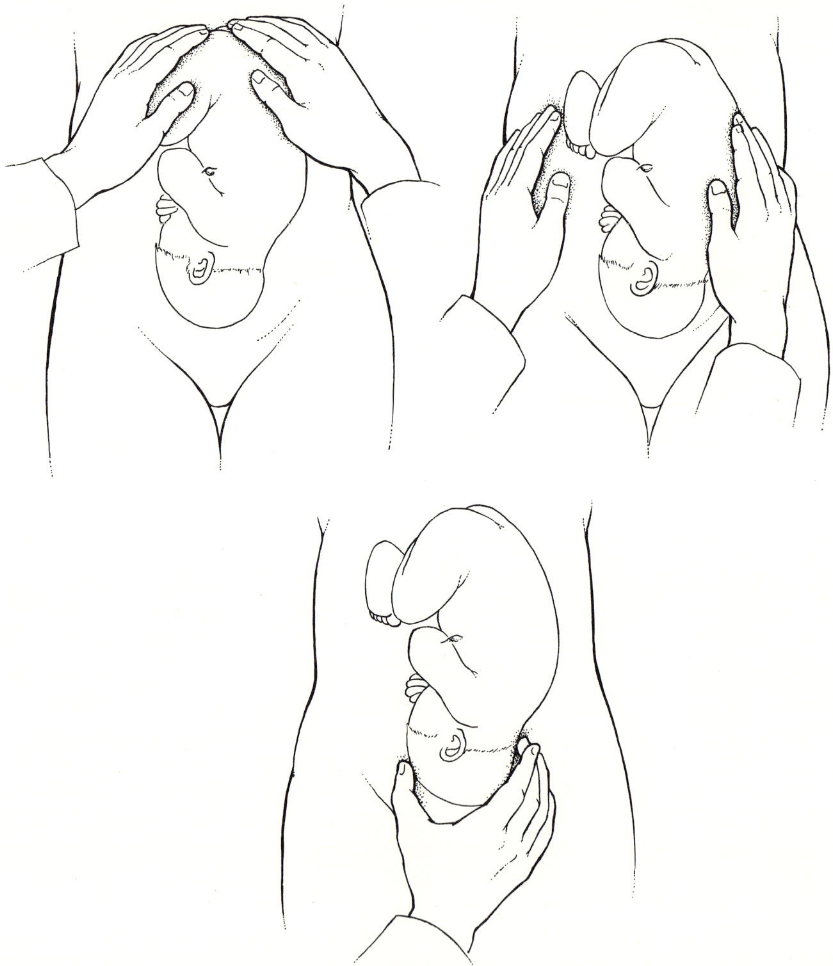

Fig. 9-4. Palpation of abdomen (Leopold's maneuver).

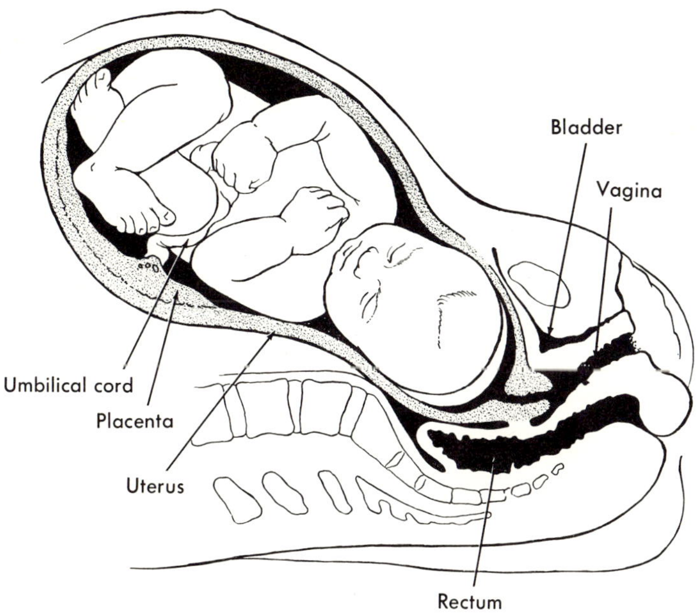

A

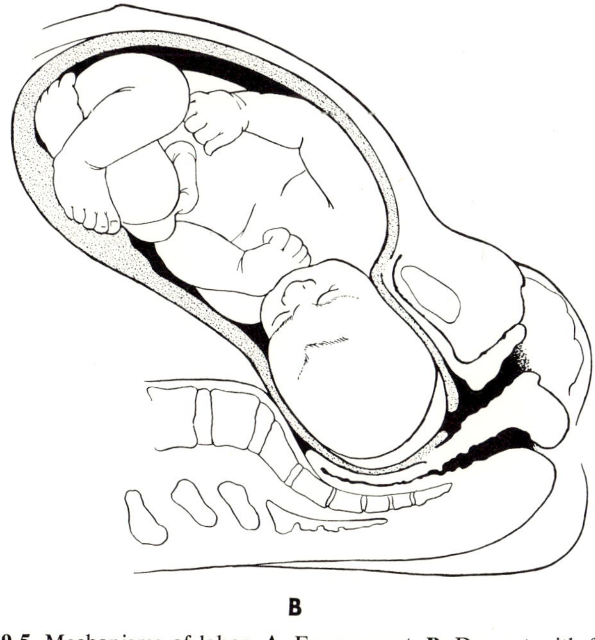

B

Fig. 9-5. Mechanisms of labor. **A,** Engagement. **B,** Descent with flexion.

Continued.

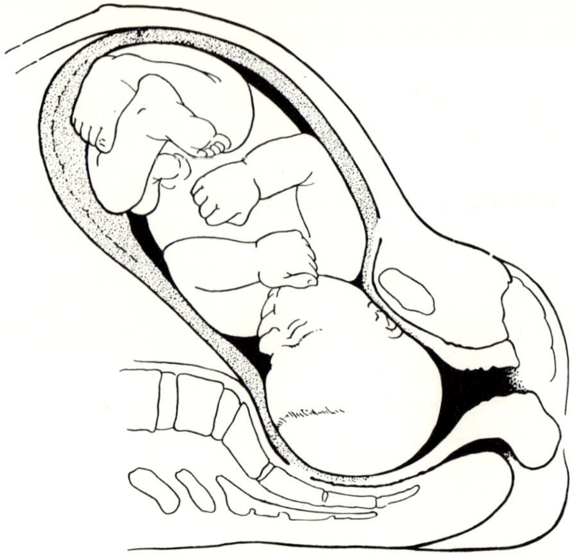

C

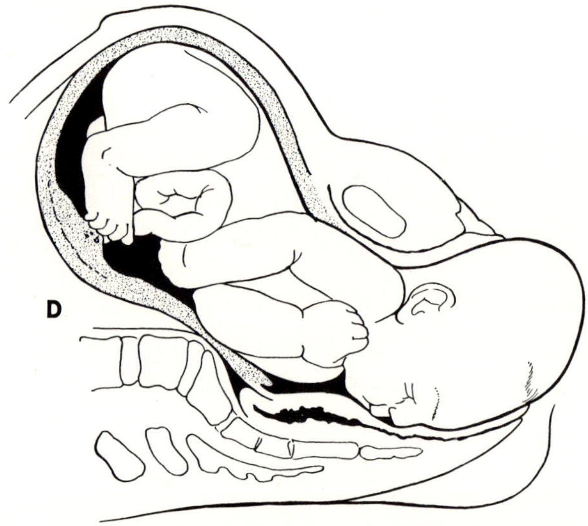

D

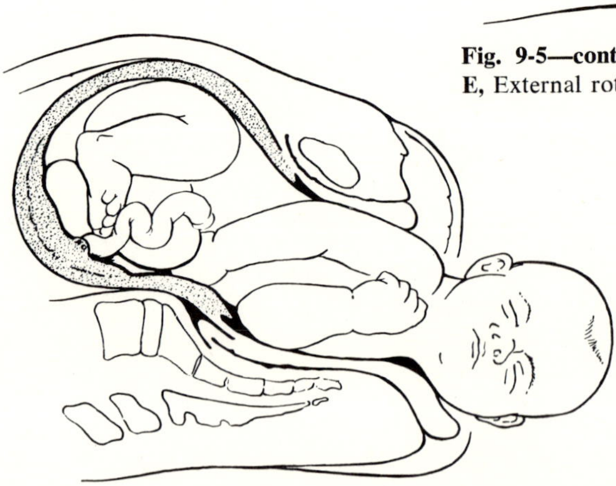

E

Fig. 9-5—cont'd. C, Internal rotation. **D,** Extension. **E,** External rotation.

breech can be balloted (moved) back and forth. In the fourth maneuver the examiner stands facing the mother's extremities, and with the tips of the first three fingers he makes deep pressure in the direction of the inlet of the true pelvis. The prominence of the head is less discernible as descent occurs into the true pelvis. If the head is not engaged in the true pelvis, the entire contour can be felt above the symphysis.

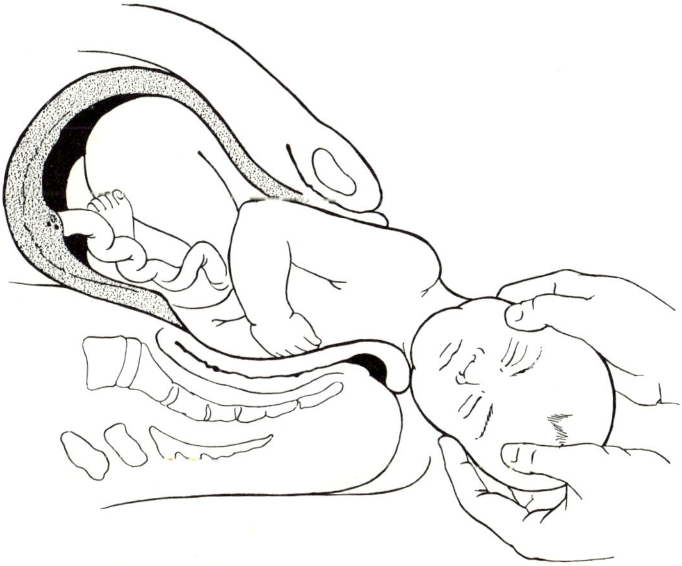

F

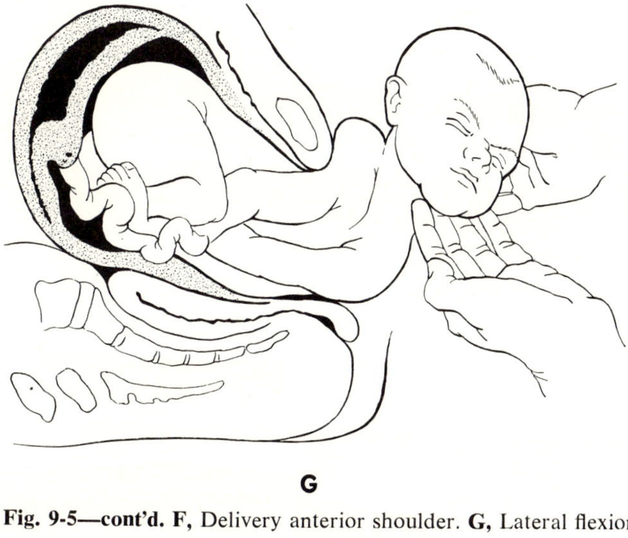

G

Fig. 9-5—cont'd. F, Delivery anterior shoulder. **G,** Lateral flexion.

Vaginal or rectal examination. During pregnancy the position of the anterior fontanel and sagittal sutures can be felt, but they are not as well palpated as in labor when the cervix is dilated.

Auscultation. Fetal heart tones are heard by means of a fetoscope placed on the mother's abdomen. When the head is presenting, the fetoscope is placed slightly below the umbilicus in the area where the baby's back had been palpated. In a breech presentation, the fetal heart tones are heard slightly above the umbilicus in the area where the hard parts (back) were felt. When the fetal heart tones are heard more laterally, a transverse position can be assumed, and in posterior position the tones are heard in the area of the mother's flank. Auscultation alone is not accurate, but together with abdominal palpation, presentation and position can be determined.

Roentgen-ray examination. The increasing perfection in roentgen-ray equipment has made possible its use when presentation and position are difficult to determine by other means. However, roentgen-ray examination still has some hazards to the gonads of the developing baby.

MECHANISMS OF LABOR

Since the true pelvis has many irregularities, the baby's head of necessity follows an orderly progression to accommodate itself for passage through the pelvis and birth canal (Fig. 9-5). These mechanisms are described in the following paragraphs in order of occurrence.

Engagement. Engagement is a mechanism by which the greatest transverse diameter of the head in vertex presentations (the biparietal diameter) enters the inlet of the true pelvis. In primigravidas engagement may occur 2 weeks prior to the commencement of labor; in multigravidas engagement may occur once labor has started. Since the transverse diameter of the inlet is wider, the vertex presents in either a transverse or right or left oblique position.

Descent. Descent is brought about by (1) pressure of the amniotic fluid, (2) direct pressure of the fundus upon the baby's buttock, (3) contractions of the abdominal muscles, and (4) the extension and straightening out of the baby's body. In the primigravida (in whom there is no pelvic disproportion) descent may not occur until labor begins; in the multigravida descent may occur with engagement.

Flexion. Flexion occurs as the descending head meets the resistance of the margins of the pelvic inlet and the pelvic floor. With this mechanism the baby's chin is in close contact with its chest, thereby allowing the shorter suboccipitobregmatic diameter rather than the suboccipitofrontal diameter (which is longer) to pass through the pelvis.

Internal rotation. As labor progresses, the force of the uterine contractions and resistance of the pelvic floor muscles move the head downward and forward until the vertex approaches the ischial spines. Internal rotation is usually complete when the head reaches the pelvic floor, the occiput impinges beneath the symphysis pubis anteriorly, and the baby's face is posterior, facing the mother's sacrum and coccyx. Sometimes rotation may not occur until the head reaches the pelvic floor; rotation before the head reaches the pelvic floor is more frequent in multigravidas than in primigravidas.

Extension. With full effacement and dilatation of the cervix, the force of the uterine muscles downward and the resistance of the pelvic floor upward bring about extension. In this stage the neck is extended so that the head is flexed toward the back. As the baby travels downward, the occiput, bregma, forehead, nose, mouth, and finally the chin pass through the vaginal canal.

Expulsion. Once the baby's head has emerged, the shoulders, which are now in a transverse position presenting in their widest diameter, must also rotate to an anteroposterior position in order to pass through the birth canal. This rotation of the shoulders brings about external rotation of the baby's head, and delivery of the shoulders follows promptly with one shoulder presenting at a time. As the shoulders are delivered, the last mechanism (lateral flexion) occurs, and the delivery of the infant's body follows.

SELECTED REFERENCES

See reference list following Chapter 13.

Questions for study

1. Define position, presenting part, and lie.
2. With a model of the female pelvis and baby, demonstrate the following: vertex presentation and breech presentation, L.O.A., R.O.P., R.S.A., and L.S.P. positions.
3. With a model of the pelvis and baby, describe the mechanisms of labor with the baby in an L.O.T. engagement.

CHAPTER 10

LABOR PROCESS

PHYSIOLOGY OF LABOR

The forty weeks in utero is a time of rapid growth and development of the baby. When the baby outgrows the uterus the labor process begins.

Labor is a physiologic and mechanical process in which the uterine muscles contract and retract rhythmically, with a gradual effacement (thinning out) and dilatation of the cervix; this process results in delivery of the baby and placenta through the birth canal. Labor is an awesome phenomenon that progresses in phases and stages; the cause for its onset is still speculative.

Labor and delivery are known as the intrapartal period. Other terms often used are accouchement, travail, confinement, and childbirth.

SIGNS AND SYMPTOMS OF EARLY LABOR

A few weeks prior to term the baby begins to descend and becomes fixed in proper position and alignment at the entrance of the true pelvis. The mother usually notices that she can breathe more easily, and she again experiences *urinary frequency*. There is a definite change in her abdominal contour as the baby descends. This process is referred to as *lightening.* Lightening occurs 1 to 2 weeks prior to delivery in the primigravida and can occur at any time as the multigravida approaches term. Mild uterine contractions known as *Braxton Hicks contractions* also occur. These are often mistaken for true labor contractions, accounting for many mothers being admitted in false labor. Braxton Hicks contractions can be differentiated from true labor contractions in that they do not become rhythmic and they do not increase in duration or intensity when the mother ambulates. They are believed to be tryout contractions for true labor. They can also occur intermittently during pregnancy, but they often go unnoticed.

Pressure of the presenting part on the rectum, bladder, and sacrum causes *backache* and *diarrhea*. The changes in hormonal levels often cause spurts of energy, and many women become quite ambitious before true labor commences. Many mothers experience an increased mucoid vaginal secretion.

SIGNS AND SYMPTOMS OF TRUE LABOR

True labor is heralded by rhythmic *contractions* of the uterus that increase in frequency, duration, and intensity. Contractions are rhythmic compressions of the muscles within the uterine fundus. As the muscles in the fundus contract and retract, the muscles in the lower uterine segment relax. Retraction is a process in which the musculature in the fundal portion of the uterus becomes thicker and thicker, while the muscles in the lower uterine segment relax and become thinner and thinner, dilating for delivery of the baby. Labor contractions are involuntary and cannot be controlled—progress once made goes on and there is no turning back. Labor is a force (contraction), exerted upon a movable object (baby), meeting resistance (cervix and pelvic floor), with a resulting give (effacement and dilatation).

Effacement is a process in which there is a thinning out and a drawing upward of the internal os of the cervix into the lower uterine segment. As the cervix becomes thinner, *dilatation* of the external os occurs. With rapid effacement and dilatation, trauma to the superficial blood vessels occurs, and a bloody *mucoid vaginal show* appears.

Tearing of the amniotic sac covering the baby, which may occur at any time following lightening, is referred to as *rupture of the membranes* (bag of waters). Occasionally this can be the first sign of labor and a forewarning that labor contractions will soon start.

STAGES OF LABOR

Labor can be divided into various stages and phases. The stages incorporate the labor and delivery process, while the phases deal with noticeable behavioral and emotional changes during the first stage.

First stage

The first stage of labor encompasses the period from the first true labor contraction to full dilatation of the cervix. The length of this stage depends upon the musculature of the uterus, the size of the baby, the effectiveness of the uterine contractions, and the resistance of the cervix in the process of effacement and dilatation. The amniotic sac, if not yet ruptured, acts as a hydrostatic bag against the cervix, aiding the labor process. In the primigravida, the cervix undergoes a process of effacement (thinning out) prior to dilatation. In the multigravida effacement and dilatation occur at the same time, since the cervix has undergone effacement previously.

Dilatation from 1 to 4 cm. (latent phase) is decidedly slower than from 4 cm. to full dilatation (active phase). The first stage of labor includes the period in which the baby is propelled through the true pelvis and made ready for expulsion. It is the longest of the three stages, lasting 6 to 18 hours in a primigravida and 6 to 12 hours in a multigravida.

Relaxation phase. When labor begins, the mother may experience mild irregular contractions and a feeling of excitement or relief that labor has started. In this early phase the cervix may be dilated from a fingertip to 2 cm., and there may or may not be a mucoid show. The mother is able to relax, cope with contractions, and continue ordinary activities. The mother should be instructed to restrict her diet to liquids during this phase, since the digestive process slows down during labor.

As the relaxation phase progresses, contractions become regular and increase in frequency, intensity, and duration; the mother's behavior changes, and she begins to concentrate on each contraction. As she progresses to the midphase, considerable and continuing effacement and dilatation of the cervix from 2 to 8 cm. occur. Relaxation on the mother's part is a great help in accelerating the labor process. The mother welcomes the presence of someone who is supporting and understanding at this time. As the contractions increase in intensity, she may need relief by administration of medications that ultimately increase her threshold for pain.

Nursing care during this phase of labor can contribute much to shortening it and making it a safe and rewarding experience for the mother. Her many needs are directly related to the physiologic changes that are occurring. She is highly perceptive to everything about her and is focusing entirely on herself and the work only she can accomplish. Constant coaching and encouragement, placing the patient in relaxation position, and having her practice abdominal breathing will help her relax and ultimately facilitate effacement and dilatation of the cervix. Keeping her informed of the progress she is making gives her the incentive to go on. Comfort measures such as back rubbing, sacral pressure during contractions, a cool cloth on the forehead, and a refreshing mouth rinse help meet her needs at this time.

Transition phase. The transition phase, the latter part of the first stage of labor, is the shortest and most uncomfortable. The cervix is now 8 to 10 cm. dilated and rapidly effacing. During this period the mother is most irritable—she feels somewhat trapped and helpless, becoming extremely agitated. She verbalizes statements she does not mean, such as "I want to go home," or "I've had it!" Constant "thereness" and encouragement to perform quick chest breathing help a great deal. Signs and symptoms of transition are burping, belching, pale ring around the mouth (circumoral pallor), diaphoresis, flushing of the face, sudden nausea or vomiting, leg cramping, and uncontrollable leg tremors. Contractions last longer and are more frequent and stronger, and at times there is a sudden rupture of the membranes. There is, however, complete relaxation and drowsiness between contractions. This phase is a highly emotional one, yet it is the shortest, lasting approximately 1 hour in the primigravida and 15 to 30 minutes in the multigravida.

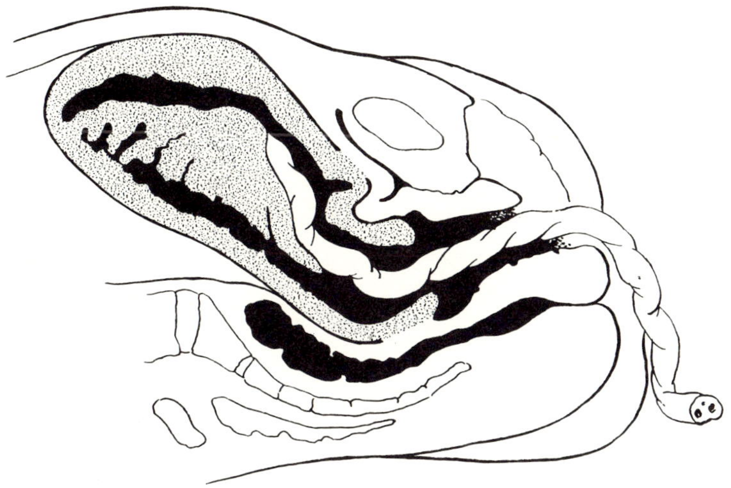

Fig. 10-1. Separation of the placenta.

Second stage

The second stage of labor starts with full dilatation of the cervix and ends with the birth of the baby. The beginning part of the second stage is one in which the mother's behavior changes from great emotional irritability to great involvement and work. With each contraction the mother now gets relief by pushing the baby through the open cervix and vaginal canal, aiding the involuntary contractions of the uterus. This phase is so involuntary that, although the mother may be heavily medicated, she inevitably pushes without coaching. However, coaching at this point shortens the second stage considerably. During this stage leg cramps are common as the mother pushes with contractions. Quick relief can be accomplished by extending the leg out straight, applying firm pressure with one hand directly over the knee, and pushing the toes forward with the other hand (Fig. 7-2).

Third stage

The third stage of labor begins following the delivery of the baby and ends with delivery of the placenta and the fetal membranes. Once the uterus is emptied, the fundus contracts downward on the placental site, facilitating separation of the placenta (Fig. 10-1) from the maternal endometrial surface. Separation of the placenta is apparent when lengthening of the umbilical cord and increased bleeding occur, and when the uterus becomes globular on palpation. The placenta is either extruded by the Schultze mechanism, in which the shiny fetal membrane causes the maternal surface to be delivered last, or it is expelled by the Duncan mechanism, in which the maternal surface is delivered first. The membranes of the placenta are eased out gently so as not to cause placental fragments to remain in the uterus, which would cause postpartal hemorrhage.

ADMISSION TO LABOR AND DELIVERY UNIT

The reception of parents begins on admission. The clerk collecting the necessary data for room assignment is just as much a part of the obstetric team as anyone else. Her sensitivity and understanding of the labor process are essential.

On admission to the labor department the nurse begins by introducing herself to the prospective parents. Especially now do parents need a kind, understanding, and confident person. The nurse quickly evaluates the mother's progress by asking, "Mrs. Jones, is this your first pregnancy?" "When did your labor begin?" "Did your water break?" "How often are your contractions?" "Do you have a bloody show?" After the mother undresses and dons a hospital gown, she is put to bed for further examination.

The manner in which the nurse proceeds depends upon her evaluation of the labor progress being made. The fetal heart tones are checked, and the mother's temperature, pulse, respirations, and blood pressure are taken.

It is now becoming common practice to eliminate shaving the pudenda prior to delivery. Studies reveal that adequate cleansing of the perineum is sufficient during labor and prior to delivery. Some doctors recommend that pHisoHex be used for perineal cleansing during the last month of pregnancy; however, this is not a universal recommendation. It has been found that a bacteriostatic agent is as effective in its ability to decrease the bacterial flora as is the traditional shave. The unshaved perineum is appreciated by the mother since there is less discomfort with the regrowth of hair. Should perineorrhaphy be anticipated, the rectal and adjacent area may be easily shaved in the delivery room. However, should a vaginal and rectal shave be ordered, soaping the pubic hair and holding the skin taut above the area to be shaved make the procedure simple. Shaving from the vaginal area toward the rectum limits contamination. Shaving should be done in between contractions for comfort of the mother.

Palpation of the abdomen, known as Leopold's maneuver, can be done by the nurse in order to feel fetal parts (Fig. 9-4). A hard, continuous surface identifies the baby's back, and small irregularities designate the baby's arms and legs. The fetal heart tones are usually heard wherever the baby's back is felt. A large abdomen with many irregularities may be indicative of a multiple pregnancy. The experienced examiner can also determine, by palpation directly above the symphysis, whether engagement of the presenting part has occurred. The presenting part that has not engaged can be felt above the symphysis; the presenting part that is already fixed in the true pelvis cannot be dislodged by the examining hand.

Identification methods vary from hospital to hospital. On admission two identical identification tags are made—one for the mother, which is applied, and the other for the baby, to be applied at the time of delivery. The correct name spelling is checked by the nurse and the mother, alleviating many of the uncertainties on identification. The baby's bracelet or necklace is checked with the mother's in the delivery room and is applied before the mother and the baby leave the unit.

THE NURSE'S ROLE DURING LABOR

The intrapartal period is a highly charged emotional time for the parents, the nurse, and auxiliary personnel. During this time the nurse must show understanding, must be empathetic and an astute observer and listener, and must have the ability to keep the mother comfortable and in full control as labor progresses.

The nurse's knowledge of the labor process and her skill in the giving of safe care are also necessary for complete effectiveness. She constantly encourages, coaches, and keeps the parents informed of the progress being made. She works closely with the physician and other members of the health team in reporting and coordinating efforts toward a safe labor and delivery.

The happenings surrounding birth are probably the most exciting, stimulating, highly charged experiences in which a family and the nurse are united. It seems, then, that the nurse's role is one in which much involvement is required in order that she be able to provide necessary support. Regardless of the preparation of the couple, there is always the need for reassurance from members of the health professions.

The nurse caring for the family during the labor and delivery period is in a unique position. She is invited to share one of the most intimate experiences between a man and his wife. Knowing this, the nurse plans her care in an effort to direct, help, encourage, communicate, and assure safe care to the entire family.

THE PAIN OF LABOR

Pain is a hurt one feels, it is subjective, it can be remembered and partly relived, and it is often a private sensation not entirely communicable. Although pain is not communicable, it is transmitted in the form of behavior. Everyone's perception of pain is unique and cannot be shared completely with another. Therefore the same painful stimulus may cause varied reactions in different people.

The varied reactions are caused by differences in nervous systems and by relationships to past experiences that result in differing attitudes toward pain.

The physiologic responses to pain affect the major body systems. Gastrointestinal motility is inhibited by the blocking of contractions, or from normal motility to slight, or by rapid contractions prior to blocking. In the respiratory system there is increased alveolar ventilation and oxygen consumption and often an increase in respirations. In the skeletomuscular system there is hypermotility of striated musculature, increased muscle tension in the area of pain stimulation, and an increase in blood flow to the muscles in that area. The response in the cardiovascular system is an increase in systolic and diastolic readings, pulse rate, stroke volume, and peripheral vasoconstriction.

Many ethnic groups, such as the Jewish and Italians, encourage pain expression, while the Americans and Irish discourage pain expression. The pain of labor may interfere with its normal progress, be it from fear, tension, or lowered pain threshold. Analgesias may serve well to the individual mother needing such relief.

Alleviation of pain of labor

Administration of an analgesic for the relief of pain during labor is considered with due respect to mother and baby. Sedation given to the mother will traverse the placenta and affect the baby, who is most vulnerable at this time. There are definite factors considered when medication is ordered for the relief of pain during labor. What effect does the analgesia have on the mother's inhaled oxygen intake? A decrease in the mother's intake with prolonged and repeated drops in blood pressure will deplete the oxygen supply to the baby. In the process of giving analgesics during prolonged labors, is there impairment in the mechanism maintaining the acid-base equilibrium? It has been proved that a drop in the mother's pH has a direct effect on the amount of oxygen transferred to the baby. If these factors are known, it is then essential for safety of mother and baby that necessary equipment such as oxygen, suction apparatus, and emergency resuscitators be available in a labor and delivery unit at all times.

Nursing care of the mother in labor is a determining factor in the amount of sedation needed. The nurse who instills confidence, gives assurance, and is aware of comfort measures can greatly reduce the amount of sedation needed. Fear has a tendency to produce much tension, and tension in turn produces and augments pain. Therefore, if fear is alleviated there will be less tension and pain. It has been proved that during normal labors the mother who is relaxed, is not fearful, and has a nurse who supports her well experiences less pain, has a shorter period of labor, and has a memorable childbearing experience. The role of the nurse during the labor and delivery process need never be underestimated.

Medications used during labor have various effects in their power to relieve pain. The method of choice is left to the discretion of the physician. In many instances the physician discusses the use of analgesia with the mother during the prenatal period.

Before medication is administered, it is important to know the quality and rate of the fetal heart tones so that changes following medication can be determined. If the patient empties her bladder before sedation is given, there is less chance that she will suffer urinary retention caused by the drug. Anxiety is lessened if the reason for the medication is explained before administration. Protection and safety measures such as using bedrails, observing respirations, and checking blood pressure, pulse, and fetal heart rate frequently are imperative. Medication helps the mother relax, making for rapid effacement and dilatation of the cervix. However, whenever medication is given too early during labor, it can slow up the labor process considerably. The time that medication is administered greatly determines the effect it will have on the progress of labor.

Medications administered

Meperidine hydrochloride (Demerol) is an analgesic, spasmolytic, and sedative for relieving or preventing severe pain. Dosage varies from 25 to 100 mg., given subcutaneously or intramuscularly, and may be repeated every 3 to 4 hours if needed. The side effects of meperidine are flushing of the face, diaphoresis, mouth dryness, and a decreased urinary output. More severe reactions are extreme weakness, hypotension, profuse diaphoresis, marked dizziness, and nausea and vomiting. These symptoms are relieved by placing the mother in a prone position. Intravenous administration of the drug may cause respiratory depression.

Scopolamine (hyoscine hydrobromide), gr. 1/100 to 1/200, is a drug that produces slower heart action (with a decrease in pulse rate), increases respirations slightly, dilates the pupils, and decreases brain activity, causing amnesia to pain. The effect of scopolamine is noticed 30 minutes to 1 hour following administration. There may be flushing of the face and dryness of the throat and mouth with extreme thirst. At times scopolamine has a tendency to excite some women; it is often combined with meperidine hydrochloride, and the resultant condition is commonly known as "twilight sleep." The nurse should darken the room and refrain from conversation with the mother, since effective communication is impossible.

Promethazine hydrochloride (Phenergan), 25 to 50 mg., is frequently given with meperidine to relieve apprehension during labor. The dose may be repeated in 3 to 4 hours whenever indicated. Since promethazine potentiates the action of central nervous system depressants, the dosage of hypnotic and analgesic drugs can be reduced.

Secobarbital sodium (Seconal Sodium), 100 to 200 mg., is a short-acting barbiturate that acts as a central nervous system depressant. Depending upon the dose given, secobarbital produces mild to profound hypnosis. In large doses it causes anesthesia; overdosage may result in respiratory depression. In obstetrics, secobarbital dosage depends upon the weight of the mother and the activity of labor. Secobarbital is given only in toxemia or when there is a history of bleeding. When it is given intramuscularly, hypnosis occurs in 7 to 10 minutes. Therefore, secobarbital is never given just prior to delivery, when the drug effect would be maximal. Secobarbital is contraindicated if the fetus is premature.

Morphine sulfate (15 mg.) is a central nervous system depressant that may be given during labor to mothers who show signs of severe toxemia. Morphine can depress the mother's respirations and in turn depress those of the baby, causing a delay in spontaneous respirations at birth. Whenever morphine is given during labor, nalorphine hydrochloride (Nalline Hydrochloride) should always be available for the newborn. When depression in the newborn is suspected, nalorphine hydrochloride can be given to the mother shortly before delivery, since it crosses the placenta readily. It can also be given to the newborn through the umbilical vein at the time of delivery to initiate respirations.

Pentazocine lactate (Talwin), 30 mg., is a new, potent, synthetic analgesic that relieves pain in 15 to 20 minutes after intramuscular or subcutaneous administration. Pentazocine lactate is not a narcotic and is as effective as meperidine or morphine.

Perphenazine (Trilafon) is a powerful and highly effective tranquilizing drug and antiemetic. The usual dose of perphenazine is 5 mg. (1 ml.), given intramuscularly.

TIMING CONTRACTIONS

The timing of contractions is significant in determining labor progress. Contractions can be felt by placing the hand directly over the fundus. Each contraction has a definite pattern—there is a rising and tightening of the uterine muscles until a peak is reached, followed by gradual relaxation. The frequency of contractions is determined by recording the time each contraction commences. The interval between contractions is the time from the beginning of one contraction to the beginning of the next. The duration of the contraction is from the beginning of the contraction until there is complete relaxation of the abdominal wall. Intensity or strength of contractions can be felt by noting the tautness of the abdominal wall as the hand is placed over the fundus. Contractions have an increasing pattern of regularity, frequency, duration, and strength.

FETAL HEART TONES

Listening to the rate, regularity, and strength of fetal heart tones gives an audioscopic picture of how the baby is faring during the labor process. Normally fetal heart tones range between 100 and 160 beats per minute. It is difficult to hear fetal heart tones during contractions. It is advisable to wait 30 seconds following contractions before attempting to obtain an accurate reading of fetal heart tones. Any changes in rate, regularity, and strength are indicative of fetal distress and need to be reported immediately. Until assistance is available, oxygen by mask may be administered to the mother. Fetal heart tones are checked and recorded every 30 minutes during the relaxation phase, every 15 minutes during transition, and every 5 minutes during beginning second stage.

In some labor and delivery units electrocardiography and ultrasonic fetal monitoring are replacing the human ear in listening to fetal heart tones. After the membranes have ruptured and dilatation of the cervix has occurred, electrodes may be placed on the fetal scalp for accurate electrocardiography.

Fetal heart tones usually become quite rapid before they become slower; tachycardia is therefore a warning of distress. A fetal heart rate that does not return to normal 1 minute following a contraction is indicative of fetal distress.

Fetal electrocardiography is used to determine fetal viability, multiple pregnancy and presentation, fetal distress, congenital heart disease, and maturity in utero. The technique is economical, nonhazardous, and simple, and results are immediately available; accuracy increases after 24 weeks gestation. In multiple pregnancy it is less hazardous than radiology. A preamplifier is connected to the maternal abdominal wall with suction cup electrodes after the skin is coated with an electrode paste similar to that used for adult electrocardiography. One electrode is placed in the midline near the umbilicus, the other close to the symphysis pubis. If fetal heart tones are not recorded, the electrodes are moved laterally. A ground electrode is attached to the patient's thigh or leg. If the patient is to be studied for a long time during labor, a stick-on-tape electrode is used since it is less traumatic to the skin, and a nondrying electrode cream is used. Other techniques such as direct application of the electrodes to the fetus transabdominally or transcervically are still being researched.

VITAL SIGNS

Maternal temperature, pulse, respiration, and blood pressure are measured every 4 hours when feasible. Any increase in pulse rate or drop in blood pressure may be indicative of bleeding with impending shock. Rises in systolic and diastolic readings are reported immediately to rule out toxemia.

Since dehydration may occur with prolonged labor, any increase in basal temperature may warrant administration of parenteral fluids. The effects of medications on maternal respirations have direct bearing on the amount of oxygen the fetus is receiving.

THE PERINEUM

The perineal area is observed frequently during labor. Any increase in bloody show is indicative of rapid effacement and dilatation. Any insidious constant trickling of blood is bleeding rather than show and should be reported immediately to the physician. Sudden rupture of the membranes may occur at any time during labor. Should this occur, it is the nurse's primary responsibility to listen immediately to fetal heart tones and to check the perineum for either umbilical cord or presenting part. With sudden rupture of the membranes the cord may become compressed or may be visible at the vaginal opening. If this occurs, the nurse should quickly elevate the mother's hips higher than the shoulders, administer oxygen to the mother, and immediately notify the physician. Any change in fetal heart tones may indicate cord compression.

Frequent washings of the perineal area ensure comfort and cleanliness; wiping from the vaginal orifice toward the rectum prevents introduction of microorganisms into the birth canal.

DIET

During labor it is advisable to withhold fluids and food since the digestive process is markedly slowed. Since there is added blood supply to the uterus to aid in the labor process, other body processes are not as efficient. Should general anesthesia be given, there is danger of aspiration of food particles into the trachea during delivery.

For the mother anticipating anesthesia, parenteral fluids are often administered when needed. Should the mother plan for regional anesthesia, fluids in small amounts may be given in early labor.

BLADDER AND BOWEL FUNCTION

Because of the anatomic position of the rectum and uterus, a full rectum may delay descent of the fetus or may cause contamination of the sterile field. When needed, a prepared carminative enema may be ordered by the physician. Should membranes be ruptured and the presenting part be high, there is always danger of a prolapsed cord; therefore a low enema would be indicated.

The proximity of the bladder to the uterus often accounts for urinary retention during labor. A full bladder can stop labor contractions and is easily detected by palpation directly above the symphysis. It is advisable to encourage frequent emptying of the bladder during labor, especially prior to medication.

CIRCULATORY CHANGES

In normal labor the pulse rate remains unchanged. Although there is little change in blood pressure during the first stage, there is a decided 5 to 10 mm. Hg change in systolic and diastolic readings during contractions. During second stage the blood pressure increases 10 mm. Hg between contractions and 20 to 25 mm. Hg during a contraction. The third stage finds systolic and diastolic readings at previous levels.

There is a decided increase of 30% to 35% in cardiac output during active labor. A leukocyte count of 15,000 is common and normal during labor.

Syncope with weakness and fainting may occur during labor because of pressure of the enlarged uterus on the aorta and vena cava. The relaxed uterus is known to obstruct venous return and cause supine hypotensive syndrome, which may also occur in the later months of pregnancy. This condition can be remedied easily by turning the mother to the Sims position, relieving pressure on the aorta and vena cava. It has also been found that there is a better blood supply to the fetus with the mother in a side-lying position.

EXAMINATIONS TO DETERMINE PROGRESS OF LABOR

Rectal examination. Rectal examination is done by insertion of a gloved index finger into the rectum. Through the rectal mucosa it is possible to feel the cervix for effacement and dilatation to determine what part is presenting and its progress in relation to the ischial spines. The relationship of the presenting part to the ischial spines is called *station.* A presenting part below the spines that is advancing toward the birth canal is designated as +1, +2, or +3. A presenting part above the spines is designated as –1, –2, or –3. Therefore a presenting part at a –3 station indicates a floating presenting part where engagement has not yet occurred, and a +3 station indicates that the presenting part is at the perineal floor and that delivery is imminent.

Vaginal examination. Vaginal examination is done by insertion of a gloved hand into the vaginal canal. This procedure makes examination findings more accurate than rectal examination. Perineal care prior to vaginal examination is essential in limiting introduction of bacteria into the vagina. When there is danger of bleeding, vaginal examination is always done in the delivery room. Whole blood should be available for administration in case of hemorrhage.

Roentgenology and roentgen-ray pelvimetry. During labor roentgen-ray films are made when progress is slow. They are valuable aids in the diagnosis of malpositions, malpresentations, multiple pregnancies, and cephalopelvic disproportion.

SELECTED REFERENCES

Bishop, E. H.: Ultrasonic fetal monitoring, Clin. Obstet. Gynec., vol. 11, no. 4, December, 1968.

Bruser, M.: A practical fetal heart monitor, Obstet. Gynec., vol. 29, no. 4, April, 1967.

Gralen, J. L. M., and others: Multipolar registration of the fetal electrocardiogram technic and comparison with bipolar method, Obstet. Gynec., vol. 31, no. 4, April, 1968.

Greenhill, J. P.: Obstetrics, Philadelphia, 1965, W. B. Saunders Co.

Langhouse, F.: Supine hypotension syndrome, Amer. J. Nurs., vol. 70, no. 6, June, 1970.

Long, A. E.: The unshaved perineum at parturition, Amer. J. Obstet. Gynec. **99:**333, 1967.

Physicians' Desk Reference, Oradell, N. J., 1969, Medical Economics, Inc.

Scott, D. B., and Kerr, M. G.: Inferior vena cava pressure in late pregnancy, J. Obstet. Gynaec. Brit. Comm. **70:**1044, 1963.

Steinback, R.: Pain, a psychophysiological analysis, New York, 1968, Academic Press, Inc.

Questions for study

1. What are the signs and symptoms of true labor?
2. What are the physiologic changes occurring in the body systems during labor? What implications does this have for nursing care?
3. Define the stages of labor.
4. Describe the behavior of mothers during the relaxation and transition phases of labor.
5. What is the purpose of a rectal examination during labor? What can be determined by rectal examination?
6. What is the purpose of vaginal examination during labor? What nursing measures are essential in preparation for vaginal examination?
7. With a model and baby describe the mechanisms that facilitate passage of the baby through the pelvis and the birth canal.
8. Mrs. Gray, a gravida I para 0 of 40 weeks gestation, is admitted to the labor and delivery unit with 5 to 8 minute moderate to strong contractions lasting 50 to 60 seconds. Fetal heart tones are 144 LLQ (left lower quadrant) and of good quality. Membranes are intact, and she has a slight bloody show. Rectal examination reveals 2.5 cm. dilatation of the cervix with slight effacement, and vertex presenting at station 0.
   a. Define gravida and para.
   b. In what phase and stage of labor is Mrs. Gray on admission?
   c. Define effacement, dilatation, vertex, and station 0.
   d. What would be your nursing responsibilities in caring for Mrs. Gray?
   e. What nursing measures would you provide in giving physical and emotional support?
9. Mrs. Brown, a gravida III para II, is admitted at 39 weeks with 3 to 5 minute strong contractions lasting 45 to 55 seconds. Fetal heart tones are 128 RLQ (right lower quadrant) and regular. Membranes are intact with a moderate bloody show. Rectal examination reveals 4 to 5 cm. dilatation with 50% effacement, vertex presenting at station +2. You are assigned to admit Mrs. Brown to the labor and delivery unit. How would you proceed?
10. What is the nurse's role during the birth of the baby?

Situations

Read the following situations and be prepared to discuss them in the next class session:

1. Mrs. Brown, a gravida I para 0, is ad-

mitted to the labor unit. Her husband is with her on admission and asks you to hurry and do something for his wife since she is having "severe pains." How would you approach Mrs. Brown? How would you evaluate the labor status of Mrs. Brown? What action would you take for her comfort?

2. Mrs. Green, a gravida IV para III, is having 3 to 4 minute contractions of moderate strength lasting 30 to 45 seconds. She has now been in active labor for 2 hours. On rectal examination the cervix is found to be 50% effaced and 2 to 2½ cm. dilated. Mrs. Green asks for a bedpan since she feels the urge to void. What measures would you take in providing safe care at this time? (Rectal examination reveals vertex presenting at a + I station, membranes ruptured at home prior to admission.)
3. Mrs. Jones, a gravida II para I, has been in labor 5 hours. Her contractions are strong q. 2 to 3 minutes lasting 50 to 60 seconds, membranes intact, bloody show. On rectal examination the cervix is 50% effaced, 7 to 8 cm. dilated. She is perspiring profusely, feels nauseous, and is having leg tremors. Evaluate her labor status.
4. Mrs. Doe, a gravida VII para VI, is admitted by stretcher to the labor and delivery unit, and delivery is imminent. She is grunting and pushing with each contraction, and on observing the perineum the baby's head is crowning. You are alone with her. How would you proceed?
5. Mr. and Mrs. Young, a white couple 21 and 18, respectively, have been married 1 year. Mr. Young is completing his senior year in college, and Mrs. Young is working as a secretary. She is 38 weeks pregnant and has been seeing her private obstetrician since the second week of pregnancy. She has gained 16 pounds, her blood pressure is 110/68, urine negative for sugar and albumin, fetal heart rate 140 LLQ regular. Mrs. Young tells her obstetrician that she has been experiencing occasional contractions and has noticed a slight mucoid vaginal discharge within the last few days. Rectal examination reveals a vertex presentation, vertex dipping into the true pelvis, L.O.T. cervix 1 fingertip dilated, no effacement, membranes intact. Mrs. Young asks you, "Do you think I'm in labor? Will I be having my baby shortly?"
   a. Considering the preceding information, how would you answer Mrs. Young?
   b. Interpret the findings revealed on rectal examination.
   c. Using the model of the pelvis and baby, describe the bony pelvis, diameters, divisions, planes, classifications, and mechanisms of labor.
   d. In light of the preceding information, how would you plan on preparing Mr. and Mrs. Young for labor and delivery?
6. Suddenly at 2:00 A.M. one morning, Mrs. Young is awakened by a sudden gush of clear fluid. She awakens Mr. Young and tells him, "I think my water broke." Mr. Young remembers the instructions given him by the nurse and gets ready to take his wife to the hospital for admission. As Mrs. Young is dressing, she begins to experience slight uterine contractions.

   On admission, Mrs. Young is examined rectally. Examination reveals a cervix with 1½ to 2 cm. dilatation with slight effacement, vertex presentation, station +1. During examination the doctor notices a slight pinkish show and seepage of amniotic fluid.
   a. With the preceding information, how would you proceed in admitting Mrs. Young to the labor and delivery unit?
   b. How would you evaluate Mrs. Young's labor status?
   c. How would you support Mrs. Young during this phase of labor? Should Mr. Young be permitted to be with his wife? How would you support them?
   d. Discuss the physiologic and emotional changes that occur as labor progresses. What measures would you institute to give safe nursing care?

CHAPTER 11

ANESTHESIA DURING LABOR AND DELIVERY

Anesthesia is usually induced during the beginning second stage of labor and at the time of delivery; in some instances anesthesia is induced during the first stage of labor as soon as labor is well established. Anesthesia can be produced by inhalation, through intravenous medication, or by local injection of anesthetic agents. Administration of anesthetic agents by a well-qualified anesthetist or nurse-anesthetist makes delivery safe and comfortable for the mother.

INHALATION ANESTHESIA

Gas anesthetics

Nitrous oxide and oxygen. Whiffs of nitrous oxide provide relief of pain during beginning second stage and delivery. It is administered in an 80% concentration with 15% to 20% oxygen. Nitrous oxide has a tendency to produce hypoxia in the fetus if given over a long period of time; it is therefore used only during delivery.

Cyclopropane. An explosive gas given by a continuous closed system, cyclopropane tends to relax the mother quickly and is commonly used for delivery and for cesarean section in a 6% to 8% concentration mixed with oxygen. It is not a safe anesthetic to give if hemorrhage is present or is anticipated. In 30% of all deliveries in which cyclopropane is used, resuscitation of the infant is necessary.

Volatile anesthetics

Volatile anesthetics are liquid vapors relatively safe but contraindicated in upper respiratory infections, pulmonary diseases, and premature labors, during fetal distress, and following the ingestion of food.

Ether. Ether (ethyl ether) is a liquid that quickly vaporizes and is highly inflammable. It is administered by the open drop method mixed with air. Ether is safe since it can be given slowly, producing light anesthesia. It does, however, cross the placenta quickly, and if given for a difficult delivery can produce narcosis in the fetus and relaxation of the uterus, with subsequent bleeding. It also has a tendency to produce nausea and vomiting and can cause aspiration of liquids if given when the stomach is full. An airway and suction apparatus should always be available when ether is administered. In emergencies, if breathing becomes embarrassed, the head is turned to the side and the chin is flexed to facilitate opening the airway. When the patient is lying supine, the head is extended backward, bringing the chin forward so that the tongue does not occlude the air passage. To protect the eye membranes and skin from ether burns, castor oil is instilled into each eye, and the face is lubricated before administration.

Trichloroethylene. Trichloroethylene (Trilene) is a blue liquid that vaporizes and when inhaled gives relief from pain. This agent can be given with each contraction during active labor. It is self-administered by a specially devised mask strapped to the mother's wrist. Once enough trichloroethylene is inhaled for relief during contractions, the mother's arm drops away from her face. It is a safe anesthetic because the mother inhales only as much as she needs for relief. It is not used as widely in the United States as it is in Canada. If used during labor, it must be continued during delivery because its use is contraindicated with gas anesthesia, in which soda lime is used.

Chloroform. Chloroform has a strong vapor, and its induction is rapid. A small overdose can be dangerous because it does not inhibit breathing as ether does—therefore, the person administering it must be skillful in observing vital signs.

INTRAVENOUS ANESTHESIA

Thiopental (Pentothal) sodium has many advantages when administered during delivery. It is rapid in induction, does not produce aftereffects of vomiting, is controllable, assures adequate oxygenation of the baby, and produces minimal bleeding following delivery. If the infant is delivered within a 20-minute period, narcosis does not occur. Oxygen by inhalation is always given during the administration of intravenous thiopental. Tachycardia and laryngospasm in the mother may occur.

LOCAL INFILTRATION

Procaine hydrochloride, 0.5% to 1%, piperocaine hydrochloride (Metycaine), 1% to 1.5%, tetracaine hydrochloride (Pontocaine), and lidocaine hydrochloride (Xylocaine), 1%, are common drugs used for local anesthesia. Local infiltration of these medications has many advantages such as the following: (1) the mortality rate is practically nonexistent; (2) there is no effect on the baby; (3) uterine contractions are not interrupted; (4) it is easy to administer and can be given by the obstetrician; and (5) toxic effects are minimal. Local anesthetics are used for cardiac patients, patients who have severe asthma, in premature deliveries, and whenever the mother has ingested food recently. For prolonged action, epinephrine (Adrenalin) in a 1:100,000 or a 1:200,000 solution is added to the anesthetic agent. Local anesthesia can be used for vaginal and abdominal deliveries.

PARACERVICAL BLOCK

With paracervical block the anesthetic agent is injected into the base of the broad ligament and lateral walls of the lower uterine segment, blocking afferent sympathetic pathways from the uterus. This anesthetic is often given during the latter half of labor, but it is short acting and may have to be repeated or supplemented with a pudendal block for delivery.

PERINEAL INFILTRATION—PUDENDAL BLOCK

Infiltration of the pudendal nerves surrounding the vulva and the perineum has many advantages. Since this method produces local anesthesia, it is the one of choice for the mother who desires to be awake and participate during delivery.

TRANSPERINEAL PUDENDAL BLOCK

In this type of block the internal pudendal nerves are injected (a point at the ischial spines) with medication, and the pudendal nerves are blocked. Injection is made midway between the anus and the ischial tuberosities in order that the area beneath the skin of the labia and the ilioinguinal nerve in the anterior portion of the vulva and clitoris is anesthetized. This technique is used when forceps delivery is anticipated.

TRANSVAGINAL PUDENDAL BLOCK

This is a much easier technique than the transperineal type. The needle is introduced into the vagina and directed through the sacrospinous ligament into the posterior areolar tissue. Although this is simpler and quicker, both methods need a skilled practitioner.

ABDOMINAL INFILTRATION

Abdominal infiltration for cesarean section is advantageous in selected mothers with toxemia, for delivery of premature infants, or whenever spinal anesthesia is not feasible. Infiltration is made into the midline below the umbilicus and through the suprapubic region. After a 10-minute waiting period the fascia is exposed, and the peritoneum and lateral rectal muscles are infiltrated. Morphine sulfate, gr. 1/4, and scopolamine, gr. 1/150, are also given 10 minutes before delivery for comfort of the mother. Local abdominal infiltration is not attempted if the mother is apprehensive and if complete relaxation is desired.

REGIONAL ANESTHESIA

Caudal anesthesia is accomplished by introducing medication into the caudal canal. The caudal canal is the lower end of the bony spinal canal formed from the nonclosure of the laminae of the last sacral vertebrae. The canal is supplied with a rich network of sacral nerves, and introduction of an anesthetic agent renders the mother free from pain during labor.

Caudal anesthesia can be continued during the second stage. The medication commonly used is piperocaine hydrochloride, 1.5%, which comes prepared in standard bottles. When labor is well established and the cervix is 3 to 4 cm. dilated, the mother is placed in Sims position. The sacral and coccygeal area is cleansed with ether and an antiseptic solution. By palpation the anesthetist identifies the sacral hiatus and injects a local anesthetic solution. The needle, usually 16 gauge 3 to 5 inches in length, is introduced into the canal at an approximate distance of 1 cm. A polyethylene catheter is then passed through the needle into the caudal canal. The needle is withdrawn; the catheter is attached to a standard medication bottle and taped to the skin so that a closed system exists. A test dose of medication is administered, and 5 minutes later the patient is examined. If there is free movement of both legs, it is ascertained that the canal has been found successfully. An additional 22 ml. of medication is continued every 40 minutes for relief from pain.

Caudal anesthesia is most advantageous and is the method of choice for the mother who is anxious and prefers freedom from pain during active labor. Caudal anesthesia does have some disadvantages such as the following: (1) it is expensive because an experienced operator must be in attendance during the entire process, and (2) it does interfere with the frequency and intensity of contractions and can lower the maternal blood pressure. When the maternal blood pressure drops below 100 mm. Hg, oxygen supply to the fetus may be impaired. Careful observation of blood pressure is imperative for prompt action. When maternal blood pressure falls, ephedrine or epinephrine should be readily available. Elevation of the mother's legs for a few minutes will restore the blood pressure to normal levels. Caudal anesthesia is contraindicated for patients who have had pilonidal sinuses, during prolonged labor, or when hemorrhage is anticipated.

SPINAL ANESTHESIA

Spinal anesthesia is accomplished by introducing an anesthetizing agent into the third and fourth lumbar interspaces, producing anesthesia from the waist downward, effective for a 2-hour to 2½-hour period. It is commonly used during cesarean section, provided hemorrhagic complications are not anticipated. It does have a tendency to lower maternal blood pressure, which in turn could cause fetal depression.

SADDLE BLOCK ANESTHESIA

Saddle block anesthesia is achieved by the introduction of a solution of dibucaine hydrochloride (Nupercaine hydrochloride), tetracaine hydrochloride, procaine hydrochloride (Novocain), or piperocaine hydrochloride to which 10% glucose is added. The medication is injected into the fourth lumbar space. This form of anesthesia is of short duration, lasting 1 to 1½ hours; therefore the time of administration depends upon the labor and delivery progress. In multigravidas it is administered prior to full dilatation, and in primigravidas it is administered when the presenting part is visible and dilatation is ascertained.

Saddle block anesthesia is administered with the mother in a sitting position. The head is flexed markedly on the chin, and the medication is introduced by the doctor into the fourth lumbar space. Thirty seconds following the administration of the medication, the patient is returned to a recumbent position, with a pillow elevating the head and shoulders. Elevation of the head and shoulders maintains anesthesia at the umbilical level. Whenever saddle block anesthesia is used there is a tendency toward a fall in blood pressure—therefore oxygen should always be available for the mother. Complaints of postpartum headache occur whenever there is leakage of spinal fluid from the injection site into the dura. Small-gauge needles for injecting the medication prevent leakage.

SPINAL EPIDURAL (PERIDURAL) BLOCK

A spinal epidural block is accomplished by injection of a local anesthetic into the epidural space. The epidural space is bounded by the dura mater and the ligaments and periosteal lining of the vertebral canal. It extends from the foramen magnum to the sacrococcygeal membrane. On their path to the periphery, the spinal nerves pass through this region, which also contains loose areolar tissue, blood vessels, and lymphatics. Anesthetic fluids may pass up and down in this space.

When the point of the needle enters the epidural space, it tents the dura mater and creates a negative pressure. This is the basis of the tests for needle position before the anesthetic is injected, for air or fluid will readily flow into the space when the needle is properly positioned.

In obstetric anesthesia, epidural blocks are most commonly administered in the lumbar or caudal region. They may be used in the late stages of labor, for delivery, or for cesarean sections. The block may be given as a single injection, or as a continuous injection through a small polyethylene catheter.

A single injection lumbar epidural block is administered through a 20-gauge blunt-tipped needle. A continuous method employs a 16-gauge needle through which a fine catheter is passed. The patient may be sitting as for a saddle block, or may be in a lateral recumbent position. Commonly used drugs are lidocaine hydrochloride (Xylocaine), mepivacaine hydrochloride (Carbocaine), or prilocaine hydrochloride (Citanest). With this type of anesthesia, the patient may maintain some degree of motor power. Some factors influencing the level of anesthesia are the dose of anesthetic, the position of the patient, and the pressure transmitted to the peridural space, that is, if the mother pushes during contractions.

Possible complications of the epidural technique are the following: (1) high subarachnoid block if the dura is inadvertently punctured, (2) hypotension, (3) toxic reaction, and (4) pain at the site of the needle puncture. As a precaution, an intravenous infusion should be started immediately whenever epidural anesthesia is given, and the vital signs of the patient and the fetal heart rate should be recorded frequently. A patient who has had an epidural block should never be left unattended. Should hypotension occur, turning the mother to her left side and administering vasopressors will help elevate the blood pressure. With chills or tremors sedation is ordered.

HYPNOSIS

Hypnosis or hypnoanesthesia is not new—it has been practiced for many centuries for relief of pain. In the middle of the nineteenth century, prior to the discovery of inhalation anesthesia, mesmerism (hypnosis) was a common practice. Hypnosis unfortunately is effective only in selected patients. It is often used with drugs and with regional anesthesias.

There are advantages and disadvantages to the use of hypnosis. Some of the advantages and benefits are the following: (1) drugs used for pain relief are minimized, many times completely eliminated; (2) it reduces fears and anxiety; (3) the mother can participate fully and aid the birth process, thereby making labor shorter; (4) it is safe to mother and baby since no sedation is given and fetal anoxia is never encountered; (5) the mother has complete control of contractions so that she can experience as much pain as she desires; (6) it is useful in premature deliveries and when food has recently been ingested; and (7) it is a gratifying emotional experience for the mother because she hears the baby cry, can hold him immediately, and can put him to breast if she so desires.

The disadvantages and contraindications are as follows: (1) it is feasible in only one of four mothers; (2) it should never be practiced by an unskilled hypnotherapist; (3) it is never selected for emotional or psychotic individuals; (4) it does take the time of skilled personnel and is expensive; and (5) it can lead to strong dependence on the therapist by the mother.

Preparation of the mother for hypnosis ideally starts early in the prenatal period, between the twelfth and sixteenth weeks of gestation. The hypnotist discusses with the mother her reasons for choosing hypnosis. Reasons that have a healthy outlook center about achieving motherhood with full memory and not being deprived of hearing the baby's first cry. A careful appraisal is therefore essential for successful hypnoanesthesia.

The training in hypnosis can be individual or by group therapy. Two or three sessions a month will determine whether or not the mother is a good candidate for hypnosis. If success is not obtained following ten sessions, there is poor promise that the mother is a good subject. In the early sessions autohypnosis (self-hypnosis) and glove anesthesia are taught. Glove anesthesia is achieved by suggesting that the hand become numb and heavy. Through postsuggestion the hand can then touch any part of the body and transfer this numbness or anesthetic state. From the beginning the mother is taught to have a pleasant outlook on the labor and delivery process, and she need experience only the amount of pain she wishes. At each session suggestions and conditioning help her reach a deeper hypnotic state, thereby raising the pain threshold.

Hypnosis in obstetrics is not a cure-all, nor can it be used exclusively or extensively. It does take time, is expensive, and takes much practice before it can be used successfully.

NURSING CARE OF THE MOTHER DURING AND AFTER ANESTHESIA

On admission to the labor and delivery unit the mother should be asked what her preference of anesthesia might be. Fears commonly associated with anesthesia are best discussed prior to the time of administration. The mother who fears inhalation or regional anesthesia may well be the one for whom that particular type of anesthesia proves ineffectual or dangerous. Often there are many misconceptions about the effects of anesthesia that the nurse may clarify in simple terms. Any marked fear of anesthesia should be reported to the obstetrician and the anesthetist.

During the administration of anesthesia, the nurse supports the patient by being nonjudgmental on the choice of anesthesia selected, by interpreting what will be done, and by helping the patient maintain the proper body position.

Nursing care of the mother during anesthesia is twofold because both the mother and the baby must be considered. During inhalation anesthesia a careful and frequent check of fetal heart tones (after each contraction) is imperative in giving safe care. When saddle block or spinal anesthesia is used, checking of the fetal heart tones and the mother's blood pressure is essential. A drop in blood pressure necessitates immediate administration of oxygen to the mother for adequate supply to the baby.

Following the administration of anesthesia many mothers experience nausea and vomiting. The nurse assures an open airway by turning the mother's head to one side and extends the chin forward to facilitate expectoration of vomitus. Suction equipment should also be available to prevent aspiration of material into the trachea.

Since anesthesia has a tendency to relax the uterine muscles, checking the fundus frequently prevents the possibility of hemorrhage. Bed rails and constant attendance until the mother is fully awake are essential for safe care at this time.

SELECTED REFERENCES

Thompson, H. G., and others: Epidural anesthesia in obstetrics, Obstet. Gynec., vol. 29, no. 5, May, 1967.

See reference list following Chapter 13.

Questions for study

1. What medications are used during labor to alleviate pain? What are the action and common dosages of each?
2. What inhalation anesthetics are used dur-

ing delivery? Give the indications and contraindications for each.

3. What emergency nursing care would you give should breathing become embarrassed following inhalation anesthesia?
4. What is local anesthesia? When is local anesthesia indicated?
5. What is spinal anesthesia? When is spinal anesthesia indicated?
6. Define hypnoanesthesia? What are the advantages, disadvantages, and indications?

CHAPTER 12

THE BIRTH OF THE BABY

The birth process necessitates preparation of a sterile field; this is facilitated by transferring the mother to the delivery or birth room, where all is in readiness for the mother and the infant.

The equipment in the delivery room (Fig. 12-1) consists of an appropriate table for adjusting the mother in lithotomy position, a heated baby's crib, anesthesia and oxygen equipment for mother and baby, adequate lighting, a supply of medications, and sterile linens and instruments for the delivery.

The vulva, rectum, and thighs are cleansed with a soap and sterile water preparation to remove surface bacteria. The mother is then draped with sterile linens to ensure further asepsis. The doctor and his assistant have scrubbed and have donned sterile gowns and gloves to assist the mother with each contraction.

With each contraction the mother pushes the baby down through the vaginal opening. As the baby's head advances (Fig. 12-2) the doctor cups his hand over the occiput to prevent sudden expulsion that may lacerate the perineum or cause trauma to the baby's head. As the head extends completely, the occiput is directed upward toward the symphysis to facilitate delivery of the baby's chin. With delivery of the head and chin the doctor feels around the neck for the umbilical cord. When the cord is loose, it is slipped over the baby's shoulder; when tight, it is clamped and cut immediately. The shoulders then rotate to accommodate their smallest diameter to the outlet, which brings about external rotation of the head. The anterior shoulder impinges under the symphysis, and lateral flexion makes possible delivery of the posterior shoulder and the rest of the body. As soon as the baby is born, a head downward position is maintained to facilitate drainage of mucus and to establish respirations. The baby cries immediately and spontaneously when the airway is patent and all is well. The baby appears cyanotic until a few vigorous cries are heard, which cause lung expansion and initiation of respirations. The Apgar scoring method is used 1 minute after birth to evaluate respiratory efforts. (See p. 138.)

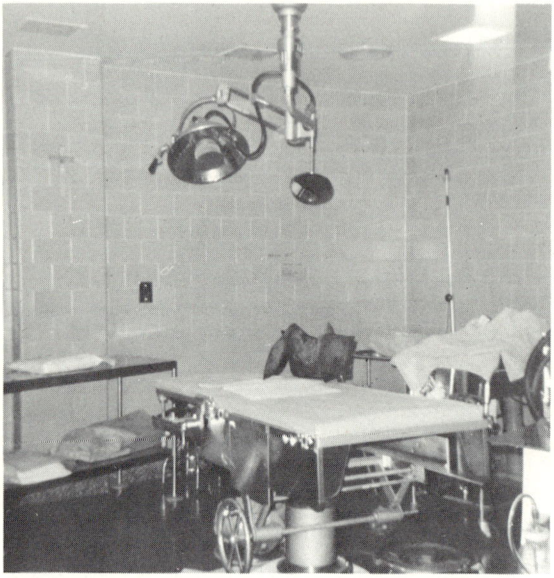

Fig. 12-1. Delivery room, Holy Name Hospital, Teaneck, N. J.

The doctor then proceeds to clamp (Fig. 12-3), cut, and tie (Fig. 12-4) the umbilical cord. Various methods are being used such as umbilical tape, small rubber band loops, or plastic lightweight clamps. The baby's eyes are treated immediately with a 1% silver nitrate preparation (2 drops in each eye) to prevent ophthalmia neonatorum (invasion of gonococcus that might have been present in the vaginal canal). The eye medication is dropped on the lower conjunctiva. This is done easily by gently pulling down the baby's lower lid. Care is taken not to drop silver nitrate on the baby's skin since the substance can cause a brown stain that may be alarming to the mother. The eyes are then flushed with either sterile water or normal saline. All preparations should flow from the inner canthus outward to prevent possible contamination from one eye to the other. Eye preparation is a requirement by state law for protection of all newborn infants.

Identification of the baby by the nurse and the doctor is done by checking the mother's wristlet and then applying an identical one to the infant. Mother and baby never leave the delivery room until identification is done. The baby is transferred to a heated crib where astute observation by the nurse includes checking for mucus, checking respirations, and keeping the baby in Sims position to maintain an open airway.

The third stage of labor is delivery of the placenta. This usually occurs 15 to 20 minutes after the birth of the baby. Should the mother be anesthetized, the doctor applies gentle fundal pressure (when he is certain the placenta has separated and is in the lower uterine segment), and the placenta is delivered.

Text continued on p. 129.

A B C D E F

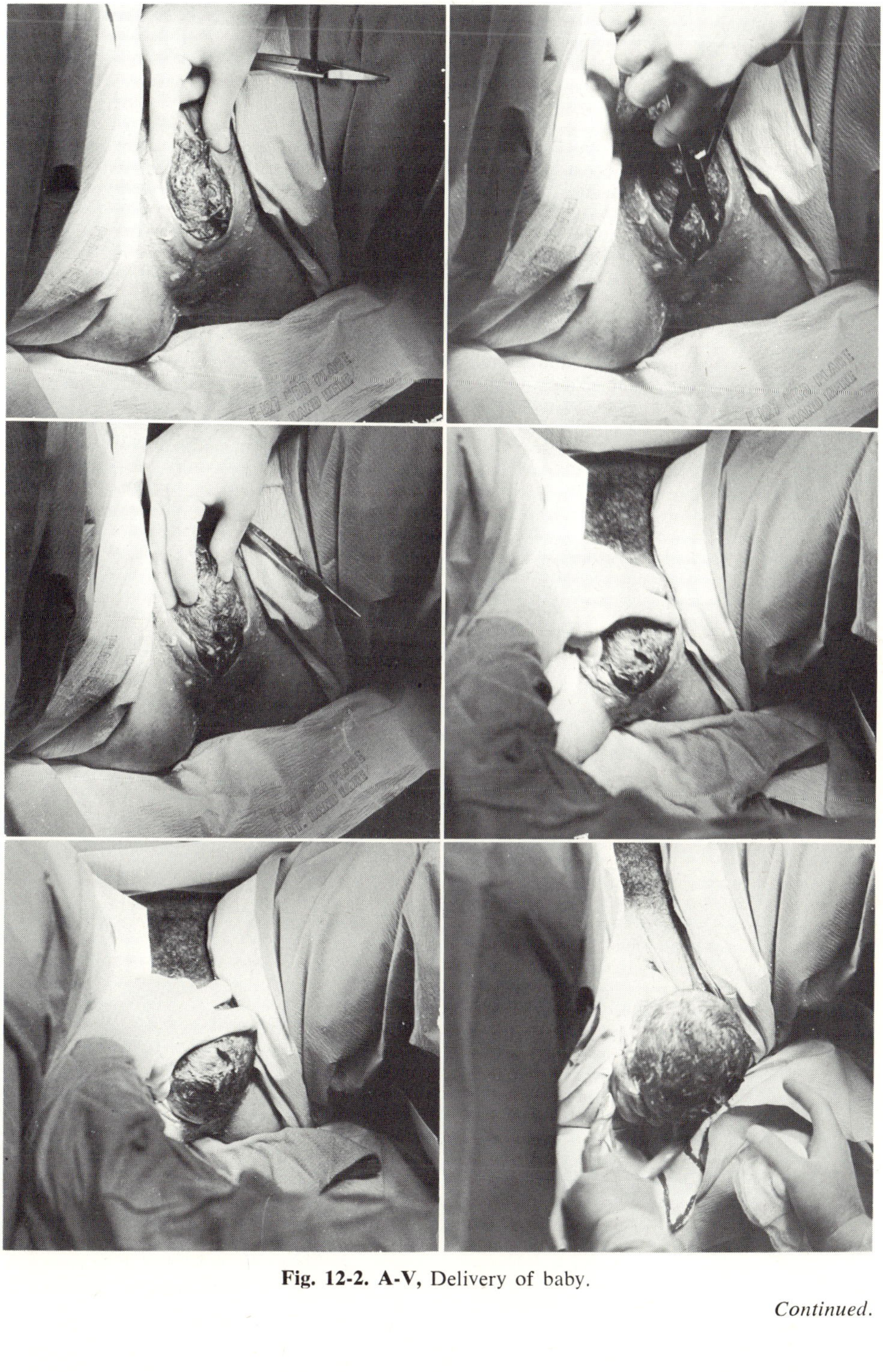

Fig. 12-2. A-V, Delivery of baby.

Continued.

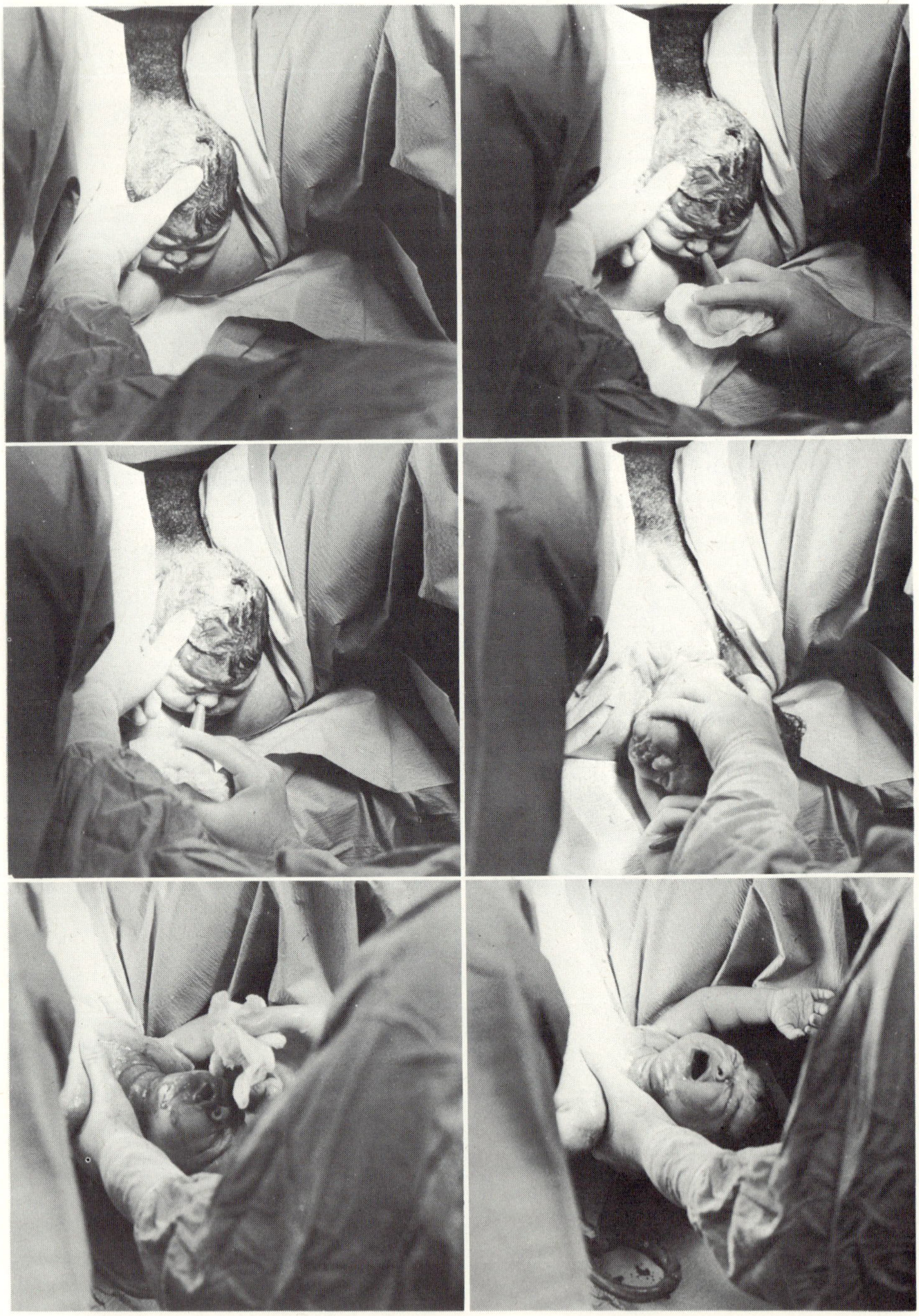
G H I J K L

Fig. 12-2, cont'd. For legend see p. 125.

M N

O P

Q R

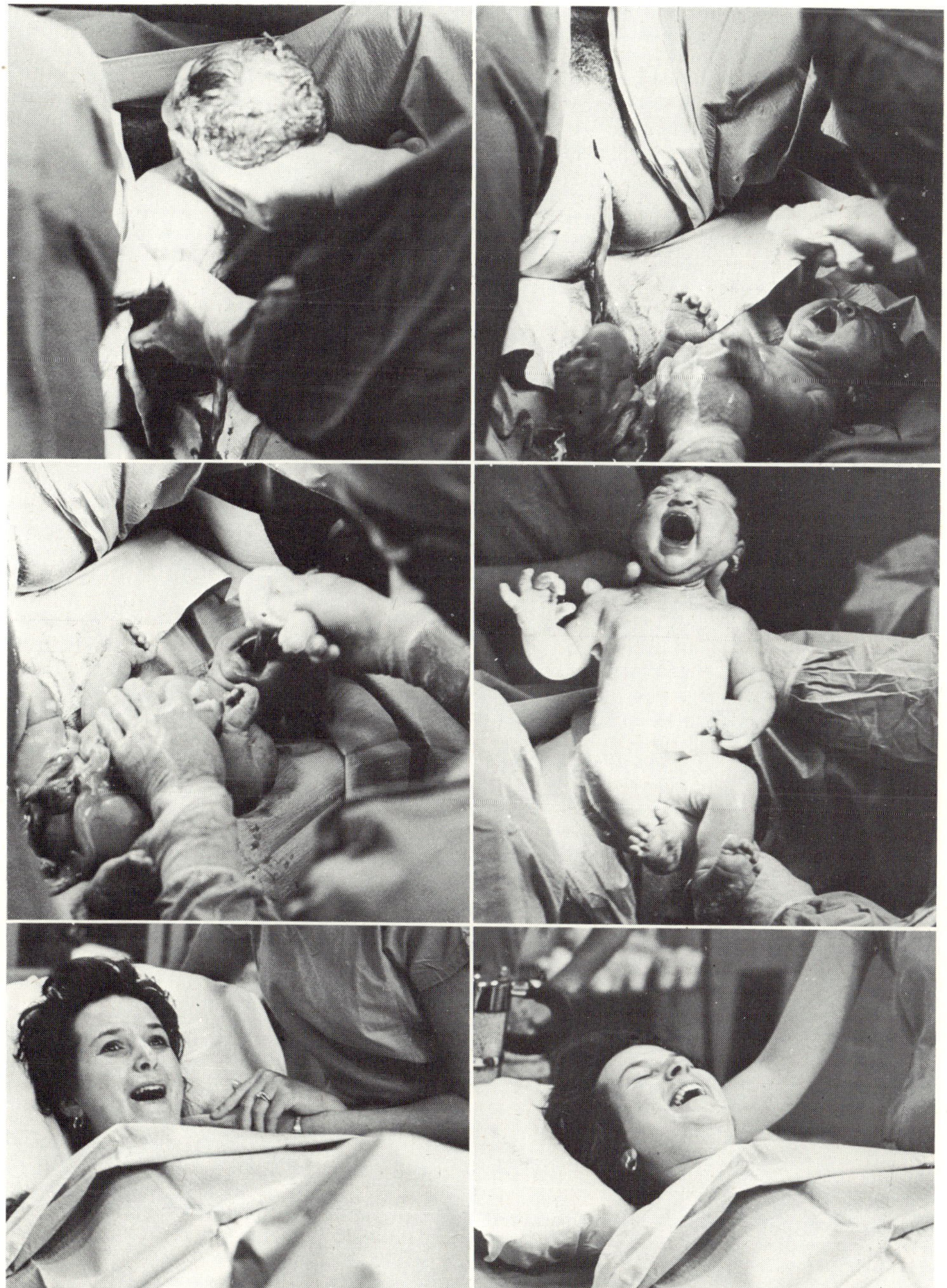

Fig. 12-2, cont'd. For legend see p. 125.

Continued.

S T
U

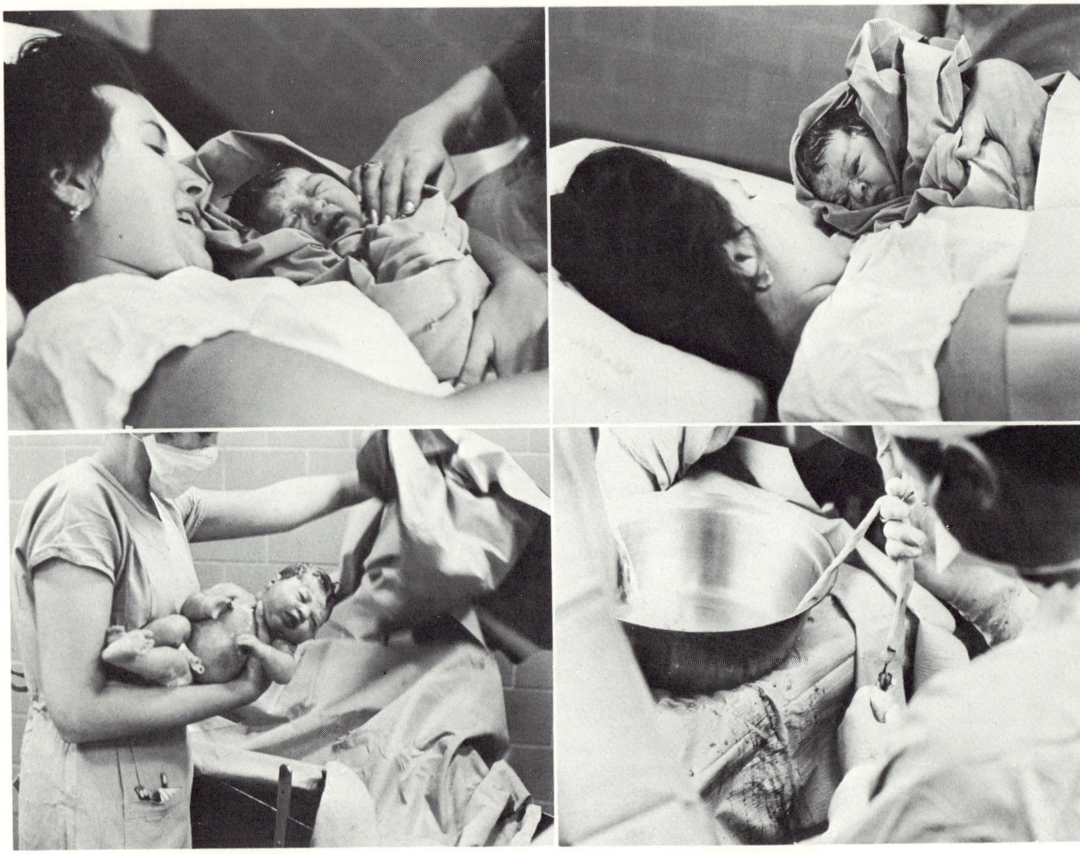

Fig. 12-2, cont'd. For legend see p. 125

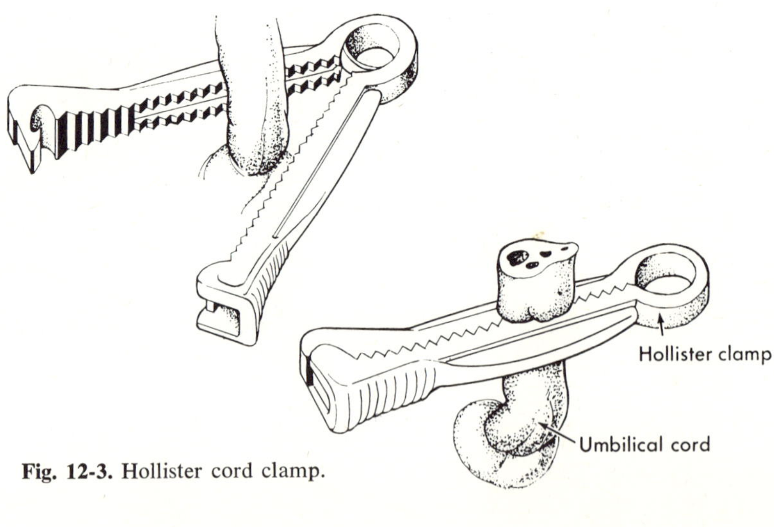

Fig. 12-3. Hollister cord clamp.

When the mother is awake she can push with a contraction to aid in delivery of the placenta (afterbirth). The placenta is always examined by the physician to ascertain the possibility of retained fragments within the uterus. Should this occur, manual exploration of the uterus is done to remove retained fragments, which can prevent effective contractions of the uterus and cause postpartum hemorrhage.

At times during the birth process just prior to delivery of the head, a small incision known as an episiotomy is made to prevent lacerations of the perineum. The incision (Fig. 12-5) is made directly downward toward the rectum (median or midline), or to the right or to the left away from the midline (right or left mediolateral). It is evident that an incision heals more rapidly when the skin edges are smooth. Rapid deliveries (know as precipitate) often produce lacerations called first, second, or third degree. Lacerations (Fig. 12-6) in which only the skin is involved are called first degree, lacerations with involvement of skin and muscles are called second degree, and lacerations with involvement of skin, muscles, and extension into the rectal sphincter are called third degree.

Oxytocics to contract the uterus during delivery are used at varying times, depending upon the physician's orders. Ergotrate, gr. 1/320 intravenously or intramuscularly, can be given after delivery of the head, after the birth of the baby, or following the expulsion of the placenta. Should the fundus have a

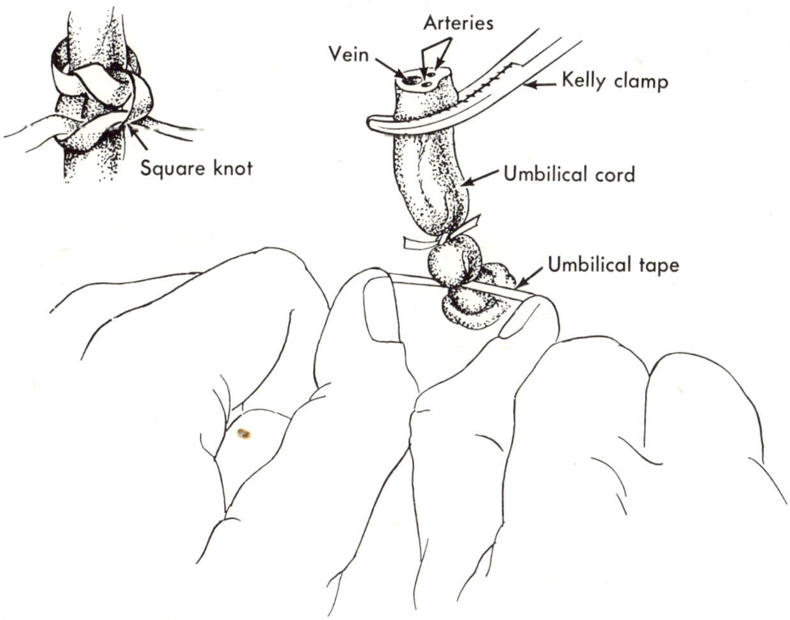

Fig. 12-4. Tying of the umbilical cord. Keeping the thumb knuckles in close approximation prevents excessive pulling on the umbilical cord.

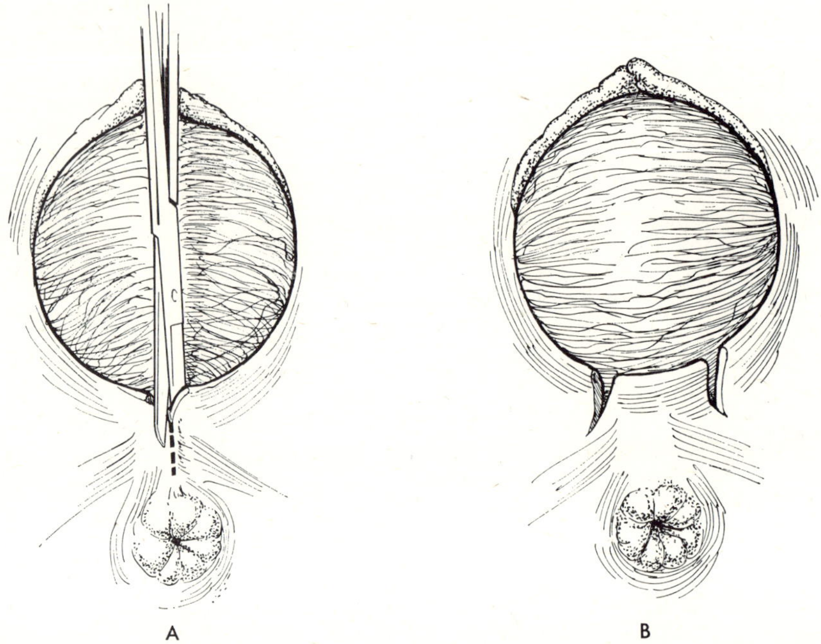

Fig. 12-5. A, Median or midline episiotomy. **B,** Right or left mediolateral episiotomy.

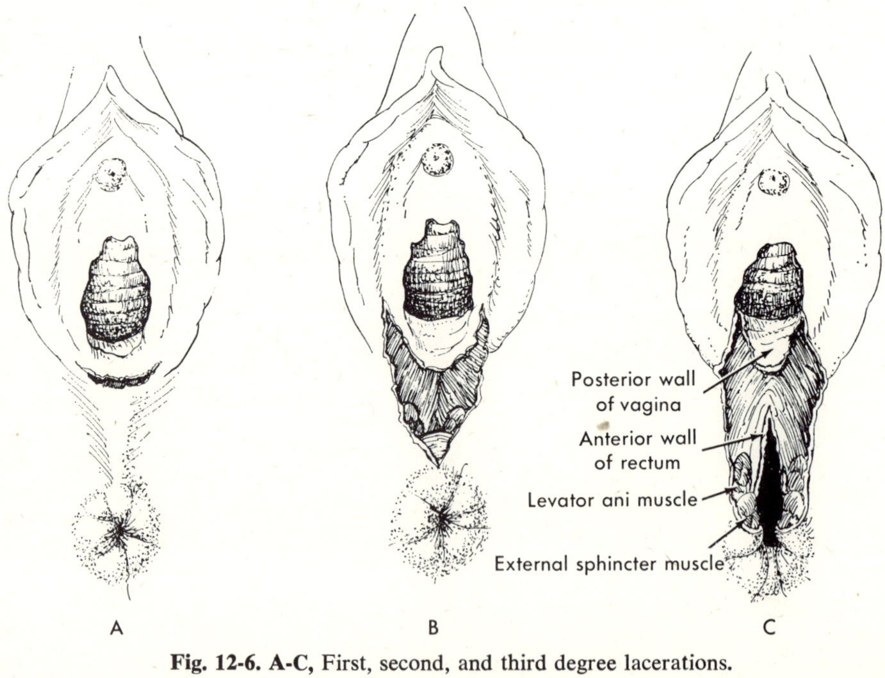

Fig. 12-6. A-C, First, second, and third degree lacerations.

tendency to relax, oxytocin (Pitocin) intramuscularly or in an intravenous dextrose solution is ordered.

Cleansing of the perineal area after delivery using aseptic technique minimizes bacterial invasion of the vulnerable reproductive tract. Sterile vulva pads are applied, and the mother's legs are lowered slowly and simultaneously to reestablish circulation. Preventing undue exposure and checking the fundus for firmness, the vaginal flow, the respirations, blood pressure, and pulse assure safe care of the mother.

Allowing the mother (and father, if he is present) to see and hold the infant will give assurance and provide satisfaction in their great accomplishment. This beginning parent-child relationship can be rewarding for the nurse who is privileged to observe so meaningful an interaction.

EMERGENCY DELIVERY

There are times when labor progresses so rapidly that the baby may be born before the physician arrives. This may happen at home or in the hospital labor room. Should a precipitate delivery occur, the nurse should stay with the mother, be calm, and give reassurance. If the head is crowning and there is no time for hand washing, proceed to help the mother.

The mother may be helped without contaminating the vaginal canal. As the head advances, instruct the mother to pant during contractions. Panting will keep the baby's head from advancing too rapidly, thus avoiding trauma to the infant and laceration of the perineum. The nurse should cup her hand over the baby's head to prevent rapid expulsion.

At no time should the head be held back with force. At no time should the mother be moved to the delivery room with the head crowning. It is better to have the mother push gently in between contractions. As the head is born by extension and external rotation, with the free hand wipe the mouth and milk the trachea. Then feel around the neck for the umbilical cord. Should the cord be present, try to slip it over the head or shoulder, whichever is feasible. Ask the mother to push down with the next contraction as the baby's head is supported.

Support the head and body, and once the baby is born, hold him by the ankles head downward to facilitate drainage of mucus. Once the airway is clear, stimulate the infant to cry by gently rubbing the back. Lay the infant in a clean area between the mother's legs and feel the fundus.

As the placenta separates, the cord will lengthen and there will be a gush of blood. Have the mother bear down for delivery of the placenta. Allow the placenta to deliver slowly by holding the lower portion to avoid tension on the membranes and possible retention within the uterus. Wrap the baby and the placenta together in a blanket until sterile equipment is available to tie and cut the umbilical cord. Gently massage the fundus to keep it firm. Often with a precipitate delivery the fundus has a tendency to relax. If this occurs and oxytocics are not available, putting the baby to breast will help the fundus contract. Keep the placenta for the doctor to inspect. Have sterile equipment ready for cord care.

Often with the excitement in this type of delivery, the nurse forgets to reassure the mother that all is well. Allowing the mother to see her baby and reassurance are paramount when anxiety is at such a peak.

CHAPTER 13

IMMEDIATE CARE OF MOTHER AND BABY

IMMEDIATE CARE OF MOTHER

The first two hours following delivery are often known as the fourth stage of labor; this is the time for astute observation of the fundus, perineum, blood pressure, and pulse.

The fundus immediately after delivery when well contracted is firm and slightly above the level of the umbilicus. At times the uterine muscles may relax, and excessive bleeding occurs. Holding the uterus (Fig. 13-1) by grasping the lower portion directly above the symphysis with one hand and holding the top of the fundus with the other hand should quickly aid in its contractile power. Failure of the uterus to contract usually results from (1) clot formation at the thrombosed placental site, (2) retained placental fragments, or (3) atony of the uterine musculature. Expression of clots by gentle manipulation of the fundus should result in a well-contracted, firm uterus. Manual removal of the placental tissue by the doctor will give the same results when indicated. Oxytocic drugs that stimulate uterine contractions are used during and after delivery to reduce blood loss following placental separation. The most common oxytocics used are ergonovine maleate (Ergotrate Maleate), 0.2 mg. or gr. 1/320, or methyl ergonovine tartrate (Methergine Tartrate), 0.2 mg. or gr. 1/320. Both can be given intramuscularly or intravenously for rapid effect. In mothers who have a tendency toward elevations of blood pressure, methylergonovine tartrate (Methergine Tartrate) is the drug of choice. Oxytocin (Pitocin), a posterior pituitary extract, can also be used in 5 or 10 unit doses. The action of oxytocin is rhythmic, and its vasopressor factor can often cause decided elevations in blood pressure.

Blood pressure and pulse are checked every 10 minutes the first hour and every 20 minutes the second hour after delivery. A decided drop in systole and diastole, with an increase in pulse rate, is indicative of hemorrhage, which at times may not be external but rather within the uterus.

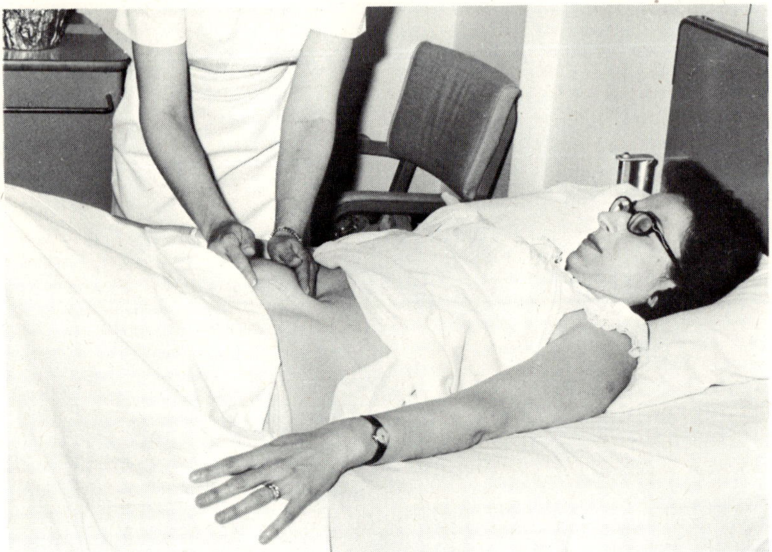

Fig. 13-1. Holding fundus of uterus.

Checking the perineum and vulva pad for excessive bleeding is accomplished by turning the mother in Sims position and separating the buttocks. A constant trickling of blood is indicative of beginning postpartum hemorrhage. When an episiotomy has been performed, observing the area for a beginning hematoma or separation of the suture line provides safe care. Although most mothers complain of pain at the episiotomy site, observation can indicate a beginning hematoma. If a hematoma is found, it should be reported immediately. Applying a sterile glove filled with ice will bring comfort until the physician arrives.

The labor process is hard work for most mothers; after full recovery from anesthesia, ingestion of fruit juice replenishes potassium loss. Diaphoresis occurs, and a partial bath and perineal cleansing provide comfort for the mother.

Occasionally some mothers are so fatigued that mild sedation may be ordered to assure rest. Many mothers are so exhilarated that they become talkative and crave food; a light diet may be given.

IMMEDIATE CARE OF THE NEWBORN INFANT

Following delivery of the baby, a rubber bulb syringe or De Lee mucus trap (Fig. 13-2) is used to aspirate mucus before the infant takes his first breath. At the time of delivery the newborn is quite cyanotic until he establishes his own circulation. When he takes his first breath, pressure builds up in the right ventricle and auricle, closing the foramen ovale; pressure on the pulmonary artery obliterates the ductus arteriosus; when the cord is clamped, cut, and tied, the ductus

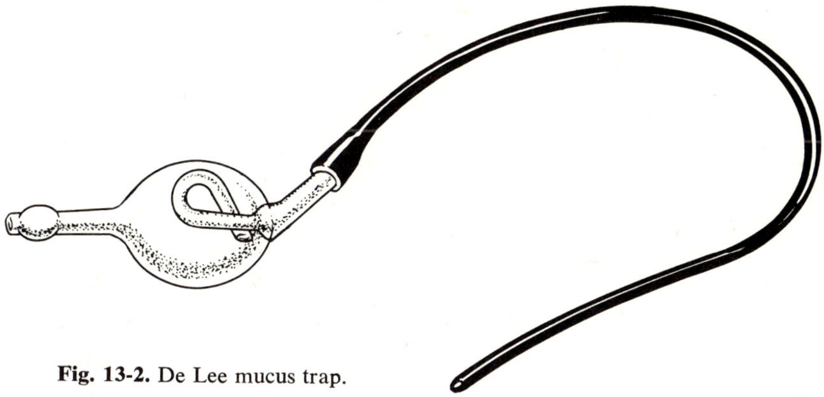

Fig. 13-2. De Lee mucus trap.

venosus becomes obliterated, eventually becoming the round ligament of the liver, and the hypogastric arteries find new routes.

The baby's eyes are treated immediately with 1% silver nitrate (two drops in each eye) to prevent ophthalmia neonatorum. Silver nitrate can produce irritation followed by redness, edema, and discharge. Care must be taken to instill the medication into the lower lid conjunctiva rather than directly on the cornea; the resultant reaction can cause concern to the mother, who may not know there is no danger involved. Local use of penicillin is discouraged because sensitivity is common.

The baby's identification band is checked with that of the mother, verified by the doctor, and applied. The baby is wrapped in warm blankets and turned on its side to facilitate the flow of mucus.

At times, because of previous sedation given the mother or because of a difficult delivery, the baby can be slow at establishing respirations. Should this occur, the air passages are freed of mucus by suctioning the infant with a suction catheter. The infant's head is extended markedly to straighten the trachea, and the nose and mouth are cleared gently so as not to injure the delicate mucous membranes. Once air passages are cleared, a few whiffs of oxygen by inhalation will usually suffice. It is important to remember that an infant should always be aspirated of mucus before any attempt is made to stimulate breathing. Should breathing be encouraged before clearing the air passages, the mucus will be inhaled into the trachea and lungs, causing atelectasis.

APPRAISAL

A quick appraisal of the newborn infant in the delivery room proves valuable for the nurse in the planning of nursing care for mother and baby following delivery (Fig. 13-3). Appraisal can be made at once with little exposure of the infant in order that his body temperature become stable.

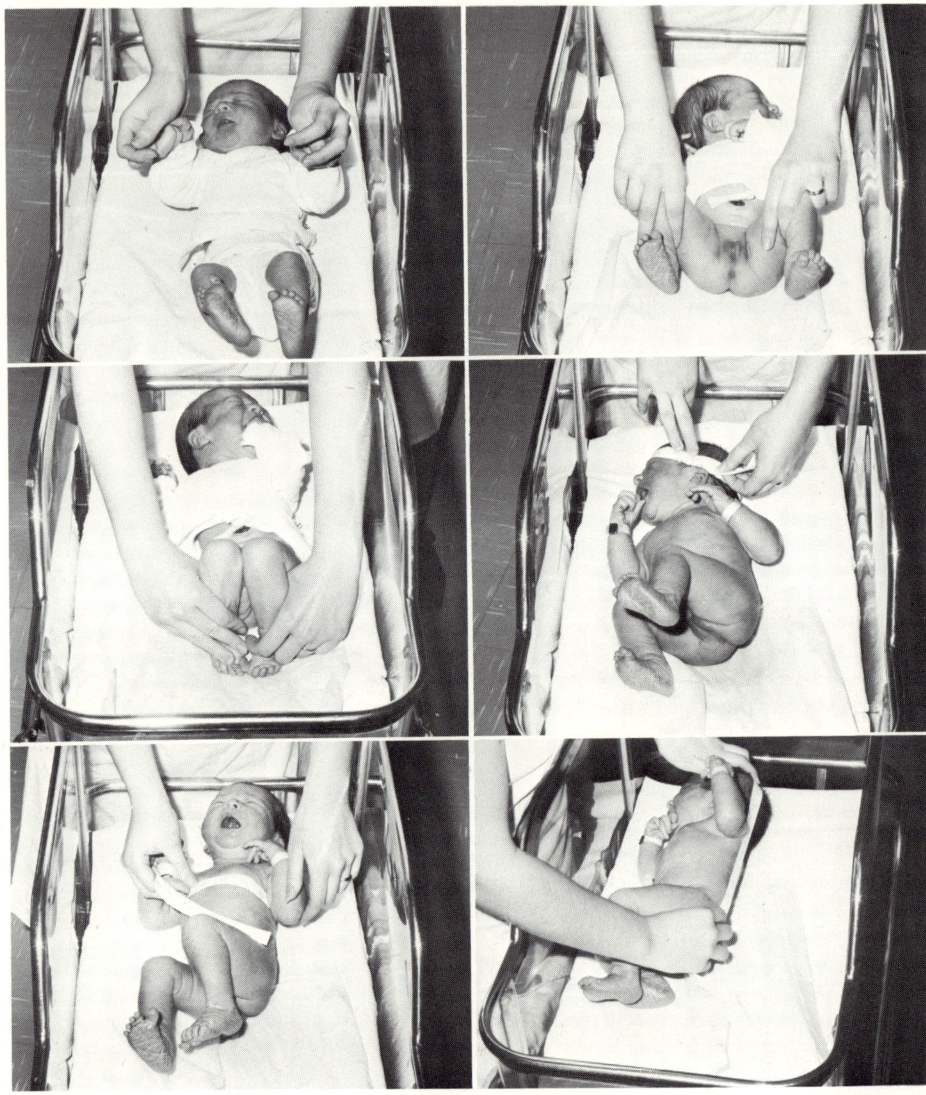

Fig. 13-3. Appraisal of newborn.

Head. Immediate observation will indicate whether or not any molding is present. To facilitate passage through the vaginal canal, there may be overriding of sutures and edema of the scalp, known as caput succedaneum. Whenever there is a fluctuating mass in any part of the skull caused by a tearing of tissue with exudation of blood, there is a resulting hematoma. Hematomas in the newborn usually absorb of themselves. If they persist, however, they may be aspirated with care, lest infection occur. The fontanels are also appraised. Is the anterior fontanel open? Is it bulging, which would indicate pressure in the spinal canal? Is the fontanel sunken, which is a sign of dehydration? Running the finger along the sagittal suture facilitates feeling for the posterior fontanel—is it slightly open? The fontanels are important in the growth and development of the infant's brain. The anterior fontanel closes between 12 and 18 months; the posterior fontanel closes between 6 and 8 weeks. Closures earlier than these would hinder adequate brain growth and development, ultimately affecting mental and intellectual ability. In normal growth and development (full-term infant), the circumference of the head and chest and the crown-rump length are practically equal.

Face. Are both sides of the face symmetric? Is the skin clear? Are the eyes clear? Nostrils patent? Does mouth inspection reveal a palate and gums that are fully cleaved? Does the tongue protrude beyond the lower gum or does it seem fixed at the frenulum? This is commonly known as tongue-tie and can interfere with a proper sucking reflex. Are the ears shaped normally, and are there auricle openings? Are the ears the same distance from the shoulders on the right and left sides? A scapula fracture could be detected easily since the distance between the ear and the shoulder would vary.

Arms and hands. Feel the arms and hands carefully for crepitation (irregularities or crackling sensations) that might be indicative of a fracture. Are fingers present and separated in both hands? Holding one hand at the shoulder joint, put both arms through normal range of motion—do you meet resistance in this maneuver? Place the thumb in the palm of the infant's hand, and with circled fingers around the baby's outer hand lift the infant slightly—does he grasp firmly when this is done? Absence of the grasp reflex is indicative of possible brain damage.

Chest and abdomen. Observe the chest and abdomen together. Are respirations irregular and abdominal, ranging between 40 and 60 per minute? This is normal in the newborn. Respirations that are regular, shallow, and labored are abnormal. Any depression at the xiphoid of the sternum is known as retraction, which is present during acute respiratory distress. Is the cord clamped off well, with no bleeding, redness, or odor?

Legs and feet. Abduct both legs well away from the body—is there resistance or interference in this maneuver that would be indicative of a congenital dislocated hip? With both feet flat and knees bent, are the knees the same height? If there are differences, this can be an added clue to congenital hip dislocation. Feel the legs and feet for crepitation, putting both legs through a normal range of motion. Check the feet by abducting, flexing, and rotating them for tightness of tendons, or resistance. If there is tightness or resistance, this can be indicative of clubbing. Move the thumb of your hand up the infant's foot from the heel to the toes. The toes should turn downward.

Genitalia. In girls check for a vagina and abnormal formations. In boys check the penis for a meatus and palpate the scrotum for testes. The testes are small marblelike organs within the scrotum that have often not made their descent from the abdominal cavity before birth. Although their absence in the scrotum at birth is normal, this should be reported and charted. Should the testes not descend before puberty, hormonal therapy or surgical intervention is indicated to prevent sterility when spermatogenesis occurs.

Back. To examine and appraise the back, turn the infant over on his abdomen. Does he have good muscle tone when he is picked up in the turning process? Is he flaccid? Does he attempt to turn his head to the side when placed on his abdomen? Normal infants have good development of the posterior neck muscles and readily turn their heads from side to side. Feel along the entire length of the spine. Have the vertebrae fused? Are there abnormal openings or protrusions? Is the anus patent? Patency of the rectum is assured when the first meconium stool has been passed.

Color. Most newborns become a delicate pink once respirations are established. The body temperature, however, takes a few days to become stabilized, and it is therefore not uncommon for the newborn to have cyanotic hands and feet for the first 24 hours.

Cry. Does the baby cry lustily? Is the cry weak, shrieky, or shrill, which might be indicative of brain damage?

Apgar scoring in appraisal of the newborn

Most babies need no assistance at birth other than to be held head down for respirations to become established. Usually there is a gasp and initial cry with ensuing respirations. Evaluation of the respiratory efforts of the newborn by a quick appraisal has been devised by Dr. Virginia Apgar. At exactly 1 minute after birth the infant is scored according to specific criteria (listed in Table 4).

In some instances it is required that the nurse check the circumference of the baby's head and chest and the crown-rump length. Normally these measure-

Table 4. Apgar scoring method*

Sign	*0*	*1*	*2*
Heart rate	Absent	Slow below 100	Over 100
Respiratory effort	Absent	Weak cry, hypoventilation	Good strong cry
Muscle tone	Limp	Some flexion of extremities	Active motion, extremities well flexed
Reflex irritability (stimulation of sole of foot)	No response	Grimace	Cry
Color	Cyanotic, pale	Body pink, extremities cyanotic	Completely pink

*Sixty seconds after birth score given for each sign. Score of 7 to 10 indicates best possible condition, score of 0 to 2 indicates severely depressed, and score of 3 to 6 indicates moderately depressed.

ments are similar for the full-term infant. Discrepancies in these measurements are found in premature infants or in infants with anomalies such as hydrocephaly or microcephaly. The average length of the full-term infant is 47 cm. (18 inches) to 53 cm. (approximately 21 inches).

Keeping the newborn infant warm is paramount for his survival. A heated crib or added blankets will help stabilize body temperature. Careful observations for an open airway and aspiration of excessive mucus will assure safe care of the newborn. Allowing freedom of motion for rooting and sucking satisfies his beginning needs.

SELECTED REFERENCES

Abramson, H.: Resuscitation of the newborn infant and related emergency procedures—principles and practice, ed. 2, St. Louis, 1966, The C. V. Mosby Co.

Eastman, N. J., and Hellman, L. M.: Williams obstetrics, ed. 13, New York, 1966, Appleton-Century-Crofts.

Willson, J. R., Beecham, C. T., and Carrington, E. R.: Obstetrics and gynecology, ed. 4, St. Louis, 1971, The C. V. Mosby Co.

Questions for study

1. What are the immediate needs of the mother following delivery?
2. What circulatory changes occur in the baby at the time of birth?
3. What are the immediate needs of the newborn?
4. How woud you appraise a newborn?
5. Define Apgar scoring in evaluating a newborn.
6. Mrs. I. is a gravida IV para III being admitted by stretcher, and delivery is imminent in the elevator on the way to the labor and delivery unit. As she pushes the baby's head is crowning. You are the nurse with her. How would you proceed in giving safe nursing care?

CHAPTER 14

PUERPERIUM AND FAMILY PLANNING

The puerperium encompasses the period immediately following delivery through 6 weeks. During this time the organs of reproduction undergo physical and physiologic changes and return to their nonpregnant state. This process is called involution. It is overwhelming when one considers the vast immediate changes that occur at delivery within a 15-minute to 30-minute period.

The mother seldom has the opportunity after delivery to share her experiences of labor and delivery; she often has a great need to discuss the strange sensations and intimate thoughts of the labor and delivery experience. The nurse may help the mother express the experience by asking questions such as the following:

"Now that you've given birth to your baby, can you tell me what you remember about labor and delivery?"

"What were some of the things that were of most comfort to you while you were in labor?"

"Is labor what you expected it to be like? In what way?"

"Try to explain how you felt when labor and delivery were all over."

"How did you feel when you first saw your baby?"

"Is there anything about labor or what happened in labor and delivery that you do not understand?"

"Do you feel that knowing what was going to happen would have helped you? Do you think it's best not to know what to expect?"

"If a friend of yours became pregnant for the first time and she came to you to find out what it is like to have a baby, what would you tell her?"

By exploring some of these questions, the professional nurse can advantageously use the information that is shared. The nurse discusses any misconceptions the mother may have that might otherwise never be resolved before another pregnancy ensues, or she may derive clues that could be applied in giving more effective support to other mothers during labor. As the mother's needs unfold, the nurse is better able to plan therapeutic nursing care.

SYSTEMIC CHANGES DURING THE PUERPERIUM

Digestive system

The organs of digestion, displaced because of enlargement of the pregnant uterus, once again return to their normal state. Many mothers experience immediate hunger following delivery as a result of their expended energies during labor. A high-protein diet with added fluids replenishes the much-needed nutriments to maintain homeostasis. Foods containing roughage help restore the peristaltic action in the bowel, relieving constipation caused by a relaxed abdominal wall. For the lactating mother, the diet is supplemented by an additional 1,000 calories to restore nutriments for an adequate milk supply.

Circulatory system

Blood volume and plasma are unstable in the early puerperium and show a slight rise. The increase in cardiac output during labor may or may not show a further rise.

The blood and metabolic changes that persisted during pregnancy usually disappear within a 2-week period following delivery. It is interesting to note, however, that there is an increase in blood fibrinogen during the first postpartal week. The leukocytes increase in number and may be as high as 30,000 if the mother has had a long labor. A leukocyte count of 15,000 after the first postpartal week is not an uncommon finding. This is a defense against possible infections and also aids in body repair. A hemoglobin reading of less than 10 mg. per milliliter and a red blood count below 3.5 million per milliliter may be found by the fourth postpartal day. A hemoglobin and red blood count repeated on the third postpartal day will determine whether or not the mother needs supplementary iron.

Excretory system

During the puerperium there is a marked increase in urinary output, the greatest increase occurring from the second to the fifth postpartal days. It is at this time that there is restoration of normal water metabolism. Approximately 3,000 ml. of fluids may be excreted daily for the first 24 hours. Retention with overflow can occur because of increased bladder capacity that exists during pregnancy. Residual urine harbors bacteria, and recording the intake and output is essential for the first 24 hours.

Lactose can be present during the first few postpartal weeks; however, this should not be confused with glycosuria, a finding in diabetes. Lactose is excreted as the breasts prepare for their lactating function.

In prolonged labors acetone in the urine is common and disappears in 3 days. In the first 24 hours 7 grams of nitrogen is excreted in the urine. On the twenty-third day 30% to 50% nitrogen may be excreted since protein materials are broken down and are either reabsorbed by the uterine wall or cast off in the urine. Nitrogen loss would have implications in planning dietary needs for both nursing and nonnursing mothers—dietary needs of necessity would be greatly increased.

Reproductive system

Uterus. Immediately following delivery the uterus weighs approximately 2 pounds; a week following delivery it weighs 1 pound; and in 6 weeks it weighs its original 2 ounces, returning once again to the pelvic cavity. With involution, autolysis of the protein of the uterus occurs with excretion. The remaining decidua of the uterus becomes differentiated into two layers. The outside layer becomes necrotic and is shed in the lochia, and the layer adjacent to the myometrium regenerates with new endometrium. The process of regeneration is rapid, and by 7 to 10 days there is epithelial formation. By the end of 3 weeks the entire endometrium is restored. The placental site, however, does not regenerate as rapidly; its regeneration takes as long as 6 weeks.

The fundus of the uterus can be felt from day to day in its process of involution (Fig. 14-1). Daily palpation (Fig. 14-2) for firmness and position of the fundus indicates whether involution is occurring. For purposes of recording this process, fingerbreadths above or below the umbilicus are used.

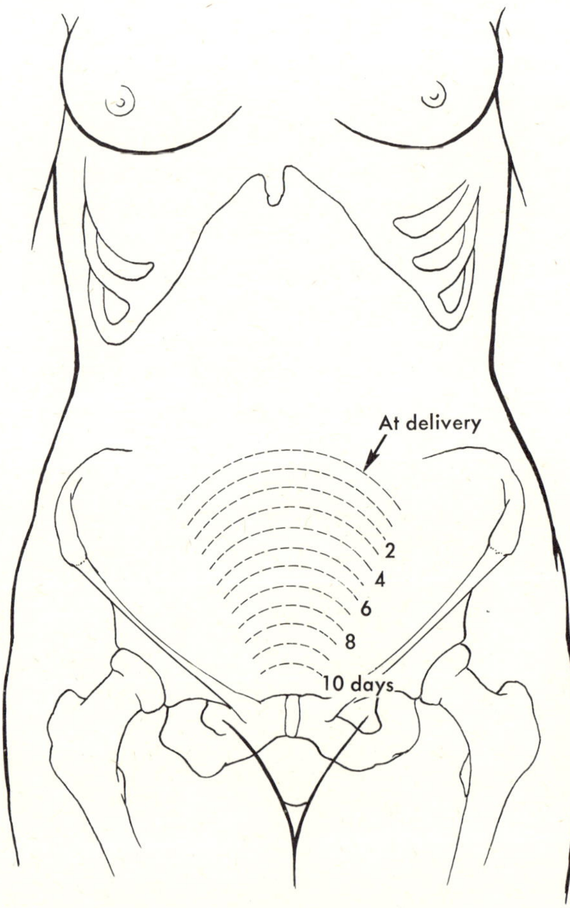

Fig. 14-1. Involution of the uterus.

Each day the fundus is felt lower in the abdominal cavity, and by the tenth day the uterus has returned to the pelvic cavity and cannot be felt above the symphysis. In the mother who is breast-feeding, the infant's sucking causes uterine contractions, which hastens involution. The fundus, which remains high and above the umbilicus, may not involute well or may be displaced by a full bladder. It is common to find a full bladder hindering proper contractility and involution of the uterus.

As involution occurs, contractions of the uterus can prove to be a great discomfort to some mothers. They are commonly referred to as aftercontractions (afterpains). Analgesics such as APC compound (acetylsalicylic acid, phenacetin, and caffeine) or codeine sulfate are usually ordered. Aftercontractions occur frequently in multigravidas, since the uterus may have lost some of its tonicity, and in mothers who breast-feed, since sucking stimulates contractions. It is well to provide a nursing mother with sedation for comfort prior to bringing the baby for feeding. A relaxed mother who is serene and comfortable is better able to meet the infant's needs.

Placental site. The placental site consists of many vascular thrombosed sinuses that eventually exfoliate, and growth of new endometrial tissue ensues. Within 6 weeks the placental site heals with no resulting scar tissue. Were there a resulting scar formation on the uterine mucosa, there would also be a diminution of endometrial lining, limiting adequate implantation sites for future fertilized ova.

Cervix. The cervical opening contracts rather slowly, and for the first few days

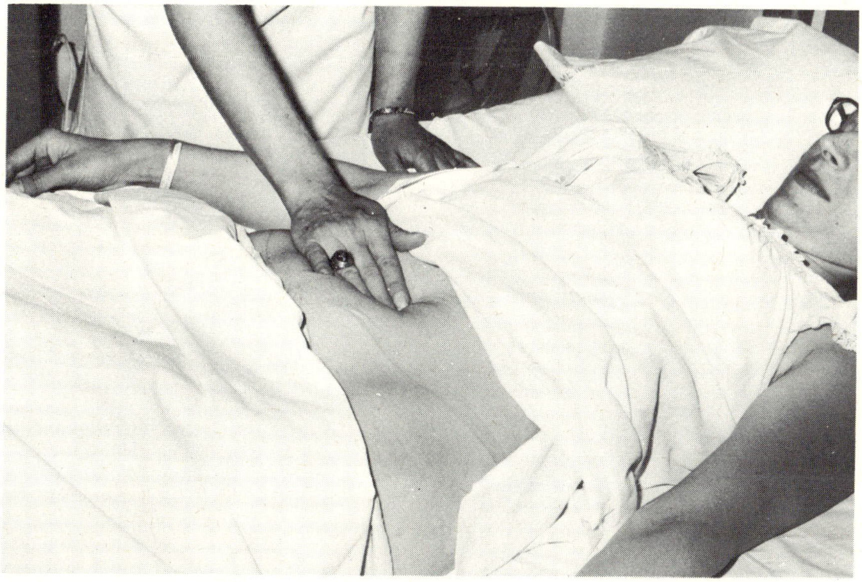

Fig. 14-2. Palpating fundus.

following delivery two fingers can be admitted. By the end of the first week, the cervical opening barely admits one finger. Although the body of the uterus involutes, the cervix forms many new cells. These muscle cells allow for healing of lacerations and tissues traumatized during the birth process.

Vagina. The vagina goes through great distensibility and rarely returns to its nonpregnant state. The rugae reappear after 3 weeks, and there is much cicatrization and healing of the soft tissues at the vaginal opening.

Abdominal wall. The abdominal wall, which has been greatly distended during pregnancy, becomes soft and flabby. The striae gravidarum become a silvery white, and after 6 weeks the muscles regain their tonicity if they have not been impaired. Many times there remains a marked separation of the abdominal rectus muscle, known as the diastasis recti. When this occurs the abdominal contents can readily be palpated through the peritoneum, fascia, and skin.

Vaginal flow. The secretions from the outer decidual lining of the uterus are cast off in the form of lochia following delivery. The lining remaining directly beneath regenerates into new epithelium within 2 or 3 days following delivery. By the latter part of the third week, the entire endometrium and the ovulatory cycle are restored.

The vaginal discharge for the first 2 days following delivery is usually red and is known as lochia rubra. In a few days the lochia becomes pinkish and is known as serosa. By the end of a week to 12 days the lochia becomes whitish and is known as alba. Lochia, which has a characteristic fleshy odor, consists of red blood corpuscles, leukocytes, epithelial cells, decidual tissue, and bacteria. It is believed there may be a decided increase in flow on the third or fourth postpartal day just before there is a sudden decrease in hormones. Any deviation from this normal pattern of lochia, such as persistent lochia rubra, a foul-smelling lochial discharge, an elevation in body temperature, or an increased flow, is indicative of retained placental fragments or beginning bacterial invasion with resulting infection.

Breasts. During pregnancy the breasts are being prepared for lactation by hormonal action. The increased amounts of estrogen and progesterone stimulate the growth of the mammary glands; the estrogens in particular develop the duct and alveolar systems. These hormones inhibit the activity of the luteinizing hormone of the anterior pituitary gland, preventing lactation. However, when the placenta is delivered, there is a release of this same hormone, which initiates lactation.

The posterior lobe of the pituitary gland secretes a hormone called oxytocin, which brings about the "letdown reflex" or ejection of milk from the lactiferous sinuses to the milk ducts of the nipple. This reflex is initiated and stimulated by the baby's sucking (Fig. 14-3). The letdown reflex is initiated through the action of stimuli to the pituitary gland, which liberates the hormone oxytocin. It is therefore inhibited by emotional factors and initiated by the baby's cry or stimulation through sucking.

In the last trimester of pregnancy, colostrum, a thick yellow-white substance, can be expressed from the nipples. Colostrum, a forerunner of milk, contains pro-

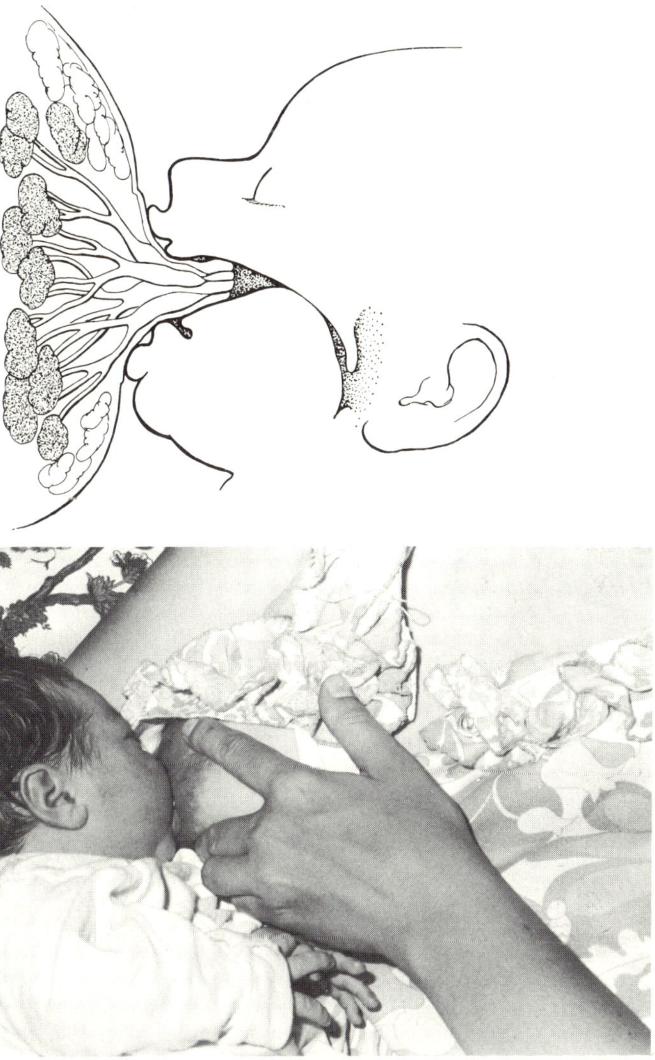

Fig. 14-3. Baby at breast. Mouth grasps nipple and areola.

teins, salts, and sugar but little fat. Although it is not very nutritious when ingested by the newborn, it acts as a cathartic in emptying the gastrointestinal tract of the baby's first stool, known as meconium. It is now recommended that 6 weeks prior to delivery the mother who anticipates breast-feeding begin by manually expressing a few drops of colostrum daily in preparation for lactation. This exercise opens the duct system, facilitating lactation following delivery. It is recommended only for mothers who feel at ease in handling their breasts—many mothers have been just as successful without this preparation.

On the second or third day following delivery there is a decided change in

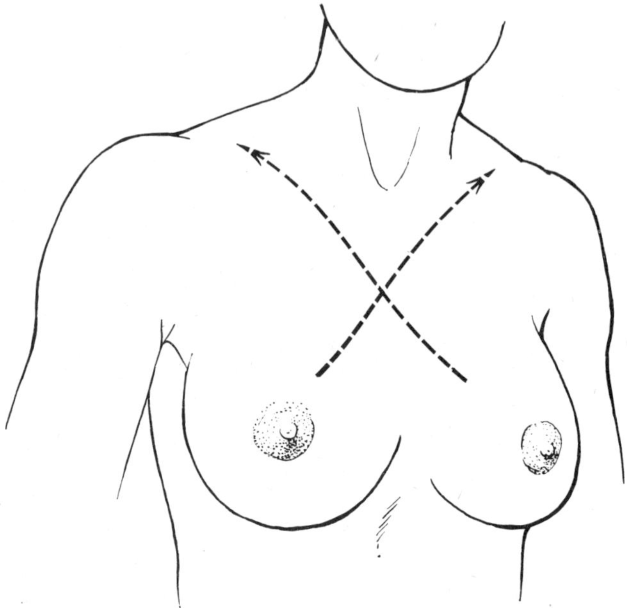

Fig. 14-4. Breast support. Broken-line arrows indicate lifting of breast toward opposite shoulder.

the breasts. They become larger and firmer, and the blood vessels may be easily discernible through the skin. The blood vessels become dilated and the breasts are heavy and uncomfortable—this is known as engorgement. Engorgement occurs with increased vascularity as the milk comes into the breasts; it is common during the second or third postpartal day. For the nonnursing mother, relief can be obtained by wearing a snug, well-fitted uplifting brassiere to support the breast tissue (Fig. 14-4). Analgesics such as APC (acetylsalicylic acid, phenacetin, and caffeine) or codeine sulfate, ½ gr., are helpful when ordered by the physician. Cold applications such as ice caps may help constrict the vessels; however, prolonged cold application produces the reverse effect, and marked dilatation may occur. Ice caps are helpful when applied for short intervals such as 10 minutes on, 20 minutes off. Explaining to the mother why engorgement occurs and that it will subside will make her less anxious. Administration of oxytocin, 0.5 ml. intramuscularly, has been found effective in bringing about the milk letdown, alleviating discomfort.

In the breast-feeding mother the areola or the entire breast becomes engorged; this not only creates discomfort but also makes it difficult for the infant to begin to suck. Often warm applications prior to breast massage and expression provide comfort for the mother. Although manual expression produces very little milk, it relieves pressure of the full, taut breast. Expression should not be a lengthy process to tire the mother. Electric pumps are discouraged since they have a tendency to injure breast tissue, causing much discomfort.

Breast milk is bluish and watery in appearance and is slightly alkaline. It is composed of 1% to 2% protein, 6.5% to 8% lactose, and 3% to 5% fat. In comparison, cow's milk contains 3.5% protein, 4.75% lactose, and 3.5% fat. Therefore protein content is higher in cow's milk, and carbohydrate and fat content is higher in breast milk; however, both cow's milk and breast milk contain 20 calories per ounce.

During lactation, the quality and quantity of breast milk depend greatly on the mother's nutrition; therefore daily intake of an additional 1,000 calories is required.

There may be marked alteration in the quality and quantity of breast milk whenever there is stress or emotional upheaval. Drugs such as those of the belladonna group dry up secretions and limit the quantity of breast milk. Large amounts of drugs such as opium, salicylates, quinine, iodides, bromides, lead, mercury, and alcohol may be transmitted to the baby through breast milk. When menstruation or a new pregnancy occurs, an increase in estrogens necessitates weaning of the baby.

It is evident that the ideal food for the newborn is breast milk. Planning for breast-feeding begins during pregnancy, with proper care of the breasts and education in the techniques of breast-feeding. The physiologic effects of breast-feeding are beneficial because they foster involution of the uterus. The psychologic benefits to the mother and the baby in developing a close mother-child relationship cannot be overemphasized.

Integumentary system

Profuse diaphoresis is apparent in many women, especially during sleep. This is one of the ways in which wastes are excreted in the immediate postpartum period. Many mothers complain of being thirsty because their body fluids need replenishment.

NURSING CARE DURING PUERPERIUM

All the body systems are affected during the puerperium as they are restored to their prepregnant state. Since the mother is now faced with responsibilities in the care of her new baby, meeting her needs will ultimately affect the way in which she will meet the baby's needs. Certainly the mother who is provided with adequate nutrition and comfort will be ready to meet the infant's needs for warmth, comfort, nutrition, and love.

Since there are so many changes occurring at an unbelievable speed during the puerperium, nursing care will center upon these changes.

Daily observation by the nurse consists of checking the breasts for engorgement and filling, the nipple tissue for cracks or fissures, and the breast tissue for masses or redness. The fundus is checked daily for proper involution; the episiotomy area is observed for ecchymosis, edema, gaping sutures, redness, and so on. With the mother in the Sims position, the color, amount, and odor of lochia are ascertained. The nurse starts her observations with the clean area of the breasts and works toward the perineum. Hand washing is essential before examination of each mother.

Personal hygiene. Following delivery most women experience diaphoresis—therefore bathing or showering is comforting and refreshing. Cleansing of the perineal area is taught as soon as the mother is able to care for her own needs, which is quite early in the postpartal period. Cleansing the perineum toward the rectum and away from the vaginal opening will prevent introduction of bacteria into the vulnerable reproductive tract. Teaching the importance of hand washing provides safety as the mother feeds, handles, and fondles her new baby.

Early ambulation. During the puerperium early ambulation has been found beneficial for the mother. Allowing mothers to be up and about early, ranging from 12 to 48 hours after delivery, is a common practice. It has been found that early ambulation improves circulation, thereby preventing blood stasis and ultimately hastening involution and restoration of normal body functions. It is not uncommon to have some mothers experience a degree of weakness when ambulating for the first time. It is well to have the mother dangle her legs for a few minutes before attempting to stand. Sitting should precede walking, and ambulatory time should be limited to the mother's tolerance.

Vital signs. The basal temperature following delivery should remain within normal limits. Any elevation above 100° orally for 24 hours is indicative of a beginning infection. The basal temperature is commonly taken orally to prevent vaginal contamination. Bradycardia is a characteristic favorable sign following delivery. Within 10 days the pulse returns to its normal rate. An elevation in pulse rate, on the other hand, should be reported immediately.

Nutrition. In the early postpartal period fluids should be ingested liberally to replace the excessive fluid loss during delivery. The diet should contain approximately 2,600 to 2,800 calories daily. A diet high in proteins, vitamins, and minerals is essential for tissue repair and the mother's well-being. The diet of the lactating mother should allow additional caloric intake to supplement the fluid and nutriments lost during the lactating process. A diet similar to that followed during pregnancy will be adequate after delivery.

Intestinal tract. During the puerperium the colon must regain its muscle tone and peristaltic action. Constipation is common following delivery. Increased intake of roughage and fruit juice is helpful. Mild laxatives that lubricate, such as mineral oil, or that increase bulk, such as senna (Senokot), may be administered. When these drugs are not effective, a cleansing soap solution or small retention enema such as sodium phosphate solution (Travad) is ordered.

Perineum. Pain at the episiotomy site may be caused by edema as healing occurs. Perineal exercise early following delivery will prevent edema by improving circulation to the area as healing progresses. Pain caused by edema is also alleviated by exposing the perineum to a heat lamp following perineal cleansing for 10 to 20 minutes several times daily. Heat improves circulation to the area, reducing edema. Commercial spray medications that soothe and act as local anesthetics can be used when ordered.

Varicosities. Dilated and tortuous veins in the lower extremities become quite pronounced during pregnancy because of pressure on the peripheral vascular system. Application of an Ace bandage before arising will prevent stasis, improve circulation, and give support, providing much comfort (Fig. 7-1). Early ambulation aids and improves circulation.

Postpartum blues. The drastic changes in all the body systems and the sudden withdrawal of hormones on the third or fourth postpartal day may cause depression or a sudden letdown feeling. It is not uncommon to find a mother crying for no reason at all. This may be frightening to the mother, who experiences the feeling without awareness of what is happening. The nurse should inform her that such a reaction is not uncommon. Early dismissal from the hospital may find the postpartum blues period occurring on the day of dismissal, adding to the vast adjustment necessary from hospital to home.

Postpartal exercises. Exercises during the postpartal period are encouraged to strengthen the abdominal and pelvic muscles. These are usually started gradually following delivery, and by the third day all may be practiced; they may be continued for 3 months at home.

Sleeping or resting position. Lying on the abdomen helps strengthen the abdominal muscles and hastens involution. Should the breasts be sensitive or full, a small pillow placed below the breasts gives comfort.

A

B

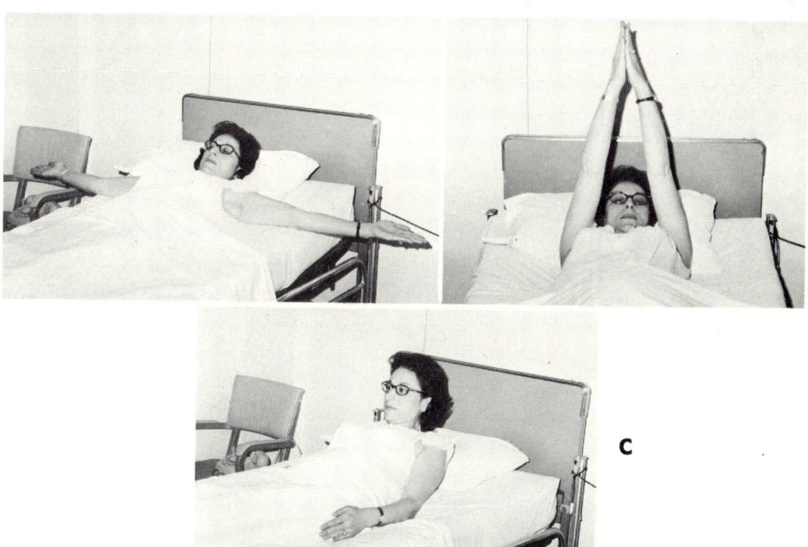

C

Fig. 14-5. A, Exercise. **B,** Exercise. **C,** Head raising.

Other exercises include the following:

1. Lying flat on her back with her arms outstretched from the sides, the mother raises her arms above her head until her hands touch; she then brings her arms down again. This may be repeated (Fig. 14-5, *A* and *B*).

2. Lying quietly and breathing deeply and slowly with the abdomen (Fig. 8-5) provides relaxation and strengthens abdominal muscles.

3. Lying flat on her back, she raises her head (Fig. 14-5, *C*) and flexes her chin forward on her chest without moving any other part of her body. This may be done five times at first and increased gradually. The mother will actually feel the pull on the abdominal muscles.

4. Lying flat on her back the mother raises one leg at a time without bending the knee (Fig. 14-6). The leg may be raised only a few inches at first and then gradually raised higher. This exercise strengthens leg muscles. Starting from the same position the mother flexes her leg, bending her knee sharply on her abdomen, allowing the heel of her foot to touch her buttock. This may be repeated with the other leg.

5. From a flat lying position and with her arms folded across her chest, the mother raises herself to a sitting position, keeping her legs outstretched.

6. The knee-chest position (Fig. 8-4) is assumed for 5 minutes twice daily a few weeks following delivery. In a kneeling position with her knees separated as widely as possible, the mother bends her body forward, bringing her chest down to the bed or floor as close to her knees as possible. Her head is turned to one side, and her back is kept straight. This exercise aids in bringing the uterus back into its prepregnant state. It is discouraged immediately following delivery since

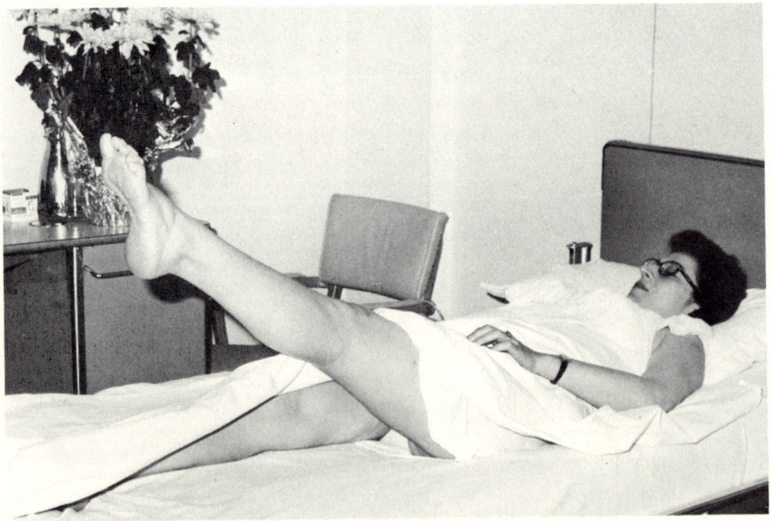

Fig. 14-6. Leg raising.

the cervix is still somewhat dilated, and there is danger of air embolism. It can safely be started 3 weeks after delivery.

Dismissal from the hospital. Dismissal from the hospital varies from 24 hours (which occurs in many overcrowded large city hospitals) to 3, 4, and 5 days after delivery. The average and common hospital stay is 4 days. Early dismissal presents many concerns for the nurse, who needs to incorporate much in supporting and guiding parents for their future parental roles. Referrals to public health services for continued health supervision are essential for mother and infant.

Teaching and guiding parents before dismissal. Individual teaching is an ongoing process that starts early in the prenatal period and continues throughout the maternity cycle. The main objective is to meet the physical and emotional health needs of families. Rehabilitation in the postpartal period is a process encompassing restoration of the mother to her prepregnant state and preparing her for care of the new infant. The primary focus is on building upon and reinforcing what the mother already knows, making her feel secure in her future responsibilities.

Group discussions of self-care and care of the newborn are valuable during the immediate postpartal period. At this time the mother is ready and willing to learn and is most perceptive. As mothers share their experiences in infant care, they become secure and confident in undertaking their new maternal roles. A bath demonstration (Fig. 14-7) may well lead to a discussion on growth and developmental patterns. Breast-feeding conferences (Fig. 14-8) incorporate bottle feeding, weaning the infant from breast or bottle to a cup and solids, and what to do about sibling rivalry.

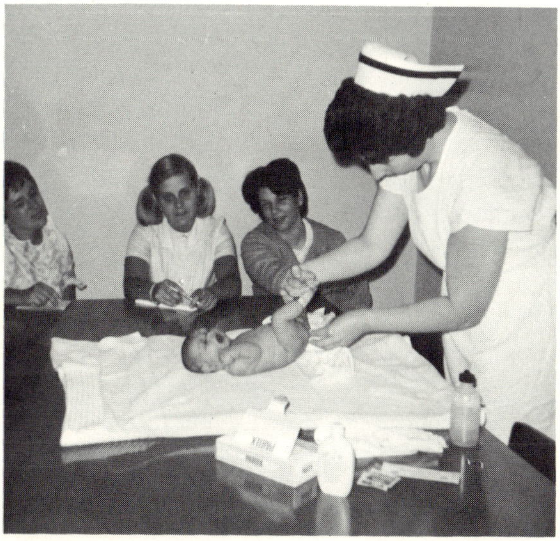

Fig. 14-7. Bath demonstration, Holy Name Hospital, Teaneck, N. J.

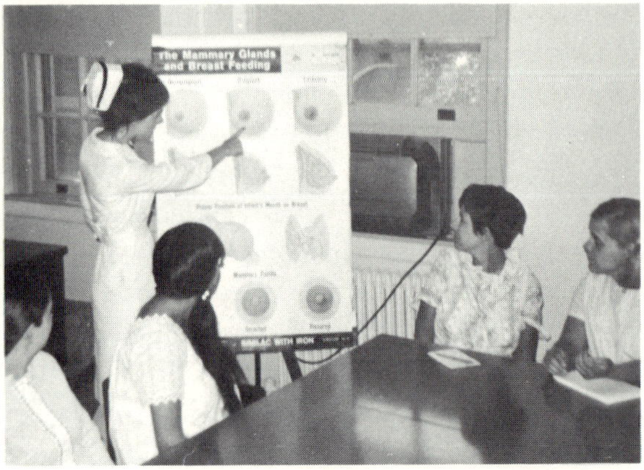

Fig. 14-8. Breast-feeding conference, Holy Name Hospital, Teaneck, N. J.

A nurse leading a group should be skilled in group dynamics; she also needs to know a great deal about maternal and child health. Interestingly, the group leader learns much from group members as she conducts conferences. Many times the group members share information with each other that is most valuable in child rearing. Informality and small group sessions encourage group discussion. Since all group members are vitally concerned with any topic that is discussed, much is covered as one question leads to another, with resulting group involvement. A group consisting primarily of primigravidas may well have to be motivated by the group leader who asks, "Have you thought about how you will manage when you get home?" This leading question will always start discussion. A heterogeneous group (with both primigravidas and multigravidas) usually encourages much interaction since previous experiences are discussed. Clues for referral to a community agency may well be identified during group discussions. Introducing mothers to services available to them fortifies their confidence as the nurse provides anticipatory guidance beyond the hospital environment. Discharge from the hospital is the beginning of a new family, and these early years are building blocks for a healthy adulthood and for contributing citizens.

Community agencies concerned with the welfare of mothers and babies are supported by city or state funds or by a private enterprise. A maternity service includes health supervision during the prenatal period and extends to the mother and the newborn after hospital discharge. The objectives of a maternity health service are as follows: (1) to visit all prospective mothers as early in pregnancy as possible, (2) to provide medical and nursing supervision throughout the maternity cycle, (3) to help parents understand the childbearing process in preparation for delivery, (4) to provide or supervise nursing care for the health of mother and baby, and (5) to teach the importance of ongoing health supervision of family members.

These objectives incorporate medical supervision and nursing care with supervision. Medical supervision may be given by a private physician, a clinic, a health center, or a midwife under the supervision of a physician or a clinic. Nursing care and supervision may be given by a public health nurse visiting the mother at home, the mother visiting the nurse at the health center, or the mother attending classes through community agencies such as outpatient clinics, Red Cross, or private organizations.

ROOMING-IN

An arrangement with facilities that allow for mother and infant to room together following delivery is known as rooming-in (Fig. 14-9). The philosophy that mother and infant are a biologic unit and that rooming-in provides for a continuing mother-infant relationship is not new. Home deliveries have always encouraged close proximity of mother and baby following delivery. As health services improved in maternal child health, hospital deliveries replaced home deliveries. The postpartal unit for the mother and the nursery for the infant seemed architecturally sound and convenient. Aseptic techniques lowered the rate of infection, and delivery in a hospital lowered the incidence of hemorrhage. With these changes, however, the family unit became separated during the mother's hospital stay.

Current trends and philosophy of maternity care focus on family-centered care (Fig. 14-10). Parents of beginning families are young and independent of the extended family. The short hospital stay presents a challenge in preparation for discharge. Rooming-in affords the mother the opportunity to become acquainted with the infant's needs and develops a beginning security in caring for the infant. The mother has a greater opportunity to observe her infant and is in a setting where the professional nurse is available for help and anticipatory guidance. Rooming-in affords the father the opportunity of participating in caring for the infant. Often a special visiting time is allotted for the beginning family to be together. Mothers who choose to breast-feed find rooming-in ideal because the baby can be fed on demand. Beginning contacts with the infant can prove valuable only after the mother's needs have been met. Should the mother have had a difficult labor and delivery, the baby's care is often done by the nurse. The mother assumes responsibility for the infant as she is ready.

Rooming-in is an optional arrangement in most hospitals, the mother privileged to choose between rooming-in or the conventional postpartal unit and central nursery. Often multigravidas choose the conventional method since they look forward to a few days of relaxation during their hospital stay.

Rooming-in may be complete, in which the mother and infant are together 24 hours daily, or partial, in which the infant is taken to a separate nursery (other than the central nursery) from 10:30 P.M. to 5:30 A.M. Newly built rooming-in units feature small glass-paned nurseries attached to each postpartum unit, so that the babies are visible. Improvised rooming-in units return the infant to the central nursery.

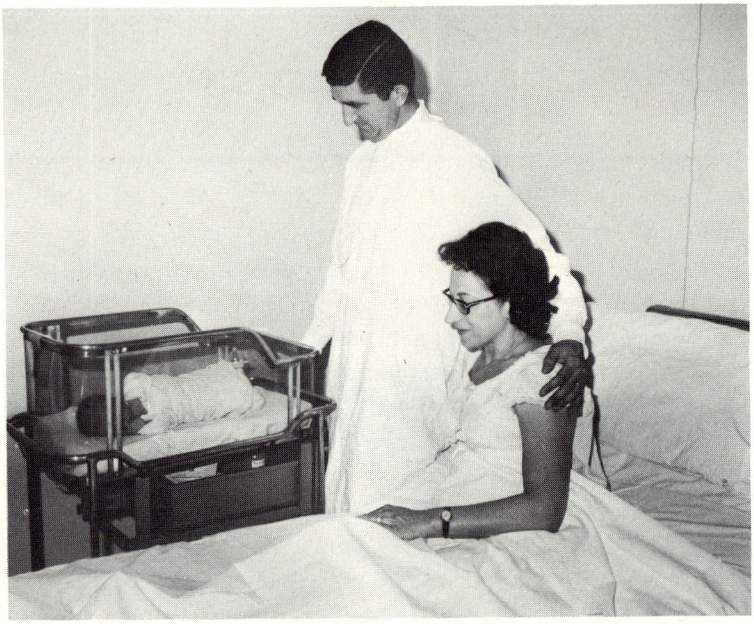

Fig. 14-9. Rooming-in.

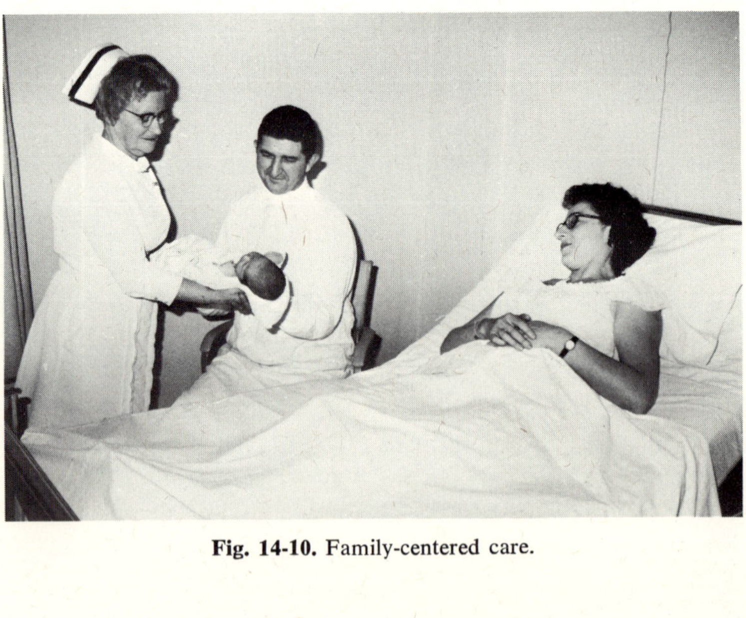

Fig. 14-10. Family-centered care.

Women who choose to room-in with their infants are instructed in proper hand washing techniques. Individual units are maintained for each infant, and transferring linens or caring for another mother's infant is discouraged in order to limit cross-contamination. The infant is cared for in his crib for safety and protection. Mothers are free to feed the infant on demand and to change and bathe the infant. During visiting hours the infant is returned to the nursery. The special visiting time for the father affords him the opportunity to feed, change, and handle the infant. Fathers wear gowns over street clothes. If the father suspects that he has a cold, he cannot visit in the unit.

Rooming-in units are staffed by professional nurses adept in the care of mothers and infants as a family unit. Nurses do far more teaching in this area when mothers and infants are together. The nurse in turn can learn much from mothers as they care for their newborn infants.

THE CENTRAL NURSERY

Every obstetric department has a central nursery, to which all babies are returned whether the mother wishes rooming-in or whether she decides to have the baby brought to her at designated hours for feeding (Fig. 14-11). Most obstetric departments are becoming quite flexible in taking the baby to the mother whenever the mother wishes her infant or if the baby is hungry at a time other than the designated feeding time.

Central nurseries are now designed in smaller units so that possibly eight babies are placed in one nursery with adequate spacing between cribs. Ideally, all cribs should be individual units, so that each infant is cared for separately with the nurse washing her hands before the care of each baby. A system in which

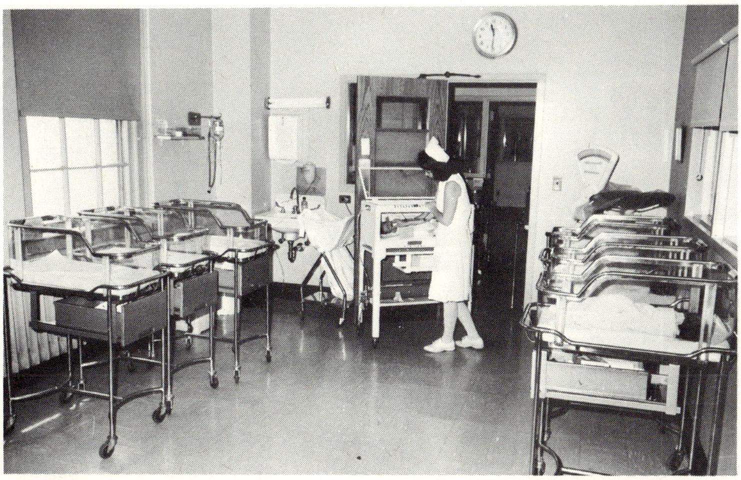

Fig. 14-11. Central nursery at Holy Name Hospital, Teaneck, N. J.

all babies in a single nursery remain together until dismissal, known as the cohort system, is valuable in controlling the spread of infection to large numbers of infants. When all eight babies are discharged, the room is cleaned thoroughly and is allowed to air for 24 hours; then a new group of babies are admitted.

Most units designate one nursery in which newborns (first 24 hours of life) are kept for intense, constant observation. All nurseries are equipped with soap and running water, a scale, and covered receptacles for soiled linen; clean linen is kept individually in each crib. In the nursery for very young newborns, suction, oxygen, resuscitation equipment, and Isolettes for warmth are essential. To control infection, nurseries are properly ventilated and are kept scrupulously clean; hand washing is mandatory. Personnel with upper respiratory infections, open skin wounds, or diarrhea are barred from working with newborns.

PLANNING FOR A FAMILY

The planning of children by young married people is a direct result of a healthier attitude toward sex in marriage. Married couples have a right to enjoy each other fully and wish to remain in optimum health to fulfill the responsibilities of parenthood. The change in the economy and new advances in science have greatly affected family life.

The population rise studied by demographers predicts soaring figures in population by the end of the century. The population growth in Africa, Asia, and Latin America is phenomenal, and the imbalance between birth and death rates finds starvation an existing problem. The highly efficient public health measures now available in developing countries have reduced the death rate, yet the problem of overpopulation still exists.

Family planning agencies around the world have been organized by the International Planned Parenthood Federation in London; there are six regional offices throughout the world. The services offered include guidance in the spacing of children, aiding childless couples with infertility problems, counseling young people in preparation for marriage, pursuing research studies on infertility and methods of birth control, supplying educational materials, and interest in the problems of the world population. Agencies operating family planning clinics are supported through government funds. The American Public Health Association and the American Medical Association have sanctioned family planning as an urgent health need.

The health of the mother is considered important if she is to care for her family. Planning for children is a combined effort on the part of both parents. The nurse's role is one of understanding and reiterating to families that all religious groups, Catholic, Protestant, and Jewish, agree on the need for responsible planned parenthood. It is the method by which family planning is accomplished that is different for various religious groups. The professional nurse needs to be familiar with the methods sanctioned by each religious group so that she may give guidance to parents when needed.

The nurse's role in family planning

The return of the mother for the 6-week postpartal examination is a time when a pelvic examination is done to ascertain a healthy reproductive system. The nurse as a member of the health team has the responsibility of case finding, education in family planning, and follow-up. Since it is the nurse with whom mothers develop confidence and friendship, she is the most approachable person with whom to discuss family planning. It is often the nurse who is attending the mother prenatally who hears, "Here I am again, hope this is the last pregnancy for awhile." It is also the nurse who reviews the history and finds the mother who has repeated pregnancies with only 1-month or 2-month spacing. The nurse is aware of the high-risk mother with diabetes, the mother with cardiac disturbances, the mother with repeated cesarean sections for pelvic disproportion, and so on. It is in these instances that she may initiate discussion by asking, "How are you feeling after having had four babies in four years?" or "Have you given any thought to planning future pregnancies?"

Once a discussion is initiated, the nurse can better assess what the mother knows about reproduction, what her plans are, her educational level, and her cultural and religious views. From these data she can set up a plan to help the family. Before the nurse can be of assistance in any family planning program, she needs to be familiar with agencies offering services, she needs to be knowledgeable in the methods used for birth control, and she needs to develop a vernacular that the mother understands. As a nurse counselor in family planning, this is an integral part of postpartum care and should be discussed early to assure effectiveness. The nurse needs to be aware of the fears mothers have about contraceptive devices such as: their effectiveness, their physical harm (as the possibility of causing cancer), their availability, their effect on sexual relationships, their cost, choice of a method, and so on.

Privacy during discussions is essential, and having the patient relate what was taught assures effectiveness. In some settings group discussions to introduce the various methods are beneficial. Visual aids and films are available (see References) and are valuable teaching tools.

The philosophy of family planning centers about family life education, which has two goals. It affords families the opportunity to decide how many children they want, and it benefits the health of the mother and children.

Family planning information is a community responsibility as well. Community organizations such as religious groups, parent-teacher associations, and social clubs are often involved in this endeavor.

In 1966 the American Nurses Association issued a statement defining the family planning responsibility of the registered nurse. Some of the salient points are the following:

1. To recognize the right of individuals and families to select and use such methods for family planning as are consistent with their own creed and mores

2. To recognize the right of individuals and families to receive information about family planning if they wish
3. To be responsive to the need for family planning
4. To be knowledgeable about state laws regarding family planning and the resources available
5. To assist in informing individuals and families of the existence of approved family planning resources
6. To assist in directing individuals and families to sources of such aid

METHODS OF BIRTH CONTROL

Contraception

Conception occurs by an orderly chain of events in which the mature ovum meets the mature sperm in the fallopian tube and successfully implants in the uterine endometrium. Contraception is intervention at any number of points in which there is a barrier that will prevent the union of ovum and spermatozoa.

An ideal contraceptive is one that is completely safe, free of side effects, reversible, easily obtainable, and inexpensive. There is no single method that meets these criteria at present.

Methods of contraception. The methods presently used are hormonal steroids (approved by the Food and Drug Administration), intrauterine devices, the diaphragm and cervical cap, chemical contraceptives (foams, jellies, creams, foaming tablets, suppositories), the condom, coitus interruptus, and the rhythm or safe period technique.

Two primary criteria are always considered in choosing a method. The method that is highly accepted by the couple is usually the most effective method; therefore acceptability and effectiveness are interdependent.

Oral contraceptives. Since 1958, oral contraceptives that consist of a synthetic progestin combined with a small amount of estrogen have been tested and marketed. Oral contraceptives, commonly known as "the pill," have wide variations in the amount of progesterone and estrogen used. Progress is being made in that reductions and modifications in dosage schedules are being introduced.

The pill is taken daily for 20 to 21 days, and following withdrawal endometrial bleeding occurs in 3 or 4 days. The hormones suppress ovulation, thereby preventing conception. It is recommended that the pill not be resumed after delivery until after the first postpartal menstrual period.

Two new methods not yet approved by the F.D.A. but being researched are the "minipill," consisting of a minute dose of a progestin only taken every day of the month, and the once-a-month and once-every-3 months injection. The once-a-month injection is a combined estrogen-progesterone combination, whereas the once-every-3 months injection consists of only progestin.

It has been found that 70% to 90% of patients accept the pill, and if taken according to instructions, it is 100% effective. Fertility is promptly restored when the pill is discontinued.

The most common side effects are nausea, weight gain, headache, breast tenderness, and breakthrough bleeding. Pelvic examination and Papanicolaou smear are always done prior to prescribing the pill. This method is contraindicated in premenopausal women with diagnosed breast cancer and in women with a history of thromboembolitic disease. Preexisting fibromas of the uterus may enlarge with the use of oral contraceptives. Pelvic examination should be repeated every 6 months. Oral contraceptives are contraindicated should the mother be breastfeeding. Doses as small as 1 mg. of norethindrone mestranol (Ortho-Novum) have demonstrated that infants had lower weight gains, and the duration of lactation was markedly decreased.

Intrauterine devices. Use of a plastic or stainless steel (spiral, loop, ring) device inserted into the uterine cavity through the cervix is very popular. The exact mechanism is not clearly understood; however, the action occurs between ovulation and implantation.

Following a pelvic examination and Papanicolaou smear, the device is inserted by the physician during the menstrual period. This is the safest time for insertion since there is assurance that pregnancy has not occurred, and, should bleeding occur upon insertion, the woman is less anxious. Although it was formerly believed that the intrauterine device was more suitable for parous women, it is now being used successfully in nulliparous women. The advantages of intrauterine devices include: (1) single insertion on the part of the woman and no further attention is needed, (2) male not required to participate, (3) inexpensive to manufacture and insert, (4) effective, surpassed only by consistent use of oral contraceptives, and (5) safe when properly inserted and managed. Side effects include: spotting, irregular bleeding, uterine cramps and pelvic pain, and spontaneous expulsion. Contraindications are pelvic inflammatory disease and large fibroids. Perforation of the uterus is a danger when inserted during the puerperium. Often hysterosalpingography can reveal the size and shape of the uterine cavity so that the proper intrauterine device may be chosen for insertion.

Intrauterine devices are less reliable than oral contraceptives and just as reliable as the diaphragm or condom. Occasionally pregnancy has occurred with the device in place; it has been found outside the membranes and at times beneath the placenta. There have been some instances in which ectopic pregnancy occurred with the device in place.

Diaphragm and contraceptive jellies or creams. The diaphragm is a circular rubber device that fits over the cervix and prevents the entrance of sperm. The diaphragm is first coated with a spermicidal jelly or cream on either side and inserted 6 hours prior to sexual intercourse. It may be left in place for as long as 24 hours. It should remain in place for 6 hours following intercourse so that there is no chance of active sperm invading the cervix and uterus. If intercourse is to be repeated, additional cream or jelly should be inserted vaginally prior to each coitus. The diaphragm is easily removed by hooking the finger behind the symphysis and grasping and removing the device. Douching following removal is not necessary. The diaphragm is washed with soap and water, rinsed, dried, and powdered with cornstarch to preserve it in between use. The diaphragm should be held to a light to check for tears prior to each insertion.

Diaphragms should be refitted following each pregnancy for efficacious use. For some women this method is repulsive; however, it is quite efficacious.

Methods not requiring pelvic examination or prescription

Condom. The condom is a rubber sheath (similar to a finger cot but larger) that covers the erect penis prior to coitus. The condom should also be tested for tears prior to use. Some couples feel safer when the woman also uses some vaginal spermicidal jelly or cream in case of breaking or slipping of the condom.

Vaginal preparations. Creams and jellies are introduced into the vagina with an applicator within 1 hour prior to coitus. Douching is forbidden until 6 hours following the last coitus.

Foaming tablets. The tablet is moistened with saliva or water and inserted deep into the vagina 5 minutes prior to coitus. A new tablet should be used prior to each coitus. Some women experience a burning sensation when the foam tablet is inserted. Foam tablets lose their effectiveness from atmospheric moisture; therefore the vial should be tightly capped. Douching is forbidden until 6 hours following the last coitus.

Sponge and foam. A special sponge is moistened with spermicidal foam liquid and inserted high into the vagina prior to coitus. The sponge should be left in place for 6 hours, and douching is permitted only following its removal.

Vaginal suppositories. Suppositories are removed from the aluminum foil and inserted a few minutes prior to intercourse. Suppositories labeled "feminine hygiene" are not necessarily effective as contraceptives.

These vaginal preparations are believed to be the least reliable of all the methods described.

Coitus interruptus. This method requires no devices or chemicals and is available at no cost. The couple proceeds with coitus until the moment of ejaculation; then the male withdraws so that the emission of sperm takes place away from the vagina and external genitalia. Some couples use this method and can still derive sexual satisfaction. However, the possibility of pregnancy is great when this method is used, because ejaculation may occur before withdrawal is complete.

Postcoital douche. This is a poor method of contraception since douching following intercourse is ineffective. It has been found that sperm enters the cervical canal seconds after ejaculation.

Rhythm and basal body temperature. The rhythm method requires temporary or periodic abstinence during the fertile period of the menstrual cycle. The first fertile day is determined by subtracting 18 from the number of days in the shortest menstrual cycle observed during a 1-year period, and the last fertile day by subtracting 11 days from the longest menstrual cycle. For example, if a woman observed cycles ranging from 27 to 30 days, her potentially fertile period (abstinence period) will extend from the ninth day (27 minus 18) through the nineteenth day (30 minus 11). This method is effective if the woman has regular cycles and is intelligent and highly motivated.

The basal body temperature is taken immediately on awakening, prior to any activity, and is recorded. A drop in temperature followed by a rise (usually around 0.7° F.) indicates that ovulation has occurred. The higher level will remain for the remainder of the cycle. Sexual relations may be resumed on the third day of sustained higher temperature.

This method calculates only the end of sexual abstinence. To calculate when abstinence should start, the woman again takes her shortest cycle figure minus 18. On that day abstinence begins. She should again start taking her temperature on awakening and recording it and continue until relations are resumed on the third day of higher temperature.

If the rhythm method is taught correctly and practiced correctly, its effectiveness is comparable to that of mechanical and chemical contraceptives. At the present time this is the only method accepted by the Roman Catholic Church.

Sterilization

Sterilization is not a contraceptive measure since it involves surgical intervention. Sterilization is voluntary in all fifty states. However, in Connecticut and Utah it is performed only for reasons of medical necessity.

In sterilization of a woman a small abdominal incision is made and the tubes are tied (tubal ligation) or cut (salpingectomy). The procedure is done in the hospital operating room.

In sterilization of a man, a small incision is made into each side of the scrotum and the vas deferens is cut and tied off, blocking passage of sperm. This procedure, known as vasectomy, can be done under local anesthesia as an office procedure.

These procedures do not affect normal potency and hormonal functioning.

SELECTED REFERENCES

Arthur, H.: The price of childbirth, Nurs. Mirror **127:**23, Nov. 29, 1968.

Burnett, C. W. F.: Is reproduction a physiological process, Part 2, Midwives Chronicles **82:**156, May, 1969.

Calderone, M. S.: An inventory of contraceptive methods adapted to public health practice, Amer. J. Public Health **52:**1712, 1962.

Calderone, M. S.: Sexual health and family planning, Amer. J. Public Health **58:**223, 1968.

Caplan, G.: Concepts of mental health and consultation, U. S. Department of Health, Education, and Welfare, Children's Bureau, 1958, Children's Bureau Publication No. 373.

Chesterman, H.: The public health nurse and family planning, Nurs. Outlook **12:**32, September, 1964.

Di Cristina, H. E.: God or man in birth control, Catholic Nurse **11:**50, September, 1952.

Di Palma, J. L.: Drugs for fertility control, RN **27:**69, January, 1964.

Eastman, N. J., and Hellman, L. M.: Williams obstetrics, ed. 13, New York, 1966, Appleton-Century & Appleton-Century-Crofts.

Editorial: The principle, not the method, Nurs. Outlook **12:**27, September, 1964.

Editorial: The story of oral contraceptives, Obstet. Gynec., vol. 31, no. 4, April, 1968.

Findlay E., and Capes, M.: Figure control

for your postpartum patient, RN **32:**38, January, 1969.
Gedda, L.: Fertility and the ethics of experiments on man, Catholic Nurse **12:**64, March, 1964.
Gelber, I.: Family planning in a growing world, Amer. J. Nurs. **64:**98, August, 1964.
Herrmann, R. O.: Expectations and attitudes as a source of financial problems in the teenager, J. Marriage & Family **27:**89, February, 1965.
Hogan, A.: The role of the nurse in meeting needs of new mother, Nurs. Clin. N. Amer. **3:**337, 1968.
Kelly, D. N.: Change is the rhythm, Catholic Nurse **13:**18, December, 1964.
Leibman, S.: Emotional forces in the family, Philadelphia, 1950, J. B. Lippincott Co.
Lynch, J. J.: The oral contraceptives, Catholic Nurse **11:**34, September, 1963.
Manisoff, M.: Family planning, a teaching guide for nurses, Planned Parenthood—World Population, New York, N. Y., 1969.
Miller, G. H., and Hughes, L. R.: Lactation and genital involution effects of a new low-dose oral contraceptive on breastfeeding mothers and their infants, Obstet. Gynec., vol. 35, no. 1, January, 1970.
Miller, R.: The nurses' role in obstetric emergencies in the hospital setting, Nurs. Clin. N. Amer. **2:**261, 1967.
Minkler, D.: Public policy in family planning, Nurs. Outlook **12:**28, September, 1964.
Tyler, E. T.: Oral contraceptives, Amer. J. Nurs. **61:**51, August, 1961.
Williams, B.: Sleep needs during the maternity cycle, Nurs. Outlook **15:**53, January, 1969.
Willson, J. R., Beecham, C. T., and Carrington, E. R.: Obstetrics and gynecology, ed. 4, St. Louis, 1971, The C. V. Mosby Co.
Yunek, M. J.: Postpartum care is more than a routine, Nurs. Outlook **17:**50, January, 1969.

Questions for study

1. Define the puerperium.
2. What are the physiologic systemic changes occurring during the puerperium and what are the implications for nursing care?
3. What are the common discomforts experienced during the puerperium? How would you plan nursing care to relieve these discomforts?
4. What are the long-range goals in nursing care for the postpartal woman?
5. Define rooming-in. What are its objectives?
6. What family planning agencies are available in your community? What services are offered to parents at the agencies?

CHAPTER 15

NEWBORN INFANT

Many of the physical and physiologic needs of the infant, such as being changed when wet, being fed when hungry, and being held when comforting is needed, relate directly to later patterns of emotional stability. Helping the mother become aware of the importance of meeting the baby's basic needs will be rewarding for the mother and the infant. It is in these beginning relationships with people that the infant develops a sense of trust in his outside world.

The newborn infant's biologic needs are closely related to his psychologic growth. Growth proceeds in an orderly fashion, and the infant gets to know the outside world through his senses of hearing, smelling, tasting, and feeling (the sense of sight is not quite developed at birth). Through a process in which his needs are repeatedly met, the infant begins to relate gratification of his wishes with someone who is separate from himself.

The needs that are basic to the infant are for food, elimination, sleep, body movement for growth, and comforting. Although many of his body systems are functioning at birth, the central nervous system is still quite undeveloped. The cry, his only defense mechanism, is so patterned that a mother soon learns whether it is a hunger cry, a pain cry, or a song that lulls her infant to sleep.

CHARACTERISTICS AT BIRTH

At birth the newborn (Fig. 15-1) looks puffy and his skin is ruddy because of retention of much fluid and a high red blood cell count. His skin, smooth and delicate to touch, may be coated with a cheesy lubricant known as vernix caseosa, or may appear wrinkled; it peels, and later becomes quite dry following exposure to the outside air. It is common to find cyanotic hands and feet (acrocyanosis) for the first 24 hours as the infant strives to maintain his body temperature and establish his own circulation. He keeps his arms and legs flexed close to his body, and the thumbs are tightly clenched in the hands. His movements are random—when jarred or unwrapped, he startles (Moro reflex) by bringing his appendages toward his body. Most newborns have excessive amounts of mucus, and occasionally the

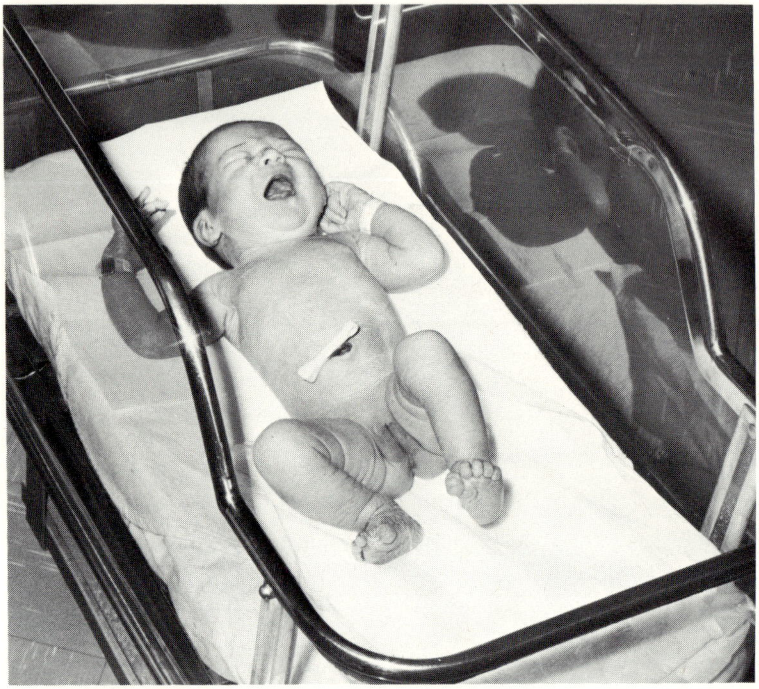

Fig. 15-1. Newborn infant.

infant gags in an effort to expel it. The mucus is tenacious, and the baby needs help by either milking the trachea (holding the baby's head down) or by using a suction bulb or a De Lee mucus trap. Immediately following birth, the infant's body temperature may be 95° to 96° F. (Fig. 15-2); keeping him warm in a heated crib until the temperature is 98° F. is essential. A cleansing bath and warm clothing fulfill the initial need for comfort.

Astute observations of the new baby cannot be overemphasized. Normally his respirations are abdominal and irregular, averaging 30 to 50 per minute. His sleep may be interrupted by his inability to swallow the mucus that accumulates during this time. The nurse's readiness to help him is imperative lest he aspirate the mucus into the trachea and lungs. When the infant is not troubled with mucus, his readiness for feeding is apparent as he roots and sucks his own hand. The sense of smell is so developed that he roots immediately when put to breast. The first attempts at feeding may be short, and his needs for food the first few days are minimal since he has been provided with stores during intrauterine life. How much will be taken at a feeding depends upon the individual newborn's needs. As he becomes satiated he sleeps fitfully for the first hour following feeding. The next 2 hours find the newborn in a lighter sleep pattern, so that by the end of the third hour he begins to stir, move, and eventually cries in order to have his hunger needs met. As the days go on, he becomes more interested in feedings, suckles for longer periods, and ingests as much as 2 to 3 ounces per feeding by the end of a week.

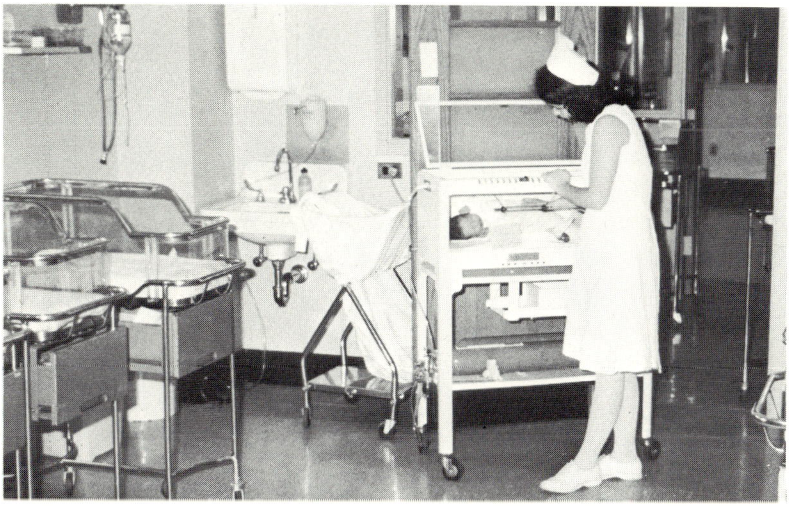

Fig. 15-2. Armstrong incubator.

Newborns void and defecate immediately after birth. As the infant begins to take nourishment, the increased peristalsis in the bowel aids in the elimination of meconium, the first stool of the newborn. Meconium consists of epidermal cells, cast-off epithelial cells, and lanugo hairs the baby swallowed while in the amniotic fluid. Meconium is greenish-black, tenacious, and often copious. Since its properties do not include digested carbohydrate, fat, or protein, it is odorless and harmless to the baby's skin and rarely irritates. By the third day the stool changes in consistency and color, becoming partially meconium and partially end products of digested milk—this is known as transitional stool. The consistency, amount, and nature of the stool depend upon the type of feeding administered to the infant. The skin of the buttocks is properly cleansed and kept dry for comfort. Irritation of the skin area around the genitals is best cared for by exposing the infant's buttocks to a heat lamp, or by coating the area with A and D ointment to protect the skin during elimination. Frequent diaper changes and care in drying the skin will avoid this problem.

Diapers that have a plastic backing may not allow for air circulation and often cause excoriation of the buttocks; when this occurs the plastic backing should be removed.

BODY SYSTEMS

Circulatory system

At birth, once the cord is tied and cut, the newborn establishes his own circulation. Although the liver is quite large, it is immature. There is a hyperbilirubinemia of 1 to 2 mg. per 100 ml. of serum, which increases in the first few days to 4 or 5 mg. when the liver cannot cope with the rapid destruction of red cells;

bilirubin levels in the bloodstream are increased, with a resulting physiologic jaundice by the third day.

The clotting mechanism of the blood is poor since there is a low concentration of prothrombin. Vitamin K, which is an essential, is usually administered to the newborn to aid in the clotting process until the infant manufactures his own. This is not possible until the infant begins to ingest food and bacteria begin to grow in the intestinal tract.

The hemoglobin is approximately 14 to 20 gm. per 100 ml. of blood, and the white blood cell count ranges from 6,000 to 22,000.

Respiratory system

Respirations in the newborn are irregular and abdominal at the rate of 30 to 50 per minute. The diaphragm is used in breathing rather than the thorax. On inspiration there is an indrawing of the lower rib cage. Normally respirations are quiet, with short periods of apnea. Respirations that become irregular and more rapid are considered abnormal.

Excretory system

Although the kidneys are immature, the newborn excretes urine within the first 24 hours. By the end of 2 weeks, the bladder empties as much as twenty times daily. Albumin is commonly present during the first week, and often urates are passed, leaving a brick red stain on the diaper. To prevent dehydration, fluids should be increased when urates are present.

Digestive system

The normal newborn digests simple carbohydrates, fats, and proteins readily. Since his stores from intrauterine life are so efficient, he takes very little nourishment for the first few days. If put to breast he roots and sucks immediately, ingesting the first milk known as colostrum. If the infant is to receive an artificial feeding, water is offered for the first 24 hours, followed by a prepared cow's milk feeding.

Integumentary system

Lanugo is the fine downy hair growth found over the entire body. It is usually lost after the first month of life. Small whitish pinpoint spots called milia may be noted over the nose. They are small sebaceous cysts that disappear in a few weeks. Mongolian spots, blue-black discolorations noted on the buttocks, back, and sacral region, are seen in white infants from dark parents and disappear in the first year.

Endocrine system

Changes in the endocrine system are metabolic and hormonal.

Metabolic changes. All newborns have a weight loss of 7 to 10 ounces by the end of the first week since the infant loses much fluid through urine and feces. However, weight is rapidly regained as the infant begins to take nourishment after the first few days.

Hormonal reactions. Many newborn infants will develop enlarged breasts during the immediate newborn period. Commonly referred to as "witch's milk," this is due to hormones transmitted to the baby in utero. The breast swelling subsides in a few days, and no treatment or care is necessary. Female infants may have a small amount of bloody mucoid vaginal discharge (menstrual flow) as hormones are passed from mother to infant. This is normal and disappears readily.

Central nervous system

At birth the central nervous system is incomplete and the brain is not yet functioning in the control of behavior. Because of this the infant needs a constant and adequate supply of oxygen and the experience of mothering activity that awakens a feeling of life. Physiologically the infant's first cry is a form of emergency breathing. As the diaphragm moves to expel fluids from the lungs in order to suck in oxygen, the sound is a result of valvelike action of the vocal cords as the air traverses them. In utero the diaphragm moves upward as the fetus practices breathing. After birth the reverse is true, as the diaphragm moves downward for respirations to continue. It is obvious in observing the newborn that there are longer periods of expirations than inhalations, yet his need for oxygen is essential. The mother can help establish adequate oxygenation by frequent handling, fondling, and allowing the infant to suck freely. Early crying is therefore a breathing exercise. However, crying for longer than 10 minutes is suggestive of air hunger. Later, the cry, his only defense mechanism, is so patterned that the mother learns to recognize whether it is hunger, pain, etc.

Respiratory independence is established with the infant's first babbling sounds. These sounds suggest that an inner balance of oxygen has been reached. A smile may often accompany the babbling. It has been found through studies that adequate, consistent mothering produces an early smile, babbling responses, and adequate speech development. There is, therefore, a close relationship between breathing, sucking, and speech.

INITIAL CARE

The infant's initial bath is most important since it introduces his beginning contact with the world about him. The baby now has more space about him and feels less protected. The purpose of the initial bath is twofold: (1) careful appraisal as already described and (2) removal of blood and mucus from the skin for comfort and warmth.

Most infants, since they would rather be clothed, cry when exposed. Keeping the infant covered while bathing will make the experience a pleasant one. A mild soap and water bath at a temperature comfortable to the adult wrist proves favorable. Hand-to-body contact while bathing gives the baby an added feeling of security and may be substituted for a washcloth. Since the newborn's skin is delicate, care should be taken to eliminate excessive rubbing, thereby avoiding eventual skin breakdown.

In dressing the infant the shirt hangs loosely from the shoulders for proper movement, and the diaper is pinned securely yet loose enough for leg movement. Pins that are inserted horizontally with points toward the back of the infant are safe should the end snap open. Wrapping the new infant snugly will make him feel secure. Placing him on his side facilitates elimination of mucus. In the nursery, daily skin care consists of cleansing the face and skin folds under the neck, arms, legs, and buttocks. The cord is left exposed to the air and cleansed daily with a 70% alcohol solution to aid in the drying process.

The infant is weighed at birth and before dismissal from the hospital. The average infant's weight depends upon the size of the parents, race, sex, maternal nutrition, and duration of pregnancy. Boys are somewhat heavier in weight than girls, and Negro infants are lighter in weight than white infants.

CIRCUMCISION

Circumcision is the surgical removal of the foreskin on the penis. Circumcision is done for hygienic purposes since most newborns have tight foreskins that cannot be retracted for cleansing purposes. A white, cheesy substance called smegma

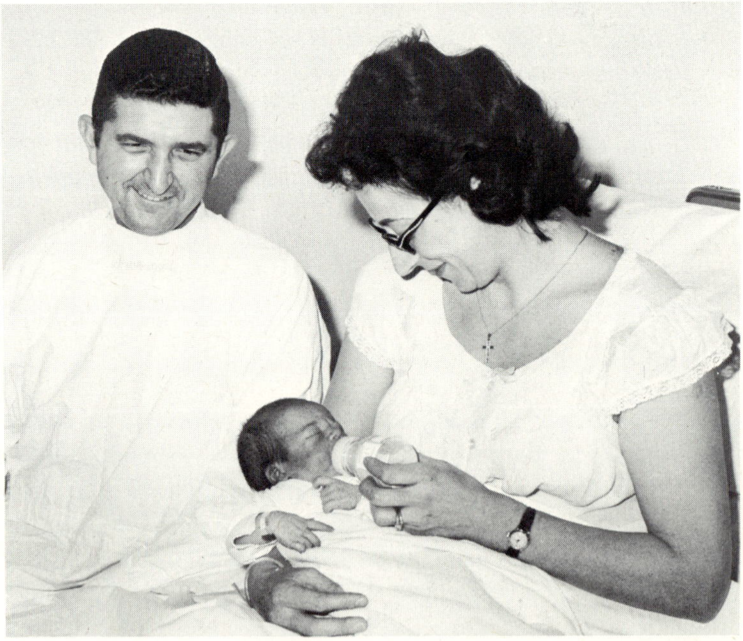

Fig. 15-3. Bottle-feeding.

accumulates around the glans penis (beneath the foreskin) and may cause irritation and infection if not cleansed properly.

Circumcision is now being done in the delivery room immediately after delivery or within the first few days of birth. Since circumcision is a surgical procedure, permission is granted by signature of the parents. The procedure is done under aseptic technique, the foreskin being freed from the glans penis with a probe. The foreskin may be removed by scalpel or by the use of a Gomco clamp, which crushes the nerve endings and blood vessels, promoting hemostasis. The infant is restrained on a circumcision board to facilitate and expedite the procedure. There is little blood loss, and a sterile gauze bandage around the penis eliminates bleeding and promotes healing. Healing is rapid and occurs within 24 hours.

Nursing measures include careful observation for bleeding and cleanliness of the area. Should the dressing become dry and adhere to the penis, removal is facilitated by using hydrogen peroxide to soften it. If a small amount of bleeding should occur when the dressing is changed, a wet bandage with an epinephrine solution (Vasodrine) will aid in constricting a small oozing blood vessel. However, if bleeding persists, the physician should be notified since a suture may be necessary.

In the Jewish faith circumcision is a religious rite performed 8 days after birth and is known as a berith. A rabbi especially prepared for this rite may perform the procedure rather than a physician.

INFANT FEEDING

The method of choice in infant feeding lies with the cooperative wishes of the parents (Fig. 15-3). The choice may be greatly influenced by the mores of a society, the cultural setting, the geographic area, and previous experiences and attitudes developed in early life. In many cultures breast-feeding is chosen simply because it is "the way of feeding"; in other cultures bottle feeding is chosen since it is "the way of feeding." Whatever the choice made, support in this beginning mother-child relationship is an integral part of the nursing care of the mother and the newborn.

The method by which the infant ingests food is through a process of sucking and swallowing. This beginning function of ingesting food not only satisfies his physiologic needs for growth and development but also his psychologic needs. As he ingests food he also begins to associate this with the world about him, which brings pleasure and a feeling of trust and security.

Sucking in the first 6 months of life is an important activity of the newborn. Not only does it provide the infant with food, but it also satisfies many psychologic needs. The first sense of security, pleasure, satisfaction, and success centers upon this mouth activity. The primary oral function is nutritional (ingestion of food), emotional (smiling and kissing), and intellectual (word making). Sucking develops the mouth, lower jaw, and lips, since the tongue lies directly over the main external carotid artery that pumps blood toward the brain. If sucking is exercised properly and frequently, it is relinquished at approximately 4 months. At 4 months the mouth muscles are then used for biting, vocalizing, and hand play.

At birth each infant is equipped with a sucking reflex. However, mouthing activity is uncoordinated, and some babies suck very vigorously, while others need to be taught the mechanism. Often the mouth needs to be opened by depressing the infant's chin, the nipple inserted well inside the mouth cavity and the chin worked up and down rhythmically. The nipple acts as a stimulus to the tongue and hard palate, and with frequent oral stimulation the infant learns to suck well.

Sucking is closely related to breathing; often the infant's respirations become deeper as sucking becomes well established. Studies reveal a minimum of 2 hours a day of oral exercise as essential for the newborn. If this minimum is provided from 1 week to 4 months following birth, there is less thumb-sucking. Therefore, each feeding (six daily) should take 20 minutes.

Although sucking time is important, handling and fondling during feedings are also necessary. Sucking without bodily contact is not beneficial. It is evident then that the infant who ingests a feeding in less than 20 minutes should be provided with a pacifier to satisfy the sucking reflex. Pacifiers are relinquished once the sucking need is met. Sucking habits found in older children are directly related to the infant who has been frustrated in early infancy. These frustrations are usually a result of inadequate mothering, or failure to satisfy the sucking reflex, producing body tension. Sucking therefore is a developmental activity that is of great importance to the infant.

Breast-feeding

Breast milk is the ideal milk for the newborn (Fig. 15-4). The first secretion, colostrum, contains a great deal of protein but little fat or carbohydrate, and it is easily digested by the newborn. It is available to the infant at the moment of birth and is replenished as the infant stimulates the breast as he suckles. It has advantages for the mother since nursing the infant causes contractions of the uterus, which limit maternal blood loss and encourage involution. Since the breast can be offered only by the mother, the closeness of infant and mother in this beginning relationship strengthens feelings of security in the infant and provides for the mother satisfaction and accomplishment in her new role.

Advantages of breast-feeding. One of the greatest advantages attributed to breast-feeding is the psychologic value it has for mother and infant. Although this is difficult to measure, for mothers who choose breast-feeding it is a most satisfying and rewarding experience in the beginning mother-child relationship.

The composition of human milk is the natural method of feeding the newborn. It is safe since it is clean, it is readily accessible to the infant from the mother's breast, its composition is of optimum nutritious value for the infant's digestive process, and it is well tolerated by all infants. Along with being the ideal food, breast milk is replenished by the infant's suckling, so his demand is met by a constant supply.

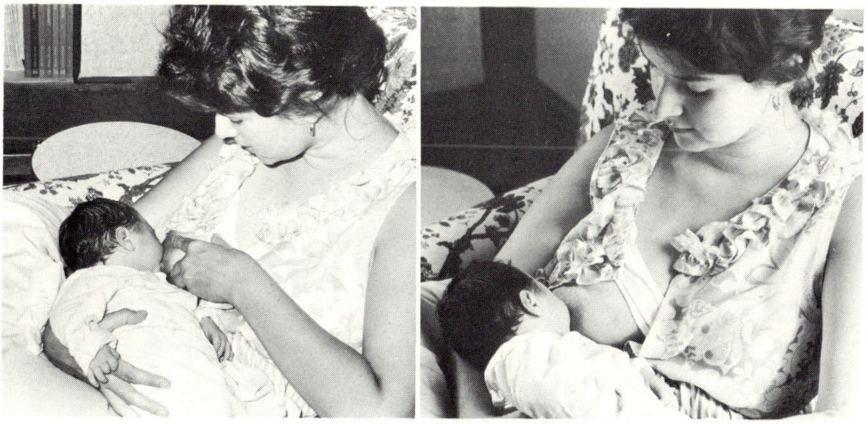

Fig. 15-4. Breast-feeding.

Letdown reflex. Lactation, a process in which milk is secreted from the breast, is primarily of hormonal and nervous control. The increase in estrogens, which have developed the mammary glands during pregnancy, plays a reverse role following delivery. The decrease in estrogens following delivery aids in initiating lactation. With the decrease in estrogens, the infant's sucking increases the production of prolactin by the anterior pituitary gland and stimulates the release of an oxytocic factor by the posterior pituitary gland. It is the release of oxytocin that makes possible the ejection or release of milk from the alveoli into the nipple ducts. This reflex is greatly affected by the emotions of the mother. Studies have shown that injections of oxytocics (such as oxytocin) or Pitocin nasal sprays will initiate the milk letdown also and give the mother sensations of pleasure and satisfaction. Worry, fatigue, and emotional stress are known to reduce milk secretions or suppress them entirely. It is common to have the letdown reflex occur during sexual relations in the nursing mother. Much anxiety and guilt are relieved when anticipatory guidance is given.

Since breast-feeding stimulates uterine contractions, nursing promotes involution. Research studies indicate that breast-feeding protects the infant from the development of allergies, and the latest dental research indicates better jaw formation and fewer oral tension habits as a result of breast-feeding.

Position. The position the mother assumes in preparation for feeding her infant depends upon access of the baby to the nipple and her comfort. At times the size of the mother's breast will determine her position. The mother with a large, pendulous breast may find lying down well over on her side ideal. The mother with a small breast may find a sitting position facilitates nursing (Fig. 15-4). Following a few feedings mother and infant work this out quite well. At times the infant is wrapped too tightly and positioning is difficult, bodily contact is interfered with, and the infant makes no attempt to nurse. Removing the outer blanket is recommended.

Environment. In order that the mother is ready to offer her breast to the infant for feeding, she must be comfortable, ready, and willing to participate. Any undue fear or outside disturbance will greatly influence the feeding session. Only after the mother's needs are met will she be ready to care for her infant.

Techniques in getting the infant to grasp the nipple. Although many babies do quite well in latching on readily, a few need some help in grasping the nipple. It is with these babies that the nurse can be helpful in teaching the mother some of the ways to help discussed in the following paragraphs.

Nipple rolling. If the nipple is not prominent, with clean hands the mother may pull the nipple out, twisting it between her thumb and forefinger. Since the nipple is made of erectile tissue, it will become prominent and the infant will latch on readily.

Rooting. A simple procedure in which a few drops of milk are expressed and appear at the nipple ducts will entice the infant to latch on and start nursing. The infant need not be forced in any way but is left free to find and root on his own accord. If this is unsuccessful, guiding the back of the infant's head in the direction of the breast and directing the nipple well into the mouth with gentle pressure under the chin stimulate the sucking reflex. Continued repeated attempts that frustrate the infant are discouraged when it is obvious that he is not hungry or is not ready for a feeding.

Full breast. When the breast is extremely full, the nipple is less prominent, and the infant finds it difficult to grasp the breast tissue. Expressing some of the milk to soften the areola makes the nipple more prominent.

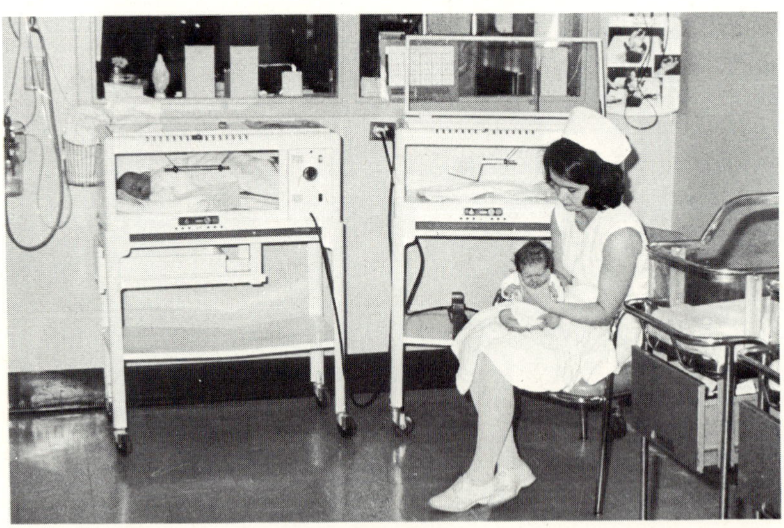

Fig. 15-5. Burping infant.

It is advisable to use both breasts at each feeding for continuous stimulation. The infant receives a large portion of his feeding the first 10 minutes at breast, since he sucks more vigorously at that time. Therefore, the second breast offered will be fuller and should be used first at the next feeding. A pin fastened to the brassiere following feedings is a good reminder. Between feedings the infant may be offered water. The baby receives the cream of the breast milk at the end of a feeding. Water following feeding helps the infant assimilate the cream.

Infants who are breast-fed are close to the mother and often do not swallow as much air as bottle-fed babies. Burping need be done only following feeding. Interrupting a feeding may cause breast tissue to break down and is not necessary.

Sleepy infant. Some infants fall asleep the minute they get comfortable and close to the mother. Turning the infant over quickly from a prone to a sitting position has been found helpful in getting the infant interested in nursing.

Crying infant. A crying infant will never latch on successfully until he is comforted and the crying ceases. Most infants cry when they are wet, are in an uncomfortable position, or are forced to take the breast. Pleasant beginning experiences at feeding time are associated with comfort and trust that are sensed by the infant. It is from this beginning satisfying relationship that he is later able to tolerate and accept a period of waiting for his feeding.

Cracked nipples. Occasionally some women develop soreness and cracking of nipple tissue. The reasons for this may be careless latching and unlatching of the infant, improper breast care, or an infant who sucks vigorously. In the latching-on process the nipple and areola should be well into the infant's mouth. In unlatching the infant, suction is released by pulling down on his chin, squeezing the fat pads of his cheeks, or inserting a finger into the corner of his mouth. Should tenderness, redness, or soreness develop, the breasts are left exposed to the air for 10 minutes following feeding. A light can also be used to augment drying. If the nipple tissue has cracked and there is tissue breakdown, a nipple shield may be used until healing occurs. For the infant who has a vigorous sucking reflex, offering a small amount of water prior to breast-feeding may alleviate the strong initial suction. Between feedings, a nipple cream or A and D ointment on a piece of wax paper will protect the nipple from adhering to the brassiere as the tissue heals. Tincture of benzoin should *never* be used, since it is painful when applied and has a sticky, adherent property that hinders healing of tissue.

Milk supply. A noticeable decrease in milk supply may occur when the mother is dismissed from the hospital. This is normal because of the excitement or the adjustment from hospital to home. Putting the baby to breast often for stimulation will increase milk production in a short time.

Approximately 3 weeks following delivery lactation is well established. Should there be days when the breasts are still full following feeding, the mother may express the milk manually or with a hand pump for comfort. The milk may be collected in a clean receptacle and stored in a freezer for as long as a month. This milk can be given to the baby by bottle when the mother is out for a social evening. Simply letting it thaw out to room temperature is all that is needed, since heating breast milk will destroy its vitamin content.

Some women experience letdown by hearing the baby cry or while away from the baby for an evening. Crossing both arms firmly over the nipple area of the breast may be done rather inconspicuously and will prevent dripping, discomfort, and embarrassment.

Menstrual cycle. The mother who breast-feeds her infant will not experience a return of the menstrual flow for 16 to 20 weeks following delivery. However, the sooner the mother introduces solid foods to the infant, the less breast stimulation there will be. The lessened stimulation of the breast by the infant results in a change in hormonal balance, which reestablishes the ovarian cycle.

Weaning. The time to wean is individual and depends upon the satisfaction being derived by mother and infant. The weaning process should be gradual, since abruptness would result in frustration and anxiety for the infant and breast discomfort for the mother.

The early introduction of solid foods satisfies some of the infant's hunger needs. As this occurs, sucking time is decreased and there is less breast stimulation. With less breast stimulation there is a diminished milk supply. With the introduction of solids, a change in hormonal balance occurs, As the hormonal balance is increased, ovulation is resumed and the mother is more likely to become pregnant.

Weaning should be accomplished slowly with the breast offered during comforting hours such as at nap time or before bedtime. It is these feedings that are eliminated last. A decrease in milk supply prior to weaning may be an indication that a new pregnancy has occurred. It is advisable to wean the infant once pregnancy is verified.

Contraindications. Any serious or debilitating disease in the mother, such as severe heart disease, and acute infections, such as tuberculosis, epilepsy, or narcotic addiction, is a contraindication to breast-feeding. A baby with a congenital deformity of cleft lip or cleft palate would need to be fed artificially.

Nutrition during lactation. The nursing mother's diet needs to be replenished in caloric and fluid intake. The many energies expended in the nursing process need to be replaced if optimum health of mother and baby is to be maintained. An additional 1,000 to 1,500 calories is added to the diet in order to maintain an adequate milk supply. Nutritious foods of added proteins and carbohydrates similar to those ingested during pregnancy are essential. Foods do not have to be eliminated from the diet unless they have an effect on the infant, such as producing loose stools, colic, etc. The importance of an adequate diet, consisting of three well-balanced meals, cannot be overstressed. The apparent slight weight increase during lactation is readily lost in due time.

Stools during lactation. Breast milk is higher in carbohydrate and more easily digested than cow's milk. Frequent bowel movements are not uncommon for the infant receiving breast milk. The stool is softer and has a peculiar characteristic odor. Staining of diapers can be controlled by soaking in a borax solution before washing. Rinsing diapers several times eliminates the presence of detergents and keeps the diapers soft against the baby's delicate skin.

Support and care of breasts. Support of the breasts with a properly fitted brassiere is essential for a good milk supply. Since the breast is composed of connective and fatty tissue, compression of the blood vessels without support would hamper proper lactation. It is important that, to keep the nipples clean and pliable, the brassiere be changed often when saturated with milk secretions. The nipples are cleansed with water only at bath time, soap having a tendency to dry out the natural secretions (sebum) supplied by the tubercles of Montgomery. The mother may be instructed to pull out the nipple tissue with clean hands and roll the nipples between the thumb and forefinger if they are not prominent (Fig. 8-8). This facilitates latching on for the infant.

Artificial feeding

Artificial feeding preparations strive toward maintaining the standard of breast milk composition. Cow's milk is lacking in simple carbohydrates and needs to be diluted for proper digestion and nourishment of the baby.

The normal newborn needs 50 calories per pound of body weight, one fifth of which should be carbohydrate for normal growth and development. The fluid intake for proper tissue hydration is 2½ ounces per pound of body weight. It is simple then to estimate that a 6-pound infant needs 300 calories, 60 calories of which should be carbohydrate, and 15 ounces in fluid intake (Table 5).

Since formulas are not as readily utilized as breast milk, the baby will not need to be fed as frequently. Formula-fed babies (Fig. 15-5) are usually on 4-hour feedings, or six feedings daily. As the infant grows older, he will need less carbohydrate as solid foods fulfill his added needs. Full-strength milk will be easily assimilated by the age of 4 months.

Many of the prepared milk sugar formulas are easy to mix since only water need be added. Prepared formulas also contain vitamins C and D, which are found in breast milk. Excessive quantities of carbohydrates cause loose stools in the infant, since they ferment in the bowel. At times an increase in carbohydrate is ordered for the infant who is having difficulty with bowel evacuation. Normally the stool of a formula-fed infant is yellow, pasty, and not as frequent as that of the breast-fed infant.

Formula preparation. Since newborns are susceptible to infections, it is important that mothers receive proper instructions on formula preparation. Many methods in teaching are used such as discussion and demonstrations with educational materials. It is preferable to ask the mother what she knows about formula preparation and proceed from the known to the unknown.

There are two methods commonly used: the terminal heat method and the aseptic method. The terminal heat method may be used in all formulas with the exception of those requiring high-protein milk. With high-protein milk formulas,

Table 5. Sample formula

Caloric value	*Protein*
20 per ounce	Whole milk
40 per ounce	Evaporated milk
10 per ounce	Skimmed milk
15 per ounce	½ skimmed milk (half of cream content in whole milk removed)
	Carbohydrate
48 per tablespoon	Cane sugar
27 per tablespoon	Dextri-Maltose No. 1
½ tablespoon	Karo syrup

Baby weight	*Daily caloric intake*	*Daily fluid intake*	*Daily carbohydrate requirement*
5 lb.	250 cal.	13 oz.	50 cal.
6 lb.	300 cal.	15 oz.	60 cal.
7 lb.	350 cal.	17 oz.	70 cal.
8 lb.	400 cal.	20 oz.	80 cal.
9 lb.	450 cal.	23 oz.	90 cal.

Example: Prepare a formula for a 6-pound infant with whole milk, cane sugar, and water:

6 lb. × 2½ oz. fluid = 15 oz.
6 lb. × 50 cal. = 300 cal. daily
1/5 carbohydrate = 60 cal. daily

Formula

Whole milk	12 oz.
Water	3 oz.
Cane sugar	1 tbsp.

Prepare a formula for a 6-pound infant with evaporated milk, Karo syrup, and water:

Formula

Evaporated milk	6 oz.		
Karo syrup	½ tbsp.	Water	9 oz.

the aseptic method is advisable to prevent coagulation of the protein in the formula.

Terminal heat method. In this method all ingredients are mixed together, using a clean technique. During the heating process, bottles and formula are made safe for feeding the infant. The procedure used is as follows:

1. Wash all bottles and nipples with mild detergent and warm water using bottle and nipple brushes. Rinse three times.

2. Wash measuring cup, mixing bowl, and utensils necessary to prepare the formula. (If powdered milk is used, an eggbeater facilitates mixing.)

3. Measure exact amount of carbohydrate, add to tap water, then add to milk

and mix thoroughly. If powdered milk sugar is used, add exact amount to tap water and mix.

4. Measure out into bottles, 6 feedings. Add 2 bottles of plain tap water for in-between feedings.

5. Invert nipples into bottles and leave screw caps loose for penetration of steam.

6. Stand bottles in 3 to 4 inches of water in a large utensil with tight cover.

7. When boiling occurs, lid will vibrate: *do not* remove lid; lower flame so boiling is slow, and time for 25 minutes.

8. When 25 minutes have elapsed, terminate heat and let pot cool.

9. When outside of pot is comfortable to touch, uncover, remove bottles, tighten caps, and refrigerate.

10. One hour before feeding remove bottle feeding from refrigerator. If heating is desired, immerse in pan of warm water. During hot weather remove bottles from refrigerator just before feeding. Studies have shown that babies have no ill effects when the formula is given unheated. However, this is a factor that differs depending upon the mother's feelings as well as upon the need of the individual infant.

Aseptic method. In this method bottles and formula ingredients are sterilized separately. The procedure is as follows:

1. Wash all equipment such as bottles, nipples, measuring cup, spoon, mixer, and tongs with mild detergent and rinse three times.

2. Invert bottles and boil all equipment except nipples for 10 minutes. Nipples are immersed into boiling water for 3 minutes. (This keeps nipples from becoming soft since rubber deteriorates easily.)

3. Water for the formula is boiled for 10 minutes. Add an extra few ounces allowing for evaporation.

4. If whole milk is used, simmer in a double boiler for 5 minutes.

5. Remove bottles after boiling, handling the outside surface.

6. Measure and mix formula ingredients, water, sugar, and milk using pot in which bottles were boiled.

7. Add formula to bottles, remove nipples with sterile tongs, invert into bottles, and screw caps on tightly.

8. Refrigerate until time for feeding.

SELECTED REFERENCES

Aldrich, C., and Aldrich, M.: Babies are human beings, New York, 1954, The Macmillan Co.

Allick, H. D.: Artificial feeding: a new concept, Nurs. Times **65**:107, Aug. 21, 1969.

Beaugard, P. A.: A newborn timer, Obstet. Gynec., vol. 35, no. 3, 1970.

Dyal, L., and Kahrl, J.: When mothers breastfeed, Amer. J. Nurs. **67**:2555, December, 1967.

Eastman, N. J., and Hellman, L. M.: Williams obstetrics, ed. 13, New York, 1966, Appleton-Century & Appleton-Century-Crofts.

Effrig, Sister Mary C.: Nursing care and success in breastfeeding, Nurs. Clin. N. Amer. **3**:345, 1968.

Eppink, H.: An experiment to determine a basis for nursing decisions in regard to time of initiation of breastfeeding, Nurs. Res. **18:**292, July-August, 1969.

Evans, R.: Needs identified among breastfeeding mothers, Nurs. Res., January-February, 1968.

Evans, R. T.: Exploration of factors involved in maternal physiological adaptation to breast feeding, Nurs. Res. **18:**28, January-February, 1969.

Gioiosa, R.: Breast feeding and child spacing, Child and Family, p. 3, Spring, 1964.

Grant, D. M.: Breast feeding may be a dying art, Canad. Nurse **64:**45, August, 1968.

Haynes, M.: Teaching continuity of care, Amer. J. Nurs. **62:**84, May, 1962.

La Leche League International: The womanly art of breast feeding, Franklin Park, Ill., 1963.

Naish, F. C.: Breast feeding, London, 1956, Lloyd-Luke.

Nichols, M. G.: Breastfeeding: a nurse-mother discovers its joys, RN **3:**50, May, 1968.

Pryor, K.: Nursing your baby, New York, 1963, Harper & Row, Publishers.

Ribble, M.: The rights of infants, ed. 2, New York, 1965, Columbia University Press.

Rubin, R.: Food and feeding: a matrix of relationship, Nurs. Forum **6:**195, 1967.

Smith, C. A.: The physiology of the newborn infant, Springfield, Ill., 1959, Charles C Thomas, Publisher.

Strand, R.: Breast is best, Midwives Chronicle **82:**85, March, 1969.

Waller, H. K.: The breasts and breast feeding, London, 1957, William Heinemann, Medical Books Ltd.

Why is breastfeeding difficult for women? RN **31:**52, May, 1968.

Yarrow, L. J.: Maternal care and infant behavior, Children, p. 33, January-February, 1963.

Questions for study

1. What are the needs of the newborn?
2. Describe development of the newborn infant's body systems; what are the implications for safe nursing care?
3. The following situations relate to breast-feeding; with added readings how would you proceed in helping mothers with the following:

   a. Mrs. P., a primigravida, is 2 days postpartum and is crying and uncomfortable when you walk in to care for her. She tells you her breasts hurt, and she dreads putting the baby to breast.

   b. Mrs. G., a multigravida, is 4 days postpartum, and her nipples are reddened and fissured. The baby has a firm grip when put to breast.

   c. Mrs. J., a primigravida, is in her last trimester of pregnancy and says, "I've been thinking about how to feed the baby and although I've read a lot about breast-feeding I'm not quite sure."

   d. Mrs. B. is ready to be discharged and has 1-year-old and 2-year-old children at home. She is concerned about how she will manage with two little ones when she has to breast-feed the new baby.

   e. Mrs. G. is doubtful about how long she will be able to nurse since she is expecting to return to work in 6 weeks. She says, "What's the use in even starting to breast-feed when I'll have to stop in 6 weeks?"

   f. Mrs. D. discusses how upset she is in that she would very much like to breast-feed, but her whole family and her husband object to the idea.

   g. Mrs. B. is 4 days postpartum and states, "I don't think I'm going to be able to continue breast-feeding because I have very little milk and the nurses tell me the baby keeps crying following feedings and is not satisfied."

   h. Mrs. D. is concerned about being able to continue breast-feeding since she doesn't like milk and feels this is an essential requirement in the diet.

   i. Mrs. F. attends a breast-feeding conference postpartally and asks, "Is it true that I will be 'safe' from becoming pregnant while I'm nursing Billy?"

   j. Mrs. J. is 1 day postpartum and tells you she is having cramplike pains while nursing. She is worried since she says there is really nothing in the breasts yet, and doesn't understand why she should bother to nurse.

   k. Mrs. T. is very concerned about what will happen with social activities while nursing. She heard that many women start leaking and find this most embarrassing. She tells you many of her friends had this problem and found it very confining.

4. Observe mother and infant during the feeding period. Record the following:
   a. Does the mother hold the infant close to her body or at a distance?
   b. Does she talk to the infant? What techniques does she use in comforting him if he cries?
   c. Does she wait for the infant's readiness for rooting and sucking or does she initiate this? If she initiates feeding, what technique does she use? How does the infant react?
   d. Does she ask questions about the baby's behavior while he is in the nursery away from her?

CHAPTER 16

MOTHER-CHILD RELATIONSHIPS

The early patterns of mother-infant relationships are significant for the biologic survival of the infant. The interchange in stimulus-response between the mother and the newborn has taken on newer dimensions with the development of the behavioral sciences. These beginning relationships result in the success or failure of the infant's development and the later social stress with which he must cope.

Mothering is a continuance of the closeness of the prenatal state—it clearly imitates conditions that existed prior to birth. The newborn needs to be carried about until he can move and coordinate his own body, which strengthens his sense of equilibrium and gives him a feeling of security. The close contact with mother provides warmth, and the holding gives reassurance. Mothering also involves showing love for the child by feeding, bathing, fondling, caressing, rocking, singing, or speaking. These all have deep significance.

The baby's greatest need is for contact with one person, a mother or mother substitute (Fig. 16-1). This need for contact is even greater than the need for food. Many mothers have difficulty in providing the necessary mothering. Often some women are so frightened by the needs of the child that they become less motherly. The infant gets to know the mother through the five senses, and her constant nearness is essential. While the infant is carried about in his mother's arms he feels a part of the moving world. If the infant is not gratified he turns to himself for comfort and uses thumb-sucking, rocking, masturbation, etc. for satisfaction.

Mothering of an infant is an inborn impulse in the personalities of many women. Infants have been known over the centuries to receive adequate mothering regardless of social, financial, and emotional stresses. Therese Benedek studied the biologic need for motherhood in observing attitudes and behavior of women during the periods of the hormonal cycle in relation to ovulation, fertilization, prenatal development, and lactation. Her findings support that biologic changes greatly enhance the development of motherliness, which increases

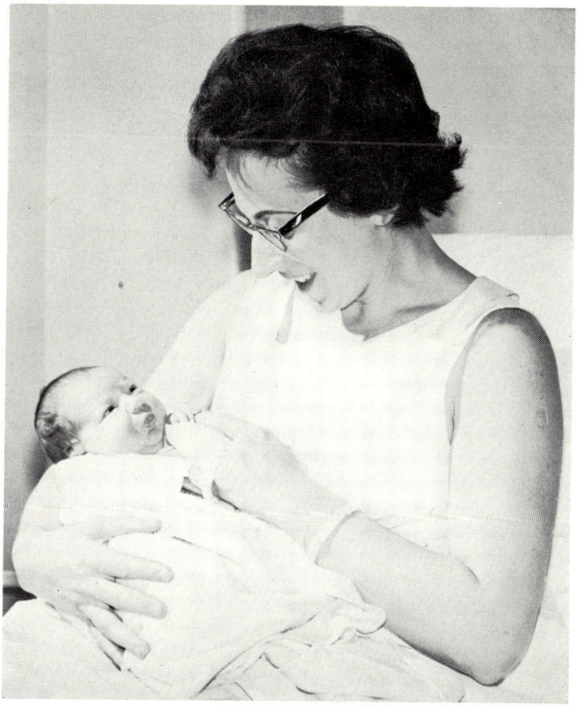

Fig. 16-1. Mother-infant relationships. (Courtesy Christ Hospital, Jersey City, N. J.)

the pleasure of childbearing and eases the discomforts of pregnancy. Helene Deutsch, in her research, found that regardless of identical social influences and similarities of reactions with various cultural influences, there still remain deep and primitive emotional relationships between mother and infant.

The ability to mother begins long before the woman is expecting her first child. It actually commences during the mother's own childhood and continues to develop as she bears and nurtures each infant. The strong basic need of women is that of reproduction, since biologically this makes her a complete woman.

From the moment of conception, when the baby begins its existence, inheritance of many traits and characteristics is carried from generation to generation. The rate of growth and development in the first 8 weeks of intrauterine life is so rapid that any interference with the maternal organism may cause irreparable damage to the fetus. Therefore, even in intrauterine life the baby is constantly struggling to survive. The separation at birth from the mother is referred to as the trauma of birth for mother and infant. At this time there is a biologic separation, but the dependency needs of mother and child are those of giving and receiving. This relationship results in a physiologic and psychologic maturing process for the mother. The mother achieves confidence in her mothering responsibilities as she feeds and cares for her infant. The infant in turn is gratified and develops a feeling of security as his needs are met.

Mother love is like food—it must be given regularly, a little at a time and frequently. Mothering is an art that differs with the need of each individual child. The father also develops fatherliness, and his experience and relationship with his wife are enhanced when rooming-in is available in the hospital unit. The birth process affects both parents in that expectations become reality, and the reality brings with it satisfactions and joys as well as worries and anxieties. The mother and father roles are developed from a series of learned experiences that, although complex, are the same experiences that occur from one generation to the next.

The interaction between mother and child begins from the moment of conception. The increased hormonal secretions during pregnancy necessary to maintain the baby implanted within the uterus give the mother a feeling of well-being. Because of this physiologic phenomenon as the infant grows and is nourished by the mother, she is prepared for her mother role.

At the time of delivery and shortly thereafter, hormonal and metabolic changes are again evident. The vast changes occurring in the immediate postpartal period interrupt the closeness of mother and infant. This separation results in the so-called postpartal blues and the depressed feelings many mothers experience. Many mothers do not feel the strong desire of love for the new baby, which may not be immediate but grows as the mother cares for the child. It is during this "emotional" period that the mother needs to receive love and mothering before she can give love to her infant. The husband and members of the health team can help the mother if they understand her behavior and help her through this trying period.

The continuation of closeness of mother and infant is inherent in the process of lactation. As the baby suckles the mother's breast, there is a closeness and a process of give and take in which mother and infant profit. The baby begins to associate his need for food as gratification from an outside source and in this way develops trust in the world about him. The mother in turn begins to develop a satisfaction in being needed, resulting in confidence and trust, a two-way process in which the mother is able to give and the infant able to receive. Any interference in this two-way relationship will affect both organisms, becoming a vicious circle.

Nursing care of the mother and the infant that is supportive in nature aids in the development of motherliness. As the nurse identifies and meets the mother's needs, the mother in turn can meet the needs of her infant.

The young teen-age mother presents a twofold need—on one hand she wishes to be dependent and free from responsibility, and on the other hand she needs to develop the ability to mother. Her husband may also be an adolescent with the same needs and may be unable to give the support needed. The professional nurse then becomes the person to give support, aiding the development of motherliness. A positive approach encouringing the young mother through early contact with the infant enhances and strengthens the mother role.

It is evident that any physical deviation in the mother or infant may play a role in the development of motherliness. The personality of the mother plays a leading role in her giving to the infant. Many mothers experience an early postpartum emotional lag due to biologic and physiologic body changes. Regression with a desire for mothering is not uncommon. The husband's relationship and awareness of the mother's needs will greatly influence the mother-infant interaction. As the mother receives love she develops trust and confidence, which ultimately strengthen her mothering role. Should the infant at birth manifest a congenital anomaly with resulting frustration, this in turn frustrates the mother. This vicious circle influences the ego organization of the infant in developing a sense of trust and influences the completion of the development of the motherliness.

SELECTED REFERENCES

Crawford, M.: Physiological and behavioral clues to disturbance in childbirth, A.N.A. Clinical Sessions, 142, 1968.

Deutsch, H.: Psychology of women, New York, 1945, Grune & Stratton, Inc., vol. 2.

Dutcher, I., and Hakerem, H.: Mother-child interaction in psychosomatic illness, Nurs. Forum **7**:17, 1968.

Hartman, C. C.: Psychotic mothers and their babies, Nurs. Outlook **16**:32, December, 1968.

Iorio, J.: Mother-infant relationships, implications for nursing. Parent-child relationships, role of the nurse, Newark, N. J., 1968, Rutgers University.

Kimball, C. D.: Mother-child relationships, Child and Family, p. 10, Summer, 1963.

McFarland, M. B., and Reinhardt, J.: Development of motherliness, Children, p. 48, March-April, 1959.

Montagu, A.: Prenatal influences, Springfield, Ill., 1962, Charles C Thomas, Publisher.

Newton, N.: Maternal emotions, New York, 1955, Harper & Row, Publishers.

Oscarson, S. E.: Hostile behavior in a maternity patient, A.N.A. Clinical Sessions **61:** 1966.

Reed, E. R. S.: Becoming a mother—nursing implications in a problem of role transition, A.N.A. Clinical Conference **204:** 1967.

Rubin, R.: Maternal touch, Nurs. Outlook **11**:828, 1963.

Rubin, R.: The neomaternal period. In Bergersen, B., and others, editors: Current concepts in clinical nursing, St. Louis, 1969, The C. V. Mosby Co.

Rubin, R.: Some cognitive aspects of childbearing. In Bergersen, B., and others, editors: Current concepts in clinical nursing, St. Louis, 1969, The C. V. Mosby Co.

Rubin, R.: Attainment of maternal role processes. Part 1, Nursing Res. **16**:237, Fall, 1967.

Rubin, R.: Models and referrants. Part 2, Nursing Res. **16**:342, Fall, 1967.

Yeaworth, R. C.: Identification and maternity nursing, Nurs. Forum **7**:249, 1968.

Yeaworth, R. C.: Mental health: a two-way street, Nurs. Outlook **16**:45, November, 1968.

Questions for study

1. While caring for mother and infant keep a daily process recording of difficulties encountered when mother and infant are together. What nursing intervention techniques were used in helping mother and infant? In retrospect evaluate the techniques used as to effectiveness or ineffectiveness.
2. Define mothering and discuss its development in early mother-infant relationships.

CHAPTER 17

PREMATURITY–THE LOW BIRTH WEIGHT INFANT

In the past the term *premature* included the newborn who was less than 37 weeks gestation or the infant who weighed less than 2,500 grams at birth. Recent research has shown that there are differences—the infant who is full term is now classified as *full size,* and the infant born prior to 37 weeks gestation is classified as *low birth weight.*

An expert committee report of the World Health Organization* has been adopted by the American Academy of Pediatrics in the revised 1964 edition of *Standards and Recommendations for Hospital Care of Newborn Infants,* which states:

> The term *premature* has been replaced by *low birth weight* (2500 gm. or less). Larger newborn infants, previously classified as *full term* are referred to as *full size* to indicate that the axis of classification is birth size. The classification of newborn infants on the basis of duration of pregnancy (premature less than 37 completed weeks, full term 37 weeks and over) is in no way precluded or discouraged by the new terminology. The new terms then make a clear distinction between birth size and gestational age at birth, a fact which in the past has often been obscured by the use of the word premature as the designation for all small newborn infants.

INCIDENCE AND CAUSES

Factors influencing the incidence of low birth weight infants are race, sex, plurality of birth, maternal factors such as age and parity, socioeconomic factors, social class, and geographic area. Premature deliveries occur in 4% to 8% of all births, the incidence being higher in the lower socioeconomic group.

Prematurity is the leading cause of neonatal death in the United States; respiratory distress syndrome is second, and congenital anomalies are third. Factors related to low birth weight infants are multiple births, toxemia, hypertensive

*WHO technical report series 1961, No. 217.

disease, placenta previa, abruptio placentae, fibroids of the uterus, cardiac failure, diabetes, thyroid dysfunction, untreated syphilis, severe infections, malformations of the uterus, incompetency of the cervix, and nutritional deficiency.

PREVENTION

Adequate early prenatal supervision is essential for prevention of prematurity. Perhaps education of young teen-agers (prior to marriage and a family) as to the importance of medical supervision during the childbearing years is a sound beginning. Education in dietary and general hygiene is imperative for the expectant mother. Since prematurity is more common in the lower socioeconomic group, alleviating overcrowding and poor housing and providing adequate clinic facilities to make services available are paramount. All community agencies are involved in lowering the rate of low birth weight infants—it is a project wherein the physician, nurse, social worker, public health agencies, and the welfare department can make great strides.

PROGNOSIS

The prognosis for infants in the higher birth weight groups (above 1,500 grams) is excellent, for infants weighing 1,000 to 1,500 grams it is good, and for those weighing 1,000 grams or less it is favorable. Survival rates have improved in recent years, more favorably in the higher birth weight infant.

Although follow-up studies of low birth weight infants are often difficult, it has been found that there is an association between cerebral palsy and premature birth. Behavior patterns of low birth weight infants have shown emotional immaturity in childhood manifested by frequency of tantrums and symptoms of withdrawal and dependency needs. Interest is growing in the course of emotional development in light of the long period of separation of mother and infant at birth. The anxiety of parents after the infant is dismissed from the hospital is another matter of real concern that needs further study.

INTRAPARTAL CARE

The care of the low birth weight infant begins with management of the mother in labor. The mother admitted prior to term or suspected of having a premature infant needs careful consideration during labor. Preanesthetic medications should be minimal for survival of the infant. Barbiturates and opiates are contraindicated since they depress respirations and deplete the infant in utero of oxygen. Regional anesthetics are safer than general anesthetics.

The practice of giving vitamin K to the mother in labor to elevate the prothrombin time in the premature infant is now contraindicated. Studies show that large doses of vitamin K may result in hyperbilirubinemia in the low birth weight infant.

The nurse is responsible for notifying the nursery that a premature birth is anticipated. This affords nursery personnel the time to heat the Isolette and have oxygen and suction equipment in readiness. The delivery room needs also to be equipped with oxygen apparatus, a warm incubator, and resuscitative equipment, including a laryngoscope for intubation if it becomes necessary. When sedation has been given the mother, 0.2 mg. of nalorphine hydrochloride (Nalline) should be available. With a depressed infant the medication is injected directly into the umbilical vein. The nurse also alerts the pediatrician so that he is available at the time of birth.

Immediately following delivery, it is a common practice to clamp the cord promptly. It was once believed that delaying the tying afforded the infant a placental transfusion of blood. Studies reveal, however, that these infants had a higher incidence of tachypnea and chest retractions; therefore early clamping is now carried out.

MANAGEMENT FOLLOWING DELIVERY

All newborns undergo some degree of asphyxia (a simultaneous decrease in both the intake of oxygen and elimination of carbon dioxide) during the process of birth. The biochemical response is one in which the blood-oxygen saturation is reduced, the carbon dioxide tension is increased, and the pH is low, resulting in a temporary respiratory acidosis. These chemical changes in the blood are important stimuli to the initiation of respirations.

The immediate care of the low birth weight infant consists of positioning the head downward to facilitate drainage of mucus and to alleviate the possibility of aspiration of blood and mucus into the lungs. With the head well extended aspiration is easily accomplished. Should respirations not be initiated within 1 minute, resuscitative measures are taken. Direct laryngoscopy, tracheal aspiration, intubation, and mouth-to-tube insufflation are safe methods of resuscitation of the low birth weight infant. Resuscitation is always accomplished by a well-qualified anesthetist or pediatrician.

Maintaining body temperature is difficult in the low birth weight infant since there is heat loss by evaporation from the skin and from the lungs when respirations become established. It is difficult at times to maintain body temperature when efforts are being made to initiate respirations; however, undue exposure should be avoided.

A careful first appraisal by the pediatrician includes observations for obvious congenital anomalies, chest auscultation, passing a rubber catheter into the stomach to aspirate fluid (a large amount, more than 30 ml., is suggestive of high intestinal obstruction and increased number of leukocytes indicative of amnionitis) to rule out choanal atresia, and passing a rubber catheter into the rectum to rule out imperforate anus. Inspection of the freshly cut umbilical cord will reveal absence of vessels indicative of diaphragmatic hernia, malformation of the gastrointestinal tract, or defects.

Transportation of the low birth weight infant from the delivery room to a nursery equipped for adequate care is essential for survival. When vital signs are well established, transfer of the infant is made safer. Many large cities have a Premature Transportation Service (such as the New York City Department of Health) equipped with an incubator carrier and a qualified nurse in attendance for transport to a center. Information concerning the pregnancy, family, and labor and delivery record should accompany the infant to provide continuity in care. It is a common practice that a specimen of the mother's blood accompany the infant for blood typing and cross matching.

The nurse accompanying the infant is adept at carrying out resuscitative measures and observes the infant during transport. The incubator provides heat and oxygen at controlled temperatures and concentrations.

CHARACTERISTICS OF THE LOW BIRTH WEIGHT INFANT

Skin and appendages

The skin of the low birth weight infant has a gelatinous appearance. The blood vessels and bony structures are visible since there is very little subcutaneous fat. Small deposits of vernix caseosa may be noticed in the skin folds. Vernix is believed to be rich in estrogens and may influence heat control. The skin is loose and wrinkled, and fine downy hairs (lanugo) are present on the forehead, sides of the face, and the extremities. The eyebrows are usually absent, and the hair on the head is scanty. The nipples and areolas of the breasts are barely visible, and breast engorgement rarely if ever occurs.

Head

The circumference of the infant's head is large in comparison to the chest. This is commonly known as pseudohydrocephalus of prematurity. The fontanels of the skull are small, and the bones are soft. The eyes of the low birth weight infant deserve frequent careful examination when the infant needs oxygen for survival. Ophthalmoscopic examination is done periodically because of the danger of retrolental fibroplasia (a blinding disease of the eye).

The ears are poorly supported by cartilage and can be folded in many positions. Asymmetric malformed ears are associated with congenital malformations of the genitourinary tract. Flaring of the nares is indicative of oxygen hunger and respiratory distress. Passing a catheter through the nose and pharynx is done at birth to rule out choanal atresia.

Observing the premature infant for mucus is imperative to maintain an open airway. Copious amounts of frothy mucus are indicative of esophageal atresia. Any vomitus that is bile-stained or brownish in nature is presumptive evidence of intestinal obstruction.

The color of the infant's skin is a good indication of the amount of oxygenation present. Low birth weight infants are either pink or red with a cyanotic hue of the hands and feet. The low birth weight infant, however, has attacks of color deviations known as harlequin color change. The color change is particularly noted when the infant is turned on his side. The upper half of the body is pale, and the lower half is pink or red with a definite line of demarcation separating each. Should the infant be turned to his opposite side or cry, the color changes reverse. Harlequin color change is a vasomotor phenomenon that is unexplained and of no particular significance in the low birth weight infant.

Activity and posture

Most infants are somnolent, while some are aroused by light cutaneous stimulation. The low birth weight infant assumes a side-lying position with upper extremities flexed, trunk slightly curved inward, and lower extremities extended with marked flexion and abduction of the thighs, commonly known as the frog-like position.

As the low birth weight infant is observed in a quiet state of semiconsciousness, contractions of the face muscles and extremities are common. Often quivering of the face muscles and random movements are apparent with the slightest stimulus and occur without crying.

Body temperature

Heat regulation is poorly developed in the low birth weight infant with a tendency toward hypothermia. Factors involved are the following: (1) poor development of the central nervous system, resulting in faulty heat regulation; (2) heat loss through radiation since there is a large skin surface area and lack of fat deposits; (3) a poorly developed respiratory center, resulting in diminished oxygen combustion causing asphyxia; (4) weak heart action with slower circulation and poor oxygenation; and (5) insufficient heat production caused by inadequate metabolism.

The incubator or Isolette provides a constant temperature, prevents cooling, and is essential for survival of the low birth weight infant. To control heat regulation, newer Isolette models are equipped with leads attached to the infant's abdomen, which automatically raise or lower the Isolette temperature as the infant's body temperature changes. Overheating is just as serious as hypothermia since dehydration, apathy, anoxia, and cyanosis may occur.

The belief that a relatively high humidity is necessary to prevent drying of the infant's mucous membranes was a result of infants' receiving high oxygen concentrations. Although high concentrations of oxygen are seldom used, high humidity is still recommended. Body temperatures of larger unclothed infants (weight over 1,500 grams) are kept between 97° and 98° F. (36.1° and 36.7° C.) with the incubator circulating air between 84° and 90° F. (28.9° and 32.2° C.) and with the relative humidity at 50% to 60%. Smaller infants need a relatively higher air temperature and higher humidity to maintain body temperature. The smaller infant needs an air temperature between 88° and 90° F. (31.1° and 32.2° C.). Should body temperature decrease, the humidity rather than air temperature is increased to prevent overheating.

Respiratory system

The lungs and rib cage of the low birth weight infant may not function efficiently at birth because of muscular weakness. Often oxygen is transmitted to the large bronchioles yet the small bronchioles may not be dilated.

Respirations in the low birth weight infant may be steady, with no pause between inspiration and expiration; they may be like the adult respiratory pattern of inspiration, expiration, pause, or there may be inspiration, pause, expiration, pause. Frequently regular breathing is interrupted with a sigh and an apneic pause. The rate of respirations is normally 40 to 60 per minute. An increase of 15 or more respirations per minute is indicative of respiratory distress. A "sinking in" at the xiphoid, known as substernal retraction, is evidence of air hunger. Grunting sounds audible on expiration are significant of severe respiratory distress (Fig. 17-1).

When periods of apnea are prolonged, the nurse may initiate respirations by elevating both of the infant's arms above the head to expand the rib cage, or by changing the position. These simple measures initiate respirations—therefore observation of the low birth weight infant is essential.

Often higher concentrations of oxygen may be necessary for short periods for survival of the smaller infant. Damage to the retina occurs when high oxygen concentrations are maintained for long periods.

Circulatory system

The heart is well developed in the low birth weight infant. The pulse rate varies from 90 to 200 per minute, the average being 120. The fluctuation in rate is a result of lack of development of the cardiac inhibitory centers. The greater tendency toward capillary fragility predisposes the infant to intracranial hemorrhage.

The red and white blood cells in the low birth weight infant are slightly lower, and anemia may develop early in the first few months of life. Since the low birth weight infant is unable to store iron in the last trimester and is depleted at birth, iron supplements are started by the third week.

Digestive system

In the low birth weight infant prior to feeding, the stomach is tubular and the pyloric musculature is well developed. Regurgitation is common since the cardiac sphincter is poorly developed.

Nutrition of the low birth weight infant is difficult, and the more immature the infant the greater the problem. Factors that interfere with feeding are the following: (1) the sucking and swallowing reflexes are absent, weak, or easily exhausted; (2) the small capacity of the stomach leads to regurgitation and vomiting; (3) the gastric acidity is low; and (4) the emptying time of the stomach is slow.

The first feeding is usually determined by the respiratory effort of the infant.

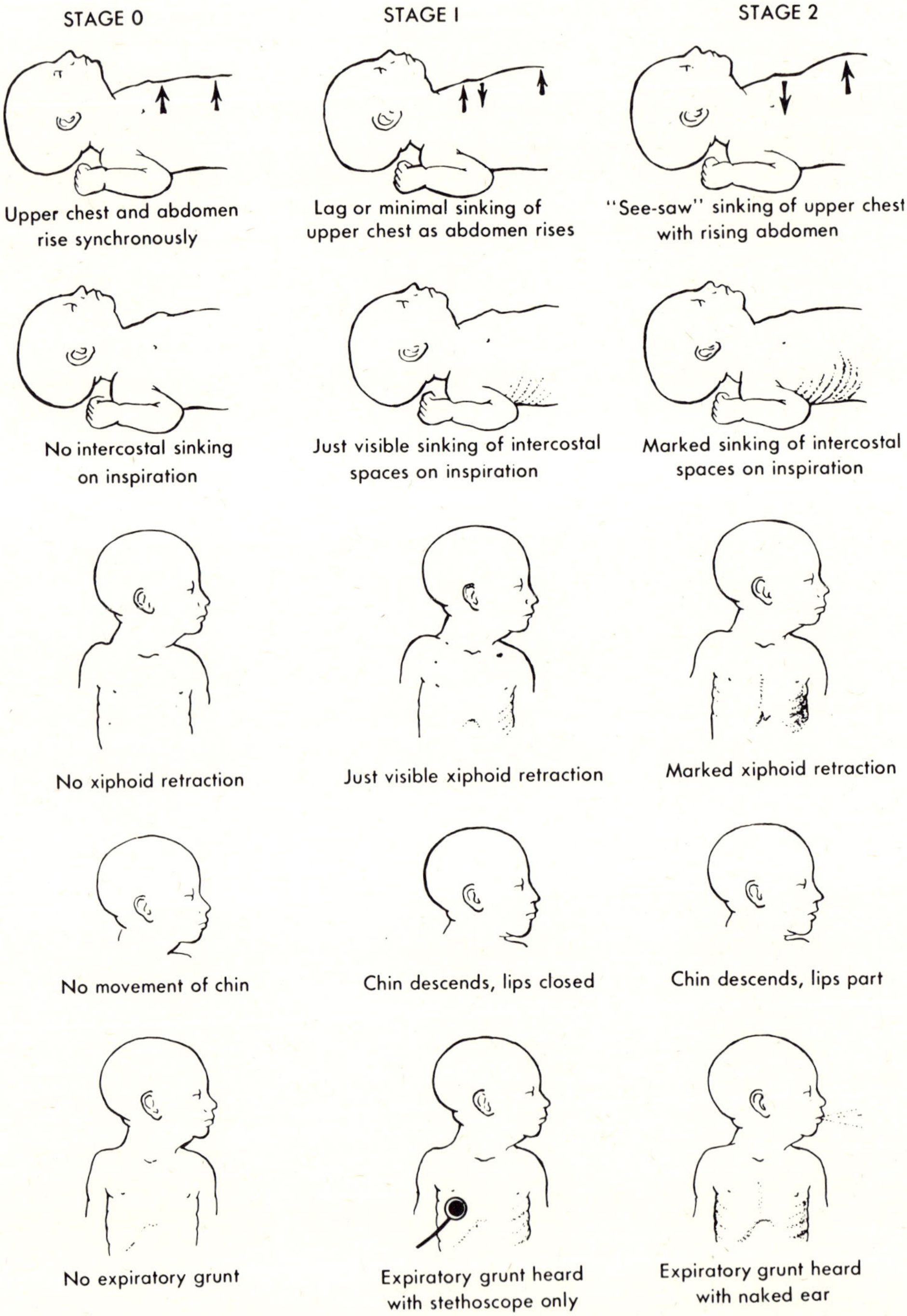

Fig. 17-1. Silverman-Anderson scoring system. A score of 0 is indicative of good expiratory effort, and a score of 10 is indicative of poor respiratory effort. (Redrawn after Silverman, W. A.: Premature infants, New York, 1961, Paul B. Hoeber, Inc.)

Certainly the infant with severe respiratory distress would be in danger if the stomach were inflated. The old belief that feeding should not be initiated until all edema disappears is long past, and studies show that the early introduction of glucose water has decreased the mortality rate. Feedings were withheld to reduce the incidence of vomiting and aspiration of fluid in the low birth weight infant. The feeding now is given with due respect to the condition of the baby and size to prevent overfeeding.

The type of feeding for the low birth weight infant is secondary to the composition. Studies show that breast milk is superior to cow's milk since the incidence of infections and the mortality rates were lower in low birth weight infants receiving breast milk. Although the larger low birth weight infants do well on breast milk, smaller infants gain weight and grow more slowly on breast milk. Therefore in the smaller infant breast milk is altered to increase the protein and caloric content.

The method used in feeding is determined by the development of the sucking and swallowing reflexes and the general condition of the infants. A weak sucking and swallowing reflex necessitates gavage feeding. Larger infants are fed by bottle and a soft nipple. If the infant's condition does not permit him to be out of the heated crib, breast milk may be pumped or manually expressed and given by bottle. Occasionally if the swallowing reflex is well developed, feeding is also accomplished by medicine dropper.

The caloric requirement of the low birth weight infant is accelerated since he ingests smaller amounts at each feeding. While the newborn requires 40 to 50 calories per pound of body weight at birth, the low birth weight infant requires 60 to 80 calories per pound in order to gain weight. At 3 weeks of age his requirements may increase to 120 calories per pound for adequate growth and development. Early first feedings contain approximately 10 to 20 calories per pound of body weight.

NURSING CARE OF THE PREMATURE INFANT

Probably one of the most important measures in nursing care of the low birth weight infant is careful observation (Fig. 17-2). The infant is housed in a transparent plastic Isolette and lies naked in the incubator so that he is visible at all times.

The Isolette protects the baby from infection and keeps his basal body temperature at about 97° F. The temperature of the Isolette is usually set at 90° F. and is regulated according to the infant's body temperature. Should the infant show such signs of anoxia as cyanosis or difficulty in breathing, he may need oxygen; therefore raising his body temperature only increases his oxygen needs.

Oxygen therapy

Oxygen is administered at levels prescribed by the pediatrician. Often the concentration does not exceed 40%. Higher levels may be given for short periods

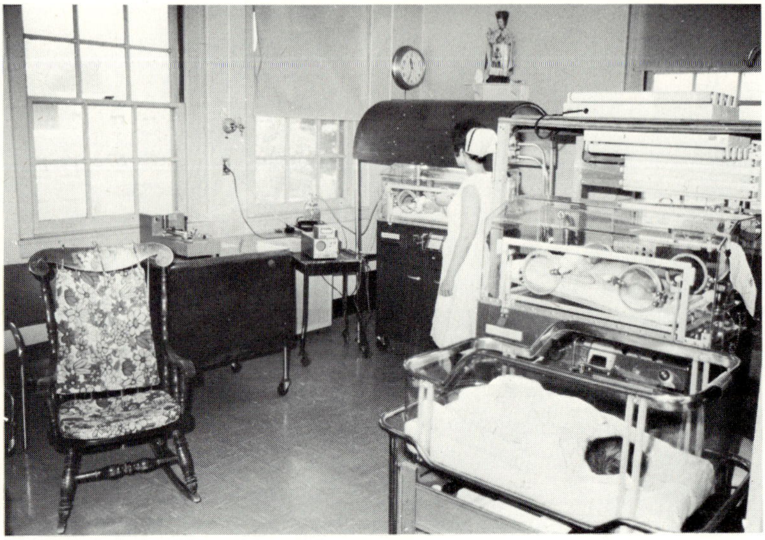

Fig. 17-2. Premature nursery.

to keep the infant alive. An oxygen analyzer is used every 4 hours to measure accurately the oxygen concentration within the Isolette. The analyzer is placed on top of the Isolette, the lead is inserted through the top opening of the Isolette, the tip is lowered to the infant's nose, and the bulb is squeezed and released three times. Then the button is pushed, and the concentration of oxygen is registered on the machine grading. High concentrations of oxygen may result in a retrolental fibroplasia resulting in blindness. All premature infants have ophthalmoscopic examinations done weekly when receiving oxygen.

Moisture

Raising the humidity within the Isolette enables the infant to be more comfortable at lower temperatures. High humidities may be ordered to the point of saturation or fogging when the infant has severe respiratory distress. Distilled water is used to provide a fine mist by vaporization.

Isolette

The Isolette provides (1) temperature control, (2) visibility, (3) humidity control, (4) freedom from clothing, (5) oxygen measured with an analyzer, (6) facilities for positioning the infant, (7) device for filtering incoming air, (8) a scale for weighing within the Isolette, (9) isolation, and (10) the latest device, a hammock suspended (as in the weighing process) that constantly rocks the infant. Studies have proved that the infant who is rocked fares better than the infant who is not rocked.

Aseptic technique

Hand washing with soap and water is essential to limit infection of the premature infant. Scrubbing the hands initially and careful washing before the care of infants is paramount. Gowns and masks are not necessary since the Isolette protects the infant. Nurses with upper respiratory infections or diarrhea are banned from caring for these infants. The nurse caring for the premature infant should not move into the normal newborn nursery. All Isolettes are thoroughly washed and aired for 24 hours before reusing. All cleaning in the room is done by wet mopping or vacuuming.

Feeding the premature infant

All premature infants are suctioned adequately in the delivery room. The stomach is also suctioned to remove excess secretions that may impede respirations.

A No. 8 polyethylene catheter is inserted through the nostril and into the stomach. With clean hands the nurse holds the tip of the catheter at the level of the nasal bridge with one hand and carries the catheter downward to the point where it lies at the level of the ensiform cartilage (the distal extremity of the sternum), marking the catheter at that point with a pencil. The tube is lubricated with sterile water and is passed through the nostril. Should the infant become cyanotic or have respiratory distress, the catheter is pinched and quickly removed. Once the tube is inserted to the pencil line (or 2 cm. beyond), the end may be inverted into a sterile water bottle. If no bubbles appear, the catheter is in the stomach. Should bubbles appear, the catheter is in the trachea and is quickly removed. Another recent method used to check for location of the tube is by ascultation with a stethoscope. If breath sounds are impaired the tube is removed, since it is in the lungs.

The feeding is started by inserting 0.5 ml. of sterile water. If the baby takes this well, the formula is given through a syringe at room temperature. It is far better to allow the feeding to flow by gravity. However, some of the very small polyethylene tubes are so narrow that the plunger of the syringe needs to be used. If so, the plunger should be turned rather than pushed to prevent too fast a feeding, and to prevent increased pressure within the stomach that may embarrass respirations. It has been found that premature infants fed too quickly develop a tachycardia with a resulting decrease in respirations. All feedings are terminated with 0.5 ml. of sterile water to clear the tubing since milk is an excellent medium for bacterial growth.

Polyethylene tubes are changed weekly or when necessary so that trauma to the nasal mucosa is minimized. The opposite nostril is then used.

Position for feeding is usually a semi-Fowler's so that there is no regurgitation of feeding with possible aspiration into the trachea. The infant is left in this position following feeding, or may be turned slightly to one side, propped by a protective roll. Burping is not necessary unless the infant is receiving more than one-half ounce at a feeding.

As soon as the infant shows signs of developing a sucking reflex, a pacifier is given during the tube feeding. As the sucking reflex improves, part of the feeding may be given through a soft nipple and the rest by gavage. The tube is left in place until the infant is able to be weaned entirely to nipple feeding.

It was once believed that premature infants should not be fed until respirations were normal. However, this proved to change the pH in the baby, with resulting acidosis. Today, parenteral sodium bicarbonate and dextrose are given through the umbilical vein until feedings may be started. Blood pH's are done frequently to prevent acidosis. A common treatment, called the Usher treatment, includes the preceding parenteral solutions given through an especially devised machine that feeds the baby through the umbilical vein slowly. Calculations are arrived at by considering the baby's body weight and general condition.

Phototherapy

Since most premature infants have immature livers, capillary fragility, etc., they often develop jaundice due to a hyperbilirubinemia. Exposure of the infant to blue or white lights, called phototherapy, breaks down bilirubin into excretable water-soluble substances. Unconjugated bilirubin, which is fat-soluble, is not excreted either in the bile or through the kidney. A liver enzyme, glucuronyl transferase, must first convert it to a water-soluble form that can be excreted in bile. Since the premature infant is usually deficient in this liver enzyme, the bilirubin level of the blood continues to rise until kernicterus occurs. Staining of brain cells results in permanent brain damage.

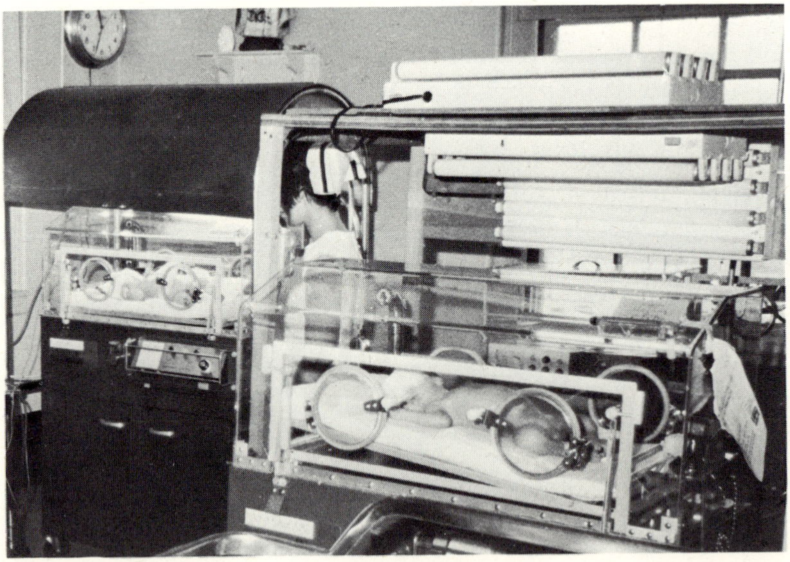

Fig. 17-3. Phototherapy.

As a preventive measure all premature infants now receive phototherapy (Fig. 17-3). The infant's eyes are covered for protection while exposed to the light, and his temperature is checked carefully. Phototherapy, along with exchange transfusion, is also being used with jaundice due either to ABO incompatibility or to Rh sensitivity.

SUPPORT OF PARENTS

When premature labor occurs, the mother has not expected the advent of labor. She is frightened and anxious since she knows small infants have a difficult time surviving outside the uterus. The mother looks for encouragement that all will go well, yet false hope cannot be given. Letting the mother know that all will be done for her and the baby will alleviate much anxiety. Since analgesias are seldom given so as not to depress the infant, added support for the mother is essential during labor. Teaching the mother abdominal and chest breathing for the first and second phases of the first stage of labor will keep her involved and will alleviate some of the discomfort. Rubbing the back or pressure in the small of the back is helpful with severe backache. Often a simple explanation as to why medication cannot be given focuses the mother on other methods for relief.

Following delivery, the baby may be far removed from the mother, yet communication between premature nursery personnel and the mother will alleviate the strains in separation of mother and infant. Allowing the mother to telephone, to participate in the care of the infant, and to have flexible visiting privileges are services most supportive to parents. Should financial problems occur, referral to a social service worker is made.

Preparation for discharge of the infant begins a week or two prior to the infant's homecoming. The mother is invited to participate more fully in the care of the infant (bathing, feeding, etc.) so that home adjustment is made easier. As the mother handles and feeds her infant, she becomes adept at meeting his needs. This gives her confidence and reassurance that her baby, although premature, is no different from the normal newborn at the time of discharge. Often the father reacts with guilt to an infant that is of low birth weight, since he cannot boast of the size of his infant. The nurse needs to be cognizant of the father's feelings and to be nonjudgmental in giving him support.

Nurses on a premature service at times become protective of low birth weight infants since they require expertness in care. The nurse, however, must always remember that her expertness may be threatening to parents who are suddenly faced with assuming this responsibility. Anticipatory guidance and involvement of parents in the care of the low birth weight infant will eliminate some of these obstacles.

SELECTED REFERENCES

Berenberg, W.: Prematurity and cerebral palsy, Ohio Med. J. **61:**1089, 1965.

Callon, H. F.: The premature infant's nurse, Amer. J. Nurs. **63:**103, February, 1963.

Canice, Sister Mary: Mothers in the nursery, Amer. J. Nurs. **64:**101, November, 1964.

Cornblath, M., Lundeene, E., Morrison, M., and Wishingrad, L.: Research and nursing care in the premature nursery, Amer. J. Nurs. **62:**92, July, 1962.

Creery, R. D. G.: The infant of low-birth-weight, Nurs. Mirror, p. 125, Oct. 20, 1967.

Erhardt, C. L., Joshi, G. B., Nelson, F. G., and others: Influence of weight and gestation on perinatal and neonatal mortality by ethnic group, Amer. J. Public Health **54:** 1841, 1964.

Farquhar, J. W.: Immediate feeding of premature infants with undiluted breast milk, Lancet **1:**550, 1965.

Ferguson, D.: The other side of the window, RN **26:**44, February, 1963.

Geddes, A. K.: Premature babies, Philadelphia, 1960, W. B. Saunders Co.

Goldstein, H., Goldberg, I. D., Frazier, T. M., and others: Cigarette smoking and prematurity, Public Health Rep. **79:**553, 1964.

Kane, S. H.: Significance of prenatal care, Obstet. Gynec. **24:**86, 1964.

Kraus, R. A.: Polyurethane foam pads, Amer. J. Nurs. **65:**98, January, 1965.

Lewis, P. M.: The premature baby, Nurs. Mirror, p. 124, April 14, 1967.

Moritz, C. R.: Preventable prematurity, a time-cost study, Obstet. Gynec. **25:**585, 1965.

Neal, M. V., and Nauen, C. M.: Ability of premature infant to maintain his own body temperature, Nurs. Res. **17:**396, September-October, 1968.

Oxygen therapy and retrolental fibroplasia, Amer. J. Public Health **58:**2009, 1968.

Peterson, W. F., Morese, K. N., and Kaltreider, D. F.: Smoking and prematurity, Obstet. Gynec. **26:**775, 1965.

Phototherapy and hyperbilirubinemia of prematurity, Nurs. Mirror **127:**45, Oct. 18, 1968.

Richardson, E. H.: A teachmobile for premature infant care, Nurs. Outlook **12:**35, June, 1964.

Silverman, W.: Dunham's premature infants, ed. 3, New York, 1961, Harper & Row, Publishers.

Struthers, J. N.: Early or late feeding of premature infants, Nurs. Times **61:**1577, 1965.

Underwood, P., Hester, L. L., Laffitte, T., Jr., and others: The relationship of smoking to the outcome of pregnancy, Amer. J. Obstet. Gynec. **91:**270, 1965.

Wortis, H., and Freedman, A.: The contribution of social environment to the development of premature children, Amer. J. Orthopsychiat. **35:**57, January, 1965.

Questions for study

1. Observe low birth weight infants of 1,200 grams, 1,500 grams, and 1,800 grams for 10 minutes each. Compare the characteristics, posture, and activity, and evaluate with textbook pictures. Compare the method of feeding for each weight group and give the rationale.
2. What are the essential components in giving safe care to the premature infant?
3. How would you prepare parents for the low birth weight infant's homecoming?
4. What facilities are available in your community for the low birth weight infant?
5. Examine an Isolette in the premature unit. Name the parts and assemble it for use should a premature infant be anticipated.

UNIT III

DEVIATIONS FROM THE NORMAL MATERNITY CYCLE

Health is the soul that animates all the enjoyments of life
which fade and are tasteless without it.

Johnson

CHAPTER 18

TOXEMIAS OF PREGNANCY

Toxemias of pregnancy are characterized by a triad of symptoms: edema, elevation in blood pressure, and proteinuria. The severity of this syndrome results in a sequela of convulsions and finally coma. In toxemias only the symptoms are treated; the specific etiology continues to be uncertain.

Toxemias occur during the third trimester of pregnancy and the early postpartal period. Only with hydatidiform mole or preexisting diabetes, hypertension, and renal disease do toxemias occur early in the first trimester of pregnancy.

The pathogenesis in toxemia is one of peripheral arteriolar vasoconstriction that causes a decreased perfusion of blood and oxygen through vital organs, with a resulting elevation in blood pressure. The resultant hypoxia and edema of the various major organ systems produce the classic syndrome of preeclampsia and eclampsia with (1) cerebral edema and hypoxia resulting in cerebral irritability ending in convulsions; (2) decreased renal blood flow with arteriolar thickening and damage to the kidneys, producing albuminuria, sodium retention, and an increase in blood pressure; (3) liver damage with tissue hypoxia and vascular stasis; and (4) reduced placental perfusion.

INCIDENCE OF TOXEMIAS

Toxemias are one of the leading causes of maternal, fetal, and neonatal deaths. The incidence is higher in young primigravidas of 13 to 16 years of age, the elderly primigravidas, daughters of toxemic mothers, and women of the low socioeconomic group.

Increased perinatal morbidity and mortality are associated with toxemia of pregnancy. Factors responsible are decreased uterine blood flow, placental ischemia, placental insufficiency, and premature placental deterioration. The fetal status is often evaluated in the following ways: (1) by fetal electrocardiography, (2) by diagnostic ultrasound to determine cessation of fetal skull growth with resulting intrauterine growth retardation, (3) amniotic fluid studies (meconium-stained fluid signifies distress; blood-stained fluid, death of the fetus), (4) ascertainment of pH of fetal blood following rupture of the membranes, and (5) determination of estriol levels, decreased levels indicating jeopardy of the fetus.

Infant mortality in all toxemias is as high as 10% to 25%. Since premature labor is a common sequela, there is a higher neonatal mortality rate resulting from intrauterine anoxia with vasospasm. Although some babies live, they may later show evidence of cerebral palsy, mental retardation, and epilepsy. Predisposing factors include multiple pregnancy, previous history of toxemia, rheumatic heart disease, diabetes, polyhydramnios, hydatidiform mole, and preexisting diseases such as ulcerative colitis, hypertension, or renal disease. Toxemias are also associated with complications such as abruptio placentae, afibrinogenemia, and hemorrhage. At times vital organs such as the adrenal glands, kidneys, and pituitary glands may be impaired. With chronic hypertensive disease, cerebral vascular hemorrhage is a common occurrence. It is therefore imperative that, following delivery, every woman with toxemia be followed for a year or two by having urine and blood pressure checked toward maintenance of optimum health.

Toxemia is present in 6% to 7% of all pregnancies. The number of infant and maternal deaths would be reduced greatly with early and continuous medical supervision during pregnancy. Early detection with prompt treatment of symptoms affords a healthy outlook for the mother and the baby.

CLASSIFICATION OF TOXEMIAS

The following classification recently revised by the American Committee on Maternal Welfare is now being widely used:

- I. Acute toxemia of pregnancy (onset after twenty-fourth week)
  - A. Preeclampsia
    1. Mild
    2. Severe
  - B. Eclampsia (convulsions or coma, usually both, when associated with hypertension, proteinuria, and edema)
- II. Chronic hypertensive (vascular) disease with pregnancy
  - A. Without superimposed acute toxemia (no exacerbation of hypertension or development of proteinuria)
    1. Hypertension known to have antedated pregnancy
    2. Hypertension discovered in pregnancy (before the twenty-fourth week and with postpartal persistence)
  - B. With superimposed acute toxemia
- III. Unclassified toxemia (data insufficient to differentiate the diagnosis)

ETIOLOGY OF TOXEMIAS

The exact etiology of toxemias is unknown; however, there is a specific nutritional deficiency involving amino acids. This results in abnormal metabolism of placental steroids, causing an electrolyte imbalance with sodium retention, vasospasm, and pathologic lesions. Many of the pathologic changes result from secondary tissue anoxia.

There is a growing impression that there is a functional derangement of vitamin B_6 metabolism in toxemias of pregnancy. The deficiency leads to failure of ingestion or absorption of pyridoxine (vitamin B_6) with further depletion as the unborn baby's demands are met. In toxemic women there has been found a marked pyridoxine deficiency in the placenta. Further studies are still being done relative to nutrition.

Human pregnancy nutrition is a field that has been researched and needs to be applied. Improving the nutrition of the poor will ultimately eliminate metabolic toxemia of late pregnancy. At the White House Conference in Washington, D. C., on December 4, 1969, President Richard Nixon stated, "Malnutrition during pregnancy is a cause of defective infants and children."

A study conducted by Dr. Thomas Brewer in Richmond, California, at the county prenatal clinic, showed a marked decrease in premature births when nutritional education was stressed. The newer trend is to discuss adequate protein, salt, and caloric intake during pregnancy.

ACUTE TOXEMIA

Preeclampsia

The signs and symptoms of toxemia are evident during prenatal visits. The first of the triad to appear is sudden and excessive weight gain during the last trimester. A gain in weight of more than 1 pound a week is significant of fluid retention in the tissues. Visible pitting edema is a sign of prolonged tissue hydration. Edema becomes apparent in the dependent body parts such as the feet and ankles. Following a period of rest, the fluid will become distributed throughout the body, resulting in puffiness of the face (especially the eyelids), hands, and fingers.

Elevation in blood pressure usually follows the edema with an increase in systolic and diastolic pressures. Increases in systolic readings of 30 mm. Hg or more and diastolic readings of 90 mm. Hg or more are definite signs of preeclampsia. The higher the systolic and diastolic readings, the more severe the preeclampsia. A finding of 140 systolic and 90 diastolic is considered borderline between a normal and an abnormal reading. However, any rise (as just stated) is equally as significant were not the 140/90 borderline reached—for example, a change from 100/60 to 130/90 would be more significant than a change from 130/80 to 140/90. Again, rises are more significant in the very young and the old during pregnancy. Change in the diastolic reading is also more important since it is a far better indication of peripheral vascular spasm. Elevations in systolic readings of more than 200 are related to hypertension existing before pregnancy.

Proteinuria, the last sign of the triad, indicates a serious disturbance in vascular physiology. The excretion of protein, normally reabsorbed in the kidney tubules, is indicative of altered permeability of the glomerular membrane.

The triad of symptoms described may go unnoticed were the mother not under medical supervision, since she may feel perfectly well. However, as time goes on, if treatment has not been instituted, there may be complaints of dizziness, with frontal or occipital headaches. As cerebral edema becomes marked, blurring of vision and scotoma (spots before the eyes) may cause temporary blindness. Ophthalmic examination reveals varying degrees of retinal arteriolar spasm and retinal hemorrhage. Epigastric pain, a serious complaint, is indicative of liver distention with subcapsular hemorrhage. Epigastric pain, hyperactive reflexes, and extreme irritability and vomiting are warnings of impending convulsions with ensuing eclampsia. Convulsions in the eclamptic mother occur with subsequent cerebral anoxia.

Eclampsia

Eclampsia, a sequela of preeclampsia, is characterized by clonic and tonic convulsions followed by a period of unconsciousness or coma. It may occur during the antepartal, intrapartal, or postpartal period—in the majority of instances (50%) it occurs during pregnancy. Eclampsia is seen more often in twin pregnancies, hydramnios, diabetes, hydatidiform mole, or extrauterine pregnancies.

The early signs and symptoms prior to a convulsion are severe epigastric pain (at times described as a tightening in the chest), extreme apprehension, irritability, and vomiting. The convulsion may occur during sleep. When awake, a fixed stare, dilated pupils, and twitching of the facial muscles about the mouth may be indicative of an imminent convulsion. A few seconds later the body becomes rigid, and all body muscles become tense and contracted for approximately 30 seconds. At the height of the convulsion, there are violent contractions and relaxations of the whole body, the teeth are tightly clenched, the face is cyanotic, and respirations cease. The convulsive stage lasts 1 to 2 minutes, is followed by a short period of apnea, and then suddenly breathing is resumed. Coma follows, and the mother remembers nothing of what occurred. Cyanosis, frothing at the mouth, and sudden vomiting may also occur.

Eclampsia is characterized by an increase in pulse and respiratory rates, exaggerated reflexes, a decrease in urinary output, and a rise in basal temperature. Convulsions may terminate in heart failure, cerebral hemorrhage, liver damage, and afibrinogenemia. The first convulsion may be a forerunner of more to follow, and often one leads rapidly into another. When convulsions continue, death ensues. In antepartal eclampsia a sudden convulsion may initiate rapid labor and delivery. The greater the number of convulsions the greater tendency toward fetal death from anoxia.

BIOCHEMISTRY VARIATIONS IN TOXEMIAS

The following variations occur in body chemistry: (1) salt and water retention over and above that of normal pregnancy; (2) edema is an entirely new change beyond that found in normal pregnancy; (3) salt retention and water retention are not connected—it is not known whether they result from a disorder of water metabolism or a disorder of sodium metabolism; (4) postpartum weight loss is greater in the mother with toxemia; and (5) decreased ability to concentrate sodium chloride above and beyond that of normal pregnancy.

It is believed that the mechanism of salt and water retention is unknown but can be explained on the basis of simple causes of edema such as increased capillary permeability or an increase in intracapillary pressure with a decrease in plasma oncotic pressure.

In normal pregnancy there is an increased rate of glomerular filtration with augmentation in tubular reabsorption. In acute toxemia, since the rate of glomerular filtration is depressed, a similar reduction or reabsorption by the distal tubules results in sodium retention. However, it is still uncertain that this is the primary mechanism.

A few days before eclampsia occurs, there are alterations in blood concentration. A rise in blood serum proteins and an increase in cell volume and hemoglobin occur as blood and plasma volumes decrease. Improvement in eclampsia is therefore associated with blood dilution, while increased levels connote severity of the condition. Rises in uric acid concentration in the blood indicate the inability of proper uric acid excretion by the kidneys. The blood chlorides and the carbon dioxide combining power of blood are reduced in eclampsia.

Following a convulsion acidosis occurs, evidenced by an increase in hydrogen ion concentration of blood. This explains the deep breathing noticed as the mother gets rid of carbonic acid. Accumulation of acids in the blood is a result of muscular activity during convulsions. As convulsions subside, organic acids are oxidized. This results in a release of sodium, which combines with water and carbon dioxide, restoring the alkali body reserve. Occasionally there are a temporary hyperglycemia and an increase in blood lactic acid following a convulsion because of muscular activity.

A urinary estriol excretion level is a simple, rapid, inexpensive method of determining various abnormalities of late pregnancy. Low levels and those dropping to 6 mg./24 hr. suggest a risk of intrauterine death within 48 hours. In toxemia, a lowered estriol level may correlate with retarded fetal growth with the presence of albuminuria between 30 and 36 weeks gestation. Estriol levels are also determined when there is a history of unexplained stillbirths or placental insufficiency.

Treatment. The primary objective in the treatment of acute toxemia is the prevention of eclampsia. Immediate treatment of the signs and symptoms assures control so that pregnancy is maintained until the baby is viable outside the uterus.

The only cure for toxemia is delivery of the fetus. Once symptoms are under control and urinary output is adequate, induction of labor is begun. Early induction prevents sustained damage to maternal tissues and improves chances of fetal survival. (For induction methods, see Chapter 20.) Should induction of labor be unsuccessful, cesarean section is performed. During delivery pudendal block, caudal block, or saddle block anesthesia is preferable so as not to depress the fetus. Administration of tranquilizing drugs and liberal use of oxygen, either by mask or nasal catheter, during labor are recommended.

In mild preeclampsia prescribed treatment is carried out by the mother at home. Weekly prenatal visits will determine subsequent treatment. Marked improvement occurs in many women who follow a low-sodium, high-protein diet, with supplemental vitamins, minerals, and added hours of bed rest. This type of diet promotes fluid tissue loss, which relieves edema. Bed rest mobilizes tissue fluid, resulting in diuresis, weight loss, and reduction in blood pressure. If signs and symptoms do not subside but become aggravated, the mother is hospitalized.

In severe preeclampsia the mother is admitted to the hospital for treatment. Along with diet and bed rest a toxemia regimen is started immediately. Complete bed rest is assured by starting barbiturates such as phenobarbital (Luminal), which is relatively long lasting, in small doses, ½ to 1 gr. three times daily.

Control of convulsions is necessary in toxemia of pregnancy. Magnesium sulfate is an anticonvulsant drug that controls cerebral irritability and also causes a lowering of blood pressure. Neuromuscular transmission is blocked, and the rate of secretion of acetylcholine liberated by motor nerve impulses is decreased. Dosage varies from 4 to 10 gm. initially (according to body weight), and a sustaining dose of 5 gm. every 6 hours is continued. Magnesium sulfate therapy warrants frequent checking of the deep tendon reflexes and urinary output. Deep tendon reflexes will disappear before respiratory paralysis occurs; therefore the drug should be discontinued if reflexes become sluggish.

Since magnesium sulfate is painful and irritating to tissues, 0.5 ml. of procaine hydrochloride (Novocain) 1% is added to each 4 gm. of magnesium sulfate and injected deep into the tissues. Deep injection is followed by massage of the area. Intravenous injections are given slowly since there may be a marked decrease in the respiratory rate, resulting in dizziness, diaphoresis, and vomiting. In high concentrations the magnesium ion depresses the myocardium. If this occurs, calcium gluconate is administered to prevent cardiac arrest. Reflexes and respirations are checked frequently and always prior to repeating a dose of magnesium sulfate. Magnesium sulfate is contraindicated when there is renal suppression and in the cardiac patient who has pulmonary edema.

Veratrum chloride in the form of Unitensen (5 mg.) is given in a 500 ml. solution of 20% glucose with hydralazine (Apresoline), 20 mg. Veratrum alkaloids cause hypotension, bradycardia, reduced renal blood flow, and reduction in renal output. Apresoline increases cerebral circulation, which is of advantage to mothers with toxemia.

Reserpine (Serpasil), the refined active principle of *Rauwolfia serpentina,* is an effective, safe, central vasodepressor that reduces vasoconstriction and hypertension and simultaneously increases organ blood and oxygen perfusion. Side effects are bradycardia and nasal congestion in the mother and the fetus. Dosage consists of 5 to 10 mg. intramuscularly or intravenously initially. This becomes effective in 30 minutes, has its maximum effect in 1 to 2 hours, and has a duration of 6 to 12 hours. The intramuscular dose of 5 mg. may be repeated every 6 hours if needed. When cerebral irritability is decreased and there is a significant drop in blood pressure, induction of labor is safe.

Paraldehyde, a safe and effective drug, keeps the eclamptic patient quiet and lowers blood pressure. Paraldehyde may be administered intramuscularly or may be mixed with equal parts of olive oil (to prevent rectal mucosa irritation). It is given as a retention enema.

Morphine sulfate (gr. ¼) is given to the severe preeclamptic patient as a central nervous system depressant. Morphine has a tendency to decrease respirations. This decrease in respirations may decrease carbon dioxide excretion by the lungs, with resulting acidosis. At times pruritus of the body (especially the nose) and vomiting occur.

A solution of 500 ml. of 20% dextrose administered intravenously has proved valuable in increasing urinary output, supplying caloric intake, and producing diuresis since this is a hypertonic solution.

Diuretics that act directly on the kidneys are used to get rid of tissue fluid, relieving excessive edema. Treatment is always given for a 3-day or 4-day period because prolonged administration of diuretics produces potassium depletion with resulting acidosis. Acetazolamide (Diamox), 250 mg., or chlorothiazide (Diuril), 0.5 to 1 gm., given daily for a 5-day period is commonly used. These drugs increase urinary output by blocking reabsorption of sodium and chlorides by the kidney tubules.

Although the preceding recommendations for control of the symptoms of toxemia are being practiced in most obstetric units, the current research by Dr. Thomas Brewer and others stresses the importance of an adequate, nutritious diet and the elimination of low-salt diets and diuretics for the prevention of toxemia. Doctors and nurses who work closely with pregnant women (especially those of the lower socioeconomic group) should stress and teach the importance of a scientific, nutritious diet. Women who are malnourished during pregnancy are more likely to develop symptoms of toxemia. The edema that normally occurs in women during the last 6 weeks of pregnancy is not to be confused with that of metabolic toxemia of pregnancy.

Nursing care. Care of the mother with toxemia requires expertness on the nurse's part in observing, planning, and evaluating the progress made through treatment. The mother with toxemia needs to understand why she is being hospitalized and the reasons for absolute bed rest, restriction of activity and visitors, and the medical regime ordered. When the mother is thus informed, she may readily accept the limitations, and there is less anxiety. Since normally pregnancy does not require hospitalization until labor and delivery are near, the apprehension and anxiety are coupled with feelings of fear of the baby's health, her own health, separation from family members that was not expected, and added financial burdens.

The alteration in diet needs to be explained as an essential part of the treatment. Perhaps food likes and dislikes and cultural food habits might be discussed with the dietitian to encourage adequate nutrition. Although the diet is limited, the importance of adequate nutrition during treatment for toxemia is essential. The mother who does not eat the food served may be depriving herself and the baby of essential nutriments.

Since many of the medications depress the central nervous system, there is also interference with vital body functions such as respirations. A rapid decrease in respirations will ultimately decrease oxygen supply to the fetus. A mother who has toxemia will give birth to an infant who has had a perilous intrauterine existence and who will have an equally perilous neonatal existence. A drop in estriol excretion is indicative of increasing severity of the maternal toxemia with a possibility of increasing fetal hypoxia. Delivery room personnel should be in readiness for the prevention of respiratory distress in the infant and for the maintenance of a normal blood pH. Oxygen administration and maintenance of body temperature are important for survival.

Fetal heart tones and vital signs are checked every 4 hours. The mother who is heavily sedated may need oxygen if the fetal heart tones decrease in rate. Provisions for adequate ventilation and quiet in the immediate environment augment the effect of sedation. If magnesium sulfate is chosen as a method of treatment, astute observation of vital signs is imperative. Respirations that become depressed should be reported immediately, and administration of calcium gluconate will prevent cardiac arrest. Extreme apprehension and irritability should be reported so that further sedation can be given to prevent convulsions and coma.

A tongue blade, oxygen apparatus, and cardiac stimulants should be readily available for emergency use. Should a convulsion occur, the tongue blade is inserted to prevent injury to the tongue and to keep an open airway. The nurse assures protection from injury by padding bedrails and loosening any tight clothing. Keeping a record of the length of time the convulsion lasts and the behavior of the mother following the attack is important. Checking the perineum is essential since a rapid labor and delivery may occur. Labor and delivery units would of necessity provide emergency sterile equipment to care for the mother and baby should delivery occur.

Nursing care of the preeclamptic and eclamptic mother requires astute observation, the reporting of exaggerated symptoms, followed by immediate administration of medication to prevent eclampsia. Following delivery the same precautions are taken since toxemia symptoms may still continue. With adequate and early treatment, however, the symptoms of toxemia subside following delivery.

SELECTED REFERENCES

Brewer, T. F.: Limitations of diuretic therapy in the management of severe toxemia, Amer. J. Obstet. Gynec. **83**:1351, 1962.

Brewer, T. F.: Metabolic toxemia of late pregnancy: a disease entity, Gynaecologia **167**:1, 1969.

Brewer, T. F.: Good prenatal nutrition prevents toxemia of late pregnancy, Postgrad. Med. **39**:119, 1966.

Brewer, T. F.: Human pregnancy nutrition: a clinical view, Obstet. Gynec. **30**:605, 1967.

Brewer, T. F.: Don't curse the darkness . . . light a candle! Reflections on the problem of maternal and infant mortality in the United States, J. Appl. Nutr. **20**:23, Summer, 1968.

Brewer, T. F.: Scientific nutrition in clinical obstetrics, Med. Tribune, July 18, 1968.

Brewer, T. F.: Why we need a new view of nutrition in human pregnancy, Curr. Med. Dig. **36**:995, 1968.

Carmichael, S. M., and others: Oral contraceptives, hypertension and toxemia, Obstet. Gynec. **35**(3):371-376, 1970

Donnelly, J. F.: Toxemias of pregnancy, Amer. J. Nurs. **61**:98, 1961.

Duhring, J. M., and Greene, J. W.: Evaluation of intrauterine fetal status, Clin. Obstet. Gynec. **9**:4, 1966.

Eastman, N. J., and Hellman, L. M.: Williams obstetrics, ed. 13, New York, 1966, Appleton-Century-Crofts.

Hassan, H. M., and Falls, F. H.: The young primipara, Amer. J. Obstet. Gynec. **88**: 256, 1964.

Heap, B.: Sodium restricted diets, Amer. J. Nurs. **60**:206, 1960.

Heap, R. F., and others: Estriol excretion in abnormal pregnancy, Obstet. Gynec. **33**:3, 1969.

Hogue, C., and Couch, K.: Care of patients with toxemia, Amer. J. Nurs. **61**:101, 1961.

Holman, G. H.: Effect of toxemia of pregnancy on the fetus and neonate, Clin. Obstet. Gynec. **9**:4, 1966.

Israel, S. L.: Teen-age obstetrics, Amer. J. Obstet. Gynec. **85**:659, 1963.

Johnson, W. D.: Malnutrition and pregnancy, Delaware Med. J. **41**:339, 1969.

Juzwiak, M.: Toxemia and prenatal care, RN **26**:69, 1963.

Klieger, J. A., Evrard, J. R., and Pierce, R.: Abnormal pyridoxine metabolism in toxemia of pregnancy, Amer. J. Obstet. Gynec. **94**:316, 1966.

McLaverty, M. P., Pavlic, R. S., and Smith, C. J.: Program for toxemia control. Amer. J. Obstet. Gynec. **92**:100, 1965.

Nyirjesy, I., and others: Clinical significance of total weight gain during pregnancy, Obstet. Gynec. **32**:3, 1968.

Palomaki, J. F., and Lindheimer, M. D.: Sodium depletion simulating deterioration in a toxemic pregnancy, New Eng. J. Med., Jan. 8, 1970.

Peckos, P. S., and Heald, F. P.: Nutrition of adolescents, Children **11**:26, January-February, 1964.

Rodman, M.: Drugs for the toxemia of pregnancy, RN **21**:67, June, 1958.

Rogers, S. F., and others: Aggressive toxemia management: pre-eclampsia and eclampsia, Obstet. Gynec. **33**:5, 1969.

Saifer, J. D.: Convulsions and coma in pregnancy, Amer. J. Obstet. Gynec. **85**:623, 1962.

Sands, R.: Obesity and pregnancy, Amer. J. Obstet. Gynec. **83**:1617, 1962.

Schwartz, L. L.: Pre-eclampsia and eclampsia early in pregnancy, Amer. J. Obstet. Gynec. **84**:1330, 1962.

Spindler, E. B.: Better diets for teenagers, Nurs. Outlook **13**:32, February, 1964.

Wohl, M. C., and Goodhart, R. S.: Modern nutrition in health and disease, Philadelphia, 1968, Lea & Febiger.

Zickefoose, M.: Nutrition during pregnancy, Delaware Med. J. **41**:121, 1969.

Questions for study

1. Mrs. J., 17 years old, is first seen for an initial prenatal visit at 32 weeks gestation. Before pregnancy she weighed 97 pounds and now weighs 131 pounds. Her urinalysis is negative, and her blood pressure is 128/88. While talking with her in preparation for the visit, she tells you she feels fine and has no complaints. Following the visit the doctor orders a 2-gm. salt 1,200-calorie diet and tells her to return to the clinic in 2 weeks. How would you proceed in helping Mrs. J. in light of the preceding history and recommended therapy?
2. When Mrs. J. returns in 2 weeks, she tells you she has not been feeling well and has experienced dizziness with headaches. Her weight is now 135 pounds, urinalysis negative, and blood pressure 148/98. The doctor orders immediate hospitalization with the following treatment:
   a. Absolute bed rest
   b. Weigh daily
   c. 2-gm. sodium high-protein 1,200-calorie diet
   d. Phenobarbital, 30 mg. t.i.d.
   e. Intake and output
   f. Vital signs q. 4 h.
   g. Check fetal heart tones daily
   h. Observe and report any signs of labor

In light of these orders, how would you proceed in admitting Mrs. J.? Explain the reasons for the orders and how you would plan her care.

3. Following a 2-week hospital stay Mrs. J. weighs 125 pounds, urinalysis is negative, blood pressure is 120/76, and she is discharged. She is now at 36 weeks gestation and is to return to the prenatal clinic in 1 week. How would you prepare her for going home?
4. Mrs. P., a gravida IV para III, is admitted at 37 weeks gestation with a severe preeclampsia. Mrs. P. has evidence of facial edema, excessive weight gain, an elevation in blood pressure of 178/110, and a 2+ albuminuria. On admission the orders read:
   a. Absolute bed rest
   b. Weigh daily
   c. Nothing P.O.
   d. Morphine sulfate, gr. ¼, stat. I.M.
   e. 1,000 ml. 20% glucose in water intravenously
   f. Magnesium sulfate, 8 gm. stat. I.M. with Novocain, 1 ml.
   g. Vital signs q. 4 h.
   h. Check fetal heart tones q. 1 h.
   i. Check urine b.i.d. for albumin
   j. Send blood to laboratory for CO_2 combining power, blood urea nitrogen in morning
   k. Watch for signs of labor

   Explain this method in treatment. How would you proceed in giving Mrs. P. safe nursing care?
5. Mrs. P. has been in the hospital 2 hours. You notice she is extremely restless, and her pressure augments and now reads 188/116. You immediately report your findings, and suddenly Mrs. P. starts to convulse. How would you proceed in giving safe care during the convulsion? Following the convulsion?
6. Mrs. G., a 17-year-old gravida I para 0, arrived at the clinic for her second prenatal visit. She is in the last trimester of pregnancy, and you observe that her face is puffy and now her legs and ankles appear quite edematous. As you talk with her she tells you she feels miserable and is having severe headaches and blurred vision, which started the day before. She stated, "Although I've been taking the water pills, I can't seem to pass much water."

   On examination her urinalysis reveals a 4+ proteinuria, weight 139 pounds, a gain of 5 pounds. Her blood pressure is 152/96.

   The doctor admits Mrs. G. to the hospital and writes the following orders:
   a. Bed rest
   b. Daily weight
   c. Low-salt, high-protein 1,200-calorie diet
   d. Phenobarbital, 30 mg. q.i.d.
   e. Intake and output
   f. Insert Foley catheter
   g. Diuril, 0.5 gm. daily
   h. B.P. and F.H. q. 4 h.
   i. T.P.R. q. 4 h.
   j. Watch for signs of labor

   Relate and discuss the purpose for each of the preceding orders and plan for nursing care of Mrs. G.
7. Mrs. Y., a gravida V para IV, arrives at the emergency room with "severe headache that won't go away" and states, "I feel real bad." She is 36 weeks pregnant and has had no prenatal care. Her blood pressure is 200/112, proteinuria 4+, she has pitting edema of the extremities, and she has had scanty urine for a few days. Mrs. Y. is immediately admitted to the labor and delivery unit. She is put in a private room, and you are assigned to care for her. Orders are as follows:
   a. Strict bed rest
   b. Morphine sulfate, gr. ¼ stat.
   c. Check B.P. and F.H. q. 2 h.
   d. Intake and output
   e. Vital signs q. 4 h.
   f. Magnesium sulfate, 8 gm. stat.
   g. 1,000 ml. of 10% glucose in water intravenously
   h. Insert Foly catheter on continuous drainage
   i. Watch for signs of labor

   Relate and discuss the purpose of the preceding orders for Mrs. Y. What other equipment on the labor and delivery unit would assure her safe care? Plan for nursing care on Mrs. Y.
8. Mrs. Gomez, of Puerto Rican extraction, is a 17-year-old making her first visit to the clinic at 32 weeks gestation. Prior to becoming pregnant she weighed 97 pounds and now weighs 121 pounds. Her urinalysis is negative for sugar, albumin, and acetone; her blood pressure is 128/88. As you talk with her she tells you she feels fine and has no complaints. Follow-

ing her visit the doctor orders a low-salt, high-protein diet.

a. In light of the preceding information and what you have read about toxemia, would you be concerned about Mrs. G.? Give scientific data to verify your suppositions.
b. How would you help her with the special ordered diet? Your plan should be based upon your knowledge of nutrition and principles of teaching.
c. To ensure a safe pregnancy for Mrs. Gomez, what other health teaching would you include in this visit?

9. Mrs. Yengo, a 37-year-old gravida II para I in her thirtieth week of pregnancy, returns for her second prenatal visit. She tells her obstetrician that she has been experiencing headaches and dizziness. She has gained 7 pounds in 1 month, her blood pressure was 120/78 and is now 148/98, and she has a +1 albuminuria. Her doctor orders immediate hospitalization with the following treatment:
   a. Bed rest
   b. Weigh daily
   c. Low-sodium, high-protein diet
   d. Phenobarbital, 30 mg. t.i.d.
   e. Diuril, 0.5 gm. daily 10 A.M.
   f. Record intake and output
   g. Check fetal heart tones daily

   Mrs. Yengo called her neighbor who was caring for 2-year-old Jane. Her neighbor agreed to care for Jane during Mrs. Yengo's hospital stay. Mr. Yengo was notified at his office of his wife's admittance.

   a. Why was Mrs. Yengo admitted for immediate treatment?
   b. With the preceding symptoms, how would you classify Mrs. Yengo's toxemia?
   c. Explain each of the preceding orders in the treatment.
   d. What nursing measures would you plan for her safe care?
   e. How woud you handle the sudden separation of Jane and her mother?

10. Mrs. Pin, a gravida IV para III, is admitted at 37 weeks gestation with a severe preeclampsia. Mrs. Pin has evidence of facial edema, excessive weight gain, a blood pressure of 178/100, and a 2+ albuminuria.

   The orders on admission follow:
   a. Absolute bed rest
   b. Nothing postoperatively
   c. Morphine sulfate, gr. 1/4 stat. I.M.
   d. 1,000 ml. 20% glucose in water I.V.
   e. Magnesium sulfate, 4 gm. stat. I.M. with Novocain, 1 ml.
   f. Vital signs q. 4 h.
   g. Urinalysis for albumin and acetone b.i.d.
   h. Blood to laboratory for CO_2 combining power, blood urea nitrogen
   i. Watch for signs of labor

   Explain the reasons for each of the preceding orders and their implications for Mrs. Pin.

   What nursing measures would you implement for safe care of Mrs. Pin and her baby?

CHAPTER 19

BLEEDING DURING THE MATERNITY CYCLE

In spite of the fact that obstetric hemorrhage continues to cause many maternal deaths, the decline in maternal mortality has been great. Maternal deaths in the United States in 1930 were 60 in 10,000 deliveries, and in 1963 there were 3.7 in 10,000 deliveries. The causes for decline in maternal mortality are the following: (1) almost all women are hospitalized for delivery; (2) there have been improvements in social conditions; (3) there are organized obstetric services that include public health; (4) there has been improvement in the standards of training of physicians and nurses who specialize in obstetrics; and (5) there has been much new scientific knowledge and research in the treatment of sepsis and the liberal use of transfusions.

Deaths from hemorrhage in the United States were 3.3 per 10,000 in 1944 and 0.59 per 10,000 in 1962. The drop in maternal death rate from hemorrhage is a result of the following: (1) any pregnant woman with bleeding is immediately hospitalized and observed; (2) all pregnant women are typed early; (3) blood is replaced immediately before a great loss occurs; and (4) hypofibrinogenemia, a causative factor, is treated with immediate intravenous injection of fibrogen.

Bleeding during pregnancy is an abnormal sign that warrants immediate medical attention. The most common causes of bleeding are either related to the cervix without interruption of pregnancy or to bleeding within the uterus that affects survival of the unborn baby.

Following is a classification of the causes of bleeding during the maternity cycle:

I. *Bleeding outside the uterus*
   A. Cervix
   B. Lacerations
   C. Erosions
   D. Polyps
   E. Carcinoma in situ

II. *Bleeding inside the uterus*
  A. Placental site
  B. Defective germ plasm
  C. Improper implantation site
  D. Detachment of placenta
III. *Bleeding during first trimester of pregnancy*
  A. Abortions (complete or incomplete)
    1. Spontaneous — Habitual, Missed
    2. Induced — Therapeutic, Criminal
  B. Ectopic pregnancy
  C. Hydatidiform mole
IV. *Bleeding during third trimester of pregnancy*
  A. Placenta previa
    1. Marginal
    2. Partial
    3. Complete
  B. Abruptio placentae
    1. Afibrinogenemia
  C. Incompetent cervix
V. *Postpartum hemorrhage*
  A. Atony of the uterus
  B. Vaginal and cervical tears
  C. Retained placental fragments

BLEEDING OUTSIDE THE UTERUS

Bleeding outside the uterus will be discussed in Chapter 27.

BLEEDING DURING THE FIRST TRIMESTER OF PREGNANCY

Abortions

Interruption of pregnancy before the baby is viable (approximately 28 weeks gestation, 1,000 grams) is called abortion. To the lay person the word *abortion* connotes an induced criminal act—therefore the term *miscarriage* is used more often. Abortions are categorized with regard to causes and the course of evolving signs and symptoms.

Spontaneous abortions follow two clinical patterns: (1) a complete abortion, in which the entire products of conception are expelled and (2) an incomplete abortion, in which a part of the products of conception is expelled.

Induced abortions are of two types: (1) therapeutic, in which there is instrumental interference to terminate pregnancy for some grave and hazardous maternal disease; and (2) criminal, in which pregnancy is interrupted without medical or legal consultation.

Of all pregnancies, 10% terminate in abortions. During the early months of pregnancy abortions are usually preceded by death of the fetus. Fetal death is a result of abnormalities of the ovum and sperm, a systemic maternal disease, or abnormalities of the reproductive tract. Of the three causes, abnormalities of the ovum and sperm are most frequent. A systemic maternal disease with severe acute infections in the mother, such as pneumonia or pyelitis, causes death as bacteria invade the developing baby.

An incidence of three consecutive abortions is known as habitual abortion. Repeated abortions are related to endocrine imbalances or may be of psychogenic origin. Abnormalities of the reproductive tract, such as displacements of the uterus, growths within the uterus, or an incompetent cervix, are infrequent causes of abortions.

A missed abortion, one in which the fetus dies and is not expelled, is characterized by periodic spotting at the time of menses and no further growth in the size of the uterus on pelvic examination.

Clinical course and treatment. First trimester bleeding may indicate threatened abortion. Absolute bed rest and astute observation of the amount and length of time bleeding persists are essential. Hormonal preparations such as thyroid and progesterone derivatives may be ordered if deficiencies are the cause. However, if bleeding persists, with the onset of uterine contractions and cervical effacement and dilatation, abortion is inevitable.

With persistent bleeding, the mother is hospitalized, and immediate blood typing, Rh, and crossmatching of blood are done. Whole blood is always available if hemorrhage ensues. As labor progresses, the products of conception are eventually expelled either completely or incompletely. With incomplete abortion, dilatation and curettage of the uterus are performed under aseptic technique. Vigilance in observing for beginning infection is imperative since lowered resistance augments the incidence of bacterial invasion.

The quantity of bleeding is difficult to measure. Recording the frequency of perineal pad changes and the amount of pad saturation gives an estimate of blood loss. Checking the blood pressure and pulse is vital to control inevitable hemorrhage and imminent shock.

Ectopic pregnancy

A pregnancy implanted outside the uterus is known as an ectopic pregnancy (Fig. 19-1). The most frequent site is within the middle or interstitial portion of the fallopian tube. Other sites are the abdomen, ovaries, or cervix. Ectopic pregnancy occurs in one out of every two hundred pregnancies and is more frequent in nonwhites than in whites. The high frequency in nonwhite people is attributed to pelvic inflammatory disease. Other causes are the following: (1) obstruction in the passage of the fertilized ovum into the uterus, such as congenital developmental anomalies; (2) infections that have caused narrowing or cicatrization (scar formation of the fallopian tube); (3) tumors pressing against the fallopian tube;

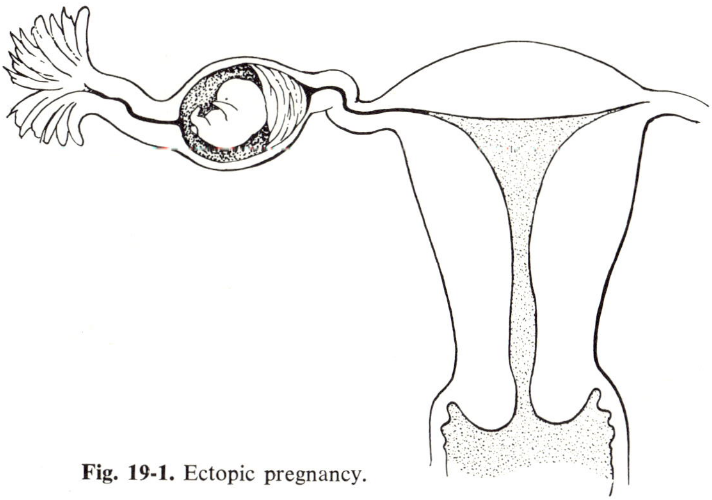

Fig. 19-1. Ectopic pregnancy.

(4) abnormal growth of the fertilized ovum in which it becomes immobilized in the tubes; and (5) previous plastic surgery of the fallopian tube.

Clinical course and treatment. Early signs and symptoms of ectopic pregnancy are usually concealed. As pregnancy progresses, death of the fetus and rupture of the tube occur, resulting in hemorrhage and shock. Early complaints of right or left ovarian pain are suggestive of a possible tubal pregnancy. Following one or two missed menstrual periods, spotting may or may not occur. Complaints of pain radiating to the shoulder following activity or heavy lifting need further investigation. A positive determining factor is the experiencing of pain when there is slight motion of the cervix on pelvic examination.

If unruptured tubal pregnancy is diagnosed, removal of the tube is indicated. Ruptured ectopic pregnancy characterized by sudden pain with abdominal tenderness is indicative of concealed bleeding with impending shock. Whole blood is immediately replaced parenterally, and surgical intervention is pursued when the mother's condition permits.

Hydatidiform mole

Hydatidiform mole is an abnormal pregnancy in which there is a benign growth (neoplasm) of the chorion. The chorionic villi become a mass of clear vesicles, and usually there is no evidence of an embryo. Occasionally when the fetus is present, the mole is a part of the placenta. Since the vesicles grow so rapidly, the pregnancy often encompasses a uterine space capacity of a 6-month or 7-month pregnancy.

Hydatidiform mole is rare, occurring once in every 2,000 pregnancies. There is a greater frequency in older pregnant women of 40 to 50 years of age and in the young women of childbearing age.

Clinical course and treatment. Bleeding characterized by spotting or profuse hemorrhage is the outstanding sign of hydatidiform mole. Spontaneous expulsion usually occurs between the sixteenth through the eighteenth weeks, pregnancy rarely going beyond 18 weeks. The rapid stretching of the uterus to accommodate the growing mole may cause pain and symptoms of toxemia before the last trimester.

The diagnosis of hydatidiform mole is ascertained with the following observations: (1) continuous or intermittent brownish-colored bleeding commencing after 12 weeks gestation; (2) excessive enlargement of the uterus not consistent with the number of gestation weeks; (3) signs and symptoms of toxemia prior to the usual third trimester; (4) difficulty in outlining and determining fetal parts by abdominal palpation; and (5) a high chorionic gonadotropin level in the serum at 12 weeks (ruling out twin pregnancy).

Dangers of hydatidiform mole are hemorrhage, infection, uterine perforation, and susceptibility to choriocarcinomas. Treatment consists of evacuation of the mole to empty the uterus and terminate bleeding. Should spontaneous evacuation not occur and bleeding become severe, evacuation with an ovum forceps is indicated. Expertness is paramount since the uterus is soft and easily perforated. At times if bleeding is not severe, oxytocics are given to evacuate the uterus. Blood and antibiotics are administered to prevent shock and infection. With spontaneous evacuation and severe bleeding, dilatation and curettage are delayed until homeostasis occurs.

Follow-up care for a hydatidiform mole is as important as the immediate treatment. Women are encouraged to avoid a new pregnancy in order that chorionic gonadotropin levels can be measured. Therefore contraceptive measures are discussed immediately following delivery so that weekly serum levels can be checked for 2 months. Should gonadotropin levels remain persistent or rise with bleeding and subinvolution, a second curettage is done. Continued rises in serum levels necessitate immediate hysterectomy (removal of the uterus). Follow-up serum levels are indicated for 1 year to rule out metastasis from a choriocarcinoma. When metastasis is present, radiation and chemotherapy are indicated.

BLEEDING DURING THE THIRD TRIMESTER OF PREGNANCY

Placenta previa

Placental inefficiencies are responsible for bleeding during the last trimester. Normally the embryo settles in the fundal portion of the uterus since the site is succulent and provides increased nourishment. At times, however, implantation occurs in the lower uterine segment close to or covering the cervix. This is known as placenta previa.

Variations of attachment are the following: (1) marginal placenta previa (Fig. 19-2, *A*) in which the placental edge is close to the internal os (yet not extending the margin) and can be palpated by the examining finger; (2) partial placenta previa (Fig. 19-2, *B*) in which the placenta partially covers the internal os; and (3) central placenta previa (Fig. 19-2, *C*) in which the placenta completely covers the internal os.

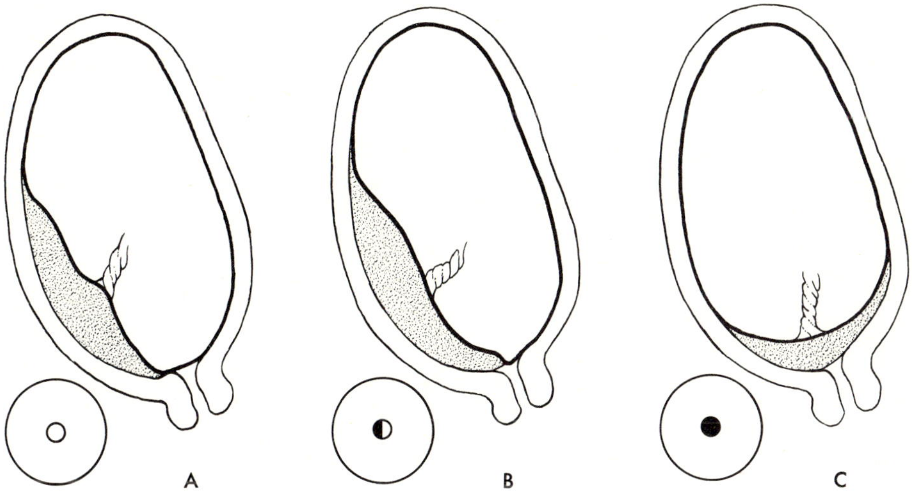

Fig. 19-2. Placenta previa. **A,** Marginal. **B,** Partial. **C,** Central.

Incidence and cause. Placenta previa occurs in approximately one in every two hundred deliveries. The marginal type is most common; the central type is least common. Placenta previa is believed to occur more frequently in multigravidas, and the incidence increases with increase in number of pregnancies. Because of atrophic changes in the endometrium, the placenta sometimes spreads out in an attempt to obtain adequate nourishment—this results in low implantation.

Diagnosis. If the mother's condition permits, amniography or placentography may be done. If amniography is done, the mother empties her bladder, and the anterior abdominal wall is cleansed with pHisoHex and a 1:1,000 tincture of merthiolate preparation. Under a 1% or 2% Xylocaine local anesthesia, amniocentesis is performed with an 18-gauge needle. A dye is injected (the amount depends upon the number of weeks gestation and the size of the fetus), and the mother is instructed to move about freely. In 30 minutes roentgenographic examination is done. Auscultation of the fetal heart is done prior to and following amniography.

In placentography an x-ray machine scans the abdomen and locates the placental site. Pelvic examination to confirm placenta previa is hazardous. If the mother's condition warrants pelvic examination, whole blood should be available, and the procedure should be performed in the operating room with preparation for either vaginal delivery or cesarean section.

Symptoms. Painless bleeding is the only symptom of placenta previa.

Treatment. In the primigravida, cesarean section is the treatment of choice. In the multigravida, with a viable fetus weighing 2,500 grams and a soft and partially effaced cervix, premature rupture of the membranes controls bleeding as the pre-

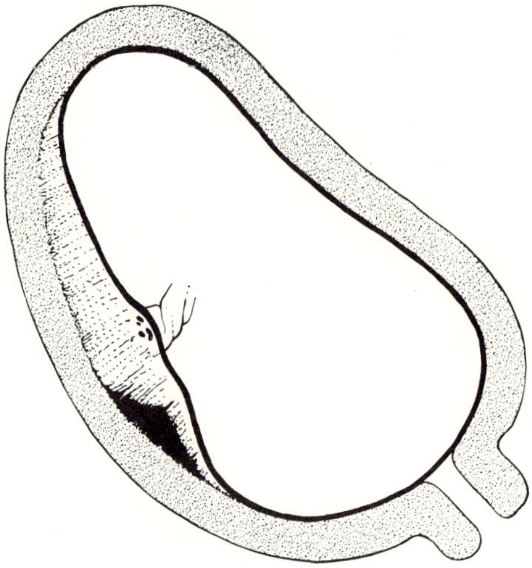

Fig. 19-3. Abruptio placentae.

senting part descends with pressure against the placenta. Usually labor commences shortly after rupture or descent of the presenting part against the placenta. With excessive bleeding, however, cesarean section is also the method of choice for the multigravida. Incision into the upper uterine segment (classical cesarean section) is done since entrance into the lower segment augments bleeding.

Abruptio placentae

Premature separation of a normally implanted placenta is known as abruptio placentae (Fig. 19-3). The clinical signs and symptoms are related to the degree of separation. A partially detached placenta causes external vaginal bleeding, whereas a totally detached placenta causes concealed bleeding. In 80% of women with abruptio placentae, bleeding is external, and in 20% bleeding is internal. The concealed type is the gravest and is seen frequently in women with hypertensive toxemia.

Abruptio placentae is more common during labor, and its symptoms can always be differentiated from those of placenta previa. In abruptio placentae the bleeding is usually concealed, and there is sharp and excruciating abdominal pain as the placenta suddenly separates. The abdomen becomes boardlike, and there is no uterine relaxation. Shock becomes imminent since the bleeding is concealed and copious.

Causes. The causes of abruptio placentae are obscure. Contributing factors may be a short cord and pressure of the enlarged uterus on the vena cava. Recent research by Hilbard indicates that a predisposing factor in 97.5% of mothers is defective foliate metabolism that occurs in the early weeks of pregnancy, causing irreversible injury to the fetus, chorion, and possibly the decidua. Multiparity is more important than age as an etiologic factor. Abruptio placentae shows a strong tendency to recur in subsequent pregnancies. A mother already predisposed to abruptio placentae may experience a recurrence when preeclampsia or chronic hypertension complicates pregnancy.

Hypofibrinogenemia is a blood clotting defect associated with abruptio placentae. It occurs in 10% of all cases of abruptio placentae and is more frequent in severe separation. Fibrinogen levels below 100 mg. per 100 ml. of blood interfere with blood coagulation. However, postpartum hemorrhage may be caused by uterine atony and not by afibrinogenemia.

In acute renal failure there is severe damage to the muscle fibers. The severe damage causes infiltration of blood, which releases myoglobin into the bloodstream. A spasm of the arterioles causes destruction of tissue in the kidney tubules, resulting in marked oliguria and renal failure.

Treatment. The immediate treatment for abruptio placentae is bed rest, replacement therapy of whole blood and fibrinogen, and then delivery. With lowered fibrinogen levels, 2 to 8 gm. of fibrinogen are added to 10% glucose in water and administered parenterally. Method of delivery depends upon the amount of bleeding and viability of the baby. Once hemorrhage is severe, the combination of replacement blood therapy and immediate cesarean section is the method of choice. However, if the baby has died in the uterus and if hemorrhage is controlled, induction of labor is attempted. Rupture of the membranes and oxytocin induction are followed by vaginal delivery. However, if there are signs of fetal distress, emergency cesarean section is performed. Cesarean section is never done until fibrinogen levels are replaced and symptoms of shock are alleviated. Vigilance following delivery is imperative since a flaccid uterus with continued hemorrhage may warrant hysterectomy.

INCOMPETENT CERVIX

Some women are unable to carry the fetus beyond the sixteenth or eighteenth gestational week because of incompetency of the internal os of the cervix. The history reveals repeated early rupture of the membranes and abortion in the middle of the second or beginning of the third trimester.

An incompetent cervix may be congenital or acquired. The acquired type may be a result of birth injury to the cervical canal or trauma during instrumental dilatation of the cervix. Dr. Shirodkar of India and Dr. Barter of the United States have devised a surgical correction by purse-string closure of the cervix. The purse-string is drawn tightly around the cervix after the first trimester of pregnancy and prior to the third trimester. At or near term the purse-string is cut so that normal labor and delivery may occur.

Another operation (devised by Lask) is done when the woman is not pregnant. Removal of a wedge of the internal cervical os and surgical closure result in a tighter canal structure.

POSTPARTUM HEMORRHAGE

Within the first 24 hours following delivery, bleeding in excess of 500 ml. is known as postpartum hemorrhage. Bleeding is the leading cause of maternal deaths, and postpartum hemorrhage is responsible for one quarter of these deaths. With blood loss there is a lowered resistance and greater susceptibility to puerperal infection. Vigilance of the nurse in checking the fundus and lochia for the first 24 hours is imperative.

Frequent causes of postpartum hemorrhage are the following: (1) atony of the uterus, (2) vaginal and cervical tears, and (3) retained placental fragments.

Atony of the uterus is the most common cause of postpartum hemorrhage immediately following delivery. Hemorrhage from retained placental fragments may occur subsequently and is usually a late cause of bleeding. A common practice is inspection of the placenta by the physician.

Contributing factors are overdistention of the uterus and multiparity. Causes that are controllable are prolonged labors, deep anesthesia, operative delivery (forceps application and episiotomy), and a difficult third stage of labor.

Postpartum hemorrhage is difficult to detect since bleeding is slow, persistent, and continuous. The usual signs and symptoms of shock such as rapid pulse, drop in blood pressure, pallor, shortness of breath, chills, air hunger, restlessness, and diaphoresis are not detected until late.

Palpation of the fundus for firmness is done often for the first few postpartum hours. Although there may be no visible vaginal bleeding, concealed hemorrhage may occur.

Treatment. Bleeding that results from the inability of the uterus to contract can be controlled. The nurse holds the uterus firmly between both hands, one hand holding it above the symphysis and the other gently massaging the fundal portion. An oxytocic, such as ergonovine maleate, gr. 1/320 (Ergotrate, 0.2 mg.), is ordered and administered intravenously. In addition, an intravenous solution of 5% glucose in water with 10 units of oxytocin continues to keep the fundus well contracted. Should these methods fail, the physician may hold the fundus firmly with one hand and compress the uterus vaginally with the other hand.

Bleeding resulting from vaginal or cervical tears is controlled by surgical repair. Fine absorbable catgut sutures are used.

Bleeding from retained placental fragments can be controlled only by manual removal. Many physicians explore the uterus routinely immediately following delivery to prevent retained fragments. Following manual removal of placental fragments, oxytocics are administered to keep the uterus firm.

Nursing care. The sight and loss of blood are of significance since they are closely related to feelings of losing life with eventual death. The many functions of blood, such as its ability to carry oxygen to the cells, to carry carbon dioxide from the cells to the lungs, to carry wastes such as nitrogen to the kidneys and digestive products to the liver, to carry sugars and proteins to cells for nourishment and survival, to carry hormones and vitamins to vital organs, to combat invasion of bacterial organisms, and to seal itself off to prevent loss, may not be entirely known, yet its essentiality for life is known universally.

Any bleeding would obviously bring about a chain of reactions such as fear, fright, worry, and anxiety. The effects in physiology due to emotional response need to be considered in the planning for nursing care. Since fright and fear produce a tachycardia with an increase in heart rate, increased blood loss occurs. The increase in epinephrine secretions in turn constricts blood vessels at a time when an attempt is being made to keep them dilated in order to replenish blood loss. The mother who asks, "Do you think I will lose my baby?" is also asking, "If I bleed long enough, will I also die?" Although many women do not verbalize these fears, they are universal.

Bleeding during pregnancy is often greater than is evident. It is an insidious flow that ultimately results in copious bleeding. Anxiety may be alleviated by explaining to the mother what will be done to help her and the baby. At times saying to the mother when she appears anxious, "I can well understand how upset you must be" will help her feel free to ventilate her feelings. It is, however, essential in emergencies to care for the blood loss immediately—yet the mother's feelings need never be forgotten.

The mother admitted for bleeding needs immediate blood work-up consisting of Rh and blood group typing, crossmatching, and available whole blood should she warrant transfusion. The nurse frequently checks vital signs. A lowering of blood pressure or an elevation in pulse is reported immediately. Blood loss is estimated by saving perineal pads and linens. Any continuous trickling of blood should be reported immediately. The rate, regularity, and strength of fetal heart tones in pregnancies beyond 20 weeks indicate the well-being of the baby. Changes in fetal heart tones are reported at once, and oxygen is administered to the mother until the physician institutes treatment. The abdomen is checked frequently for tenderness, tenseness, or any increase in size or irritability of the uterus. Complete bed rest in Trendelenburg position is enforced if bleeding has occurred. If bleeding is followed by the onset of labor, the constant "thereness" of the nurse is essential when a premature delivery is anticipated since sedation is withheld or used rather sparingly. Physical and emotional support by the medical team is paramount.

Operative intervention is preceded by shaving the abdominal wall from beneath the breast line and including the perineal area. If spinal anesthesia is to be administered, the lumbar area is also shaved in preparation. Preoperative medications are ordered with due respect for size and condition of the unborn baby. At times atropine sulfate is administered to dry up secretions prior to inhalation anesthesia and is given one-half hour prior to surgery. Parenteral therapy is begun with an 18-gauge needle so that blood may be administered if needed. When a premature or low birth weight infant is anticipated, preparation is made for an Isolette and for adequate aspiration and resuscitative measures. A pediatrician is also in attendance to care for the infant so that the obstetrician may devote entire attention to the mother.

Symptoms of shock include pallor, weakness, clammy skin, lowered blood pressure, and rapid weak pulse. Intravenous fluid equipment should be available at the bedside. Hypertonic solutions such as 6% dextran are ordered to keep the vessel open until whole blood is crossmatched. These solutions are known as plasma expanders since they stay in the vessel to prevent irreversible shock.

Postoperative care consists of vigilance in observing and checking vital signs, maintaining asepsis to prevent bacterial invasion, observing the abdominal dressing and vaginal area for excessive bleeding, and providing comfort and reassurance for the mother. It is well to remember that bleeding usually is noted on either side of the wound and often is not directly over the incisional site. Vaginal bleeding often goes unnoticed since the perineal pad may be only spotted—yet there may be trickling and continuous blood loss beneath the mother.

Postpartum hemorrhage in which the uterus fails to contract necessitates grasping the uterus between both hands just above the symphysis with gentle massage at the fundal portion. Oxytocics are ordered to aid in contracting the uterine muscles if the cause is loss of contractile power.

Since any bleeding necessitates hospitalization, the financial means of the family need to be considered. Many times this is a great worry to the already anxious mother, and the nurse makes referral to a social worker so that the family is alleviated of some of the financial responsibilities. Provisions for homemaker service may also help keep the family together if the father needs to work.

Spiritual care of mother and infant. In times of emergency spiritual attendance can be most comforting to the mother who is fearful and anxious about herself and her baby. She should be offered spiritual attendance regardless of religion. For the Roman Catholic, spiritual attendance before surgery relieves much anxiety associated with the fear of death. A minister or rabbi known to a Protestant or Jewish mother will give added strength and faith in times of stress.

Every nurse should be familiar with the procedure in administering the sacrament of Baptism to the baby of Roman Catholic or Christian parents. If the baby is in danger of death at birth, anyone, regardless of his own religious beliefs, may administer the sacrament of Baptism. The procedure is a simple one. At the same time water is poured over the infant's forehead, the words "I baptize thee in the name of the Father, and of the Son, and of the Holy Spirit" are spoken. It is also essential that this be charted and made known to the parents. When time permits a priest may be summoned. If the mother aborts early in pregnancy, the water is poured over the products of conception because the forehead may not be discernible.

Baptism is also administered in like manner to Protestant infants in danger of death.*

---

*Presbyterians, Methodists, Baptists, and Disciples of Christ believe that the child who dies unbaptized is immediately received into the presence of God; therefore to these infants the administration of the sacrament is meaningless. (Phillips, C.: RN, p. 61, April, 1966.)

SELECTED REFERENCES

Barter, R. H., Dusbabek, J. A., Riva, H. L., and Parks, J.: Surgical closure of incompetent cervix during pregnancy, Amer. J. Obstct. Gynec. **75**:511, 1958.

Berner, H.: Amniography, an accurate way to localize the placenta, Obstet. Gynec., vol. 29, no. 2, 1967.

Cianfrani, T., and others: Ectopic pregnancy, Amer. J. Nurs. **63**:93, April, 1963.

Eastman, N. J., and Hellman, L. M.: Williams obstetrics, ed. 13, New York, 1966, Appleton-Century & Appleton-Century-Crofts.

Goodrich, F.: Obstetric hemorrhage, Amer. J. Nurs. **62**:96, November, 1962.

Greenhill, J. P.: Obstetrics, ed. 13, Philadelphia, 1965, W. B. Saunders Co.

Hilbard, B. M.: Abruptio placentae, Obstet. Gynec. **27**:2, February, 1966.

Phillips, L. L., Skrodelis, V., and Taylor, H. C., Jr.: Hemorrhage due to fibrinolysis in abruptio placentae, Amer. J. Obstet. Gynec. **84**:1447, 1962.

Planned Parenthood Federation of America. Abortion in the United States, New York, 1958, Harper & Row, Publishers.

Shirodkar, V. H.: A new method of operative treatment of habitual abortion, Antiseptic **52**:299, 1955.

Taylor, H. C., Jr.: The management of obstetrical hemorrhage in the United States, Bulletin of the Sloane Hospital for Women, vol. 10, Spring, 1964.

Taylor, S. E.: Essentials of gynecology, Philadelphia, 1965, Lea & Febiger.

Tucker, J. M.: Nursing care in obstetric hemorrhage, Amer. J. Nurs. **62**:98, November, 1962.

Questions for study

1. Define spontaneous, induced, complete, incomplete, therapeutic, criminal, missed, and habitual abortion.
2. What are the causes of abortion?
3. Define ectopic pregnancy and the immediate course and treatment.
4. Define placenta previa and abruptio placentae. Compare the variation in signs and symptoms. What is the treatment for placenta previa and abruptio placentae?
5. Define postpartum hemorrhage. Give causes and treatment.
6. What are the nursing responsibilities if bleeding occurs during the maternity cycle?
7. Mrs. G., a gravida I para 0, has missed two menstrual periods and suspects she is pregnant. Two weeks following her second missed period she suddenly notices some spotting and calls her doctor. He orders strict bed rest and tells her he will pay her a visit rather soon.
   a. Mrs. G. is having
      (1) A missed abortion
      (2) A threatened abortion
      (3) A complete abortion
      (4) A placenta previa
   b. Strict bed rest is ordered
      (1) To prevent further bleeding
      (2) To replenish blood supply
      (3) To prevent labor
      (4) To keep her calm

   Twenty-four hours later Mrs. G. reports to her doctor that she has continued to bleed and has passed a large clot. He tells her to save the clot for his examination and sends an ambulance for Mrs. G.'s admittance to the hospital.

   c. Mrs. G. is immediately scheduled for an emergency dilatation and curettage. Mrs. G. has probably
      (1) Completely aborted
      (2) Incompletely aborted
      (3) Spontaneously aborted
      (4) Induced abortion
   d. Following surgery it is *most* important for the nurse to observe and check
      (1) Vital signs
      (2) Color
      (3) Amount of vaginal bleeding
      (4) The fundus
      (5) The restlessness
         (a) 1, 2, and 4 are correct
         (b) 1 and 3 are correct
         (c) 1, 2, 3, and 5 are correct
         (d) All are correct
   e. A common complication with bleeding is
      (1) Tremors
      (2) High blood pressure
      (3) Anemia
      (4) Infection
8. Mrs. J. was delivered at 3:00 A.M. by low forceps of a living baby boy. At 4:00 A.M. on checking the lochia you notice she is bleeding profusely. In order to give safe nursing care you would first
   a.
      (1) Put her in Trendelenburg position
      (2) Grasp the fundus firmly between both hands

(3) Notify the doctor
(4) Check her blood pressure and pulse

b. The doctor ordered Ergotrate, 0.2 mg. stat. intravenously. Ergotrate is a
(1) Hormone derivative
(2) Synthetic oxytocin
(3) Iron preparation
(4) Vasodilator

c. Although these things are done, bleeding continues, and Mrs. J. goes into shock. Symptoms of shock are
(1) Flushed face and profuse diaphoresis
(2) Profuse diaphoresis, paleness, and tremors
(3) Lowered blood pressure, increased pulse rate
(4) Increased blood pressure, decreased pulse rate

d. After a few hours Mrs. J. has stopped bleeding, and her condition improves. However, she keeps frantically calling for the nurse every 10 minutes. When you arrive to answer her call, she tells you she feels she is going to hemorrhage again. You would answer
(1) "You needn't worry about hemorrhage anymore since the medication we gave you guarantees against further bleeding."
(2) "You feel you're going to hemorrhage again?"
(3) "I can understand how frightened you must be, but I will be in to check you often, Mrs. J."
(4) "Once you've stopped bleeding you need not worry about starting up again."

9. Mrs. Brown, your neighbor, calls you by phone and says that she is having some vaginal bleeding. You are aware that she has missed two periods and has made one visit to an obstetrician in town. You ask whether she is experiencing any contractions, and she says "No, but do you think I will lose my baby?" You relate that you will be right over to help her.
How would you proceed in helping Mrs. Brown?
How do you feel you could give safe care until you got in touch with her obstetrician?
What might be some of the possible outcomes with spotting in the first trimester?

10. Mrs. Greene has two children, John, 5 years old, and Mary, 3 years old, and is now pregnant a third time. John is in school, and Mary is attending nursery school. She has missed two periods, and while shopping she suddenly experiences sharp abdominal cramping and begins to have some spotting. She is admitted by ambulance to the hospital close by.
With the preceding symptoms, can you think of what the diagnosis may be?
What are the measures for safe care of Mrs. Greene if you were the nurse admitting her?
What would your plans be for her two children?
What are some of the possible outcomes with interruption of this pregnancy?

11. Mrs. James, a gravida IV para III, is admitted with moderate vaginal bleeding at 29 weeks. On admission she gives a history of an uneventful pregnancy and has been receiving prenatal care for 4 months. There is no pain with the bleeding, and fetal heart tones are regular, 140 RLQ.
In view of the preceding history, what kind of diagnosis would probably be given to Mrs. James?
Orders:
a. Complete bed rest
b. Blood typing and crossmatching stat.
c. C.B.C.
d. Have 500 ml. of whole blood available
e. No rectals or vaginals
f. Phenobarbital, gr. ½ t.i.d. p.o.
g. Watch for signs of labor
h. Check B.P. and P.Q. 2 hr.
i. F.H.Q. day
Explain each of the preceding orders in giving safe care to Mrs. James.

12. Mrs. Zero, a gravida VI para V, is admitted to labor with 8-minute to 10-minute contractions of moderate strength lasting 40 to 50 seconds. Membranes are intact, no show. Rectal examination reveals 5 cm. dilatation, vertex presenting at a +1 station. Suddenly she experiences sharp abdominal pain, and the fundus does not relax for a full 75 seconds. There is no show vaginally.
What do you feel is occurring at this point with Mrs. Zero?
What action would you take?
What might be the possible outcomes with Mrs. Zero?

CHAPTER 20

PATHOLOGY OF LABOR

DYSTOCIA

A long or difficult labor is referred to as dystocia. Dystocia may be caused by ineffectual uterine contractions (functional), abnormalities in size or position of the fetus, and/or lacerations in the structure of the birth canal (mechanical).

Uterine dysfunction (functional)

During normal labor, early uterine contractions are irregular and last only a few seconds, but as labor continues contractions increase in frequency, duration, and strength. In women with uterine dysfunction, contractions never become normal, they may continue to be irregular, and they last only a short time. Although the contractions are quite uncomfortable, there is no change in effacement and dilatation of the cervix. This is referred to as dysfunctional latent phase of labor. If some women progress beyond the latent phase, one of the following may occur: (1) the active phase may be normal, (2) the active phase may be slow with the cervix dilating 1 cm. every hour, continuing until delivery, or (3) the active phase may begin but progress may cease prior to complete dilatation.

In normal labor the force of the contractions is from the fundus to the cervix, with the upper segment becoming shorter as the muscle fibers become thicker with retraction. The cervix is pulled upward around the presenting part, which is pushed through the enlarging cervical opening. In uterine dysfunction, one of these mechanisms is altered and does not occur.

Etiology. Uterine dysfunction is usually encountered in primigravidas with cephalopelvic disproportion, overdistention of the uterus by polyhydramnios, multiple pregnancy, anomalies of the uterus, postmaturity, and growths such as fibromyoma or cicatrization of the cervix as a result of a previous delivery or gynecologic problem.

With prolonged labor that is ineffectual, intrauterine infection, fetal death, and postpartum hemorrhage are frequent complications.

Management. Dysfunctional labor can usually be suspected during the first 6 to 8 hours of labor. Management consists of evaluation by vaginal examination or roentgen-ray pelvimetry to determine the cause. If the cause is mechanical as in cephalopelvic disproportion or abnormal position or presentation of the fetus, surgical intervention is necessary. If the cause is uterine inertia, stimulation of the uterus with drugs may be the mode of treatment.

Drugs such as preparations of promethazine hydrochloride (Phenergan) or promazine (Sparine) may be given to relax and ease tension without altering uterine contractions. To prevent infection, antibiotics such as penicillin, 1,200,000 units, and streptomycin, 0.5 gm., are given every 12 hours. To keep the mother well hydrated, parenteral fluids are administered.

Stimulation of labor may be started by artificial rupture of the membranes. If this does not strengthen contractions after a 2-hour period, an intravenous drip of 5% dextrose in water with 5 units of oxytocin may be started at 15 drops per minute. The doctor, in order to be able to time contractions, should remain with the mother while oxytocin is being given. Contractions that are prolonged and strong, lasting 2 minutes or more, are dangerous since they decrease uterine blood flow and oxygen supply to the fetus. If tetanic contractions occur, the infusion is discontinued. Pulse and blood pressure are checked carefully every 15 minutes. The infusion is continued for at least 1 hour following delivery to reduce post-partum bleeding. Sparteine sulfate (Tocosamine, 75 to 150 mg., I.M.) is often used to stimulate dysfunctional labor; however, its effect is unpredictable. It is sometimes used for a dysfunctional latent phase. Should sparteine be given during the active phase, uterine atony, tetanic contractions, and fetal bradycardia often occur.

When stimulation brings little progress, without further effacement or dilatation and with ineffectual contractions and irregular fetal heart tones, surgical intervention is imperative. Regional anesthesia is the method of choice for delivery, since it does not alter uterine tone.

Constriction ring dystocia

A constriction ring is a tetanic band of smooth muscle that occurs at any level in the wall of the uterus. The ring is stationary and is so tight around the baby that it prevents descent.

Although rare, a constriction ring occurs when contractions are irregular and uncoordinated from the beginning of labor. The cervix and lower segment hang ahead of the presenting part and are quiescent as the fundus contracts. The baby is actually pulled upward rather than pushed down with each contraction. Diagnosis is usually made by vaginal examination, in which the band may be felt, or a deep depression over the ring may be ascertained on abdominal palpation.

If diagnosis is made during labor prior to complete cervical dilatation, morphine and intravenous glucose alleviate the condition. In some women, 5 minims of 1:1,000 epinephrine hydrochloride given intramuscularly will relax the constriction ring. If treatment is ineffectual, cesarean section is performed. If the

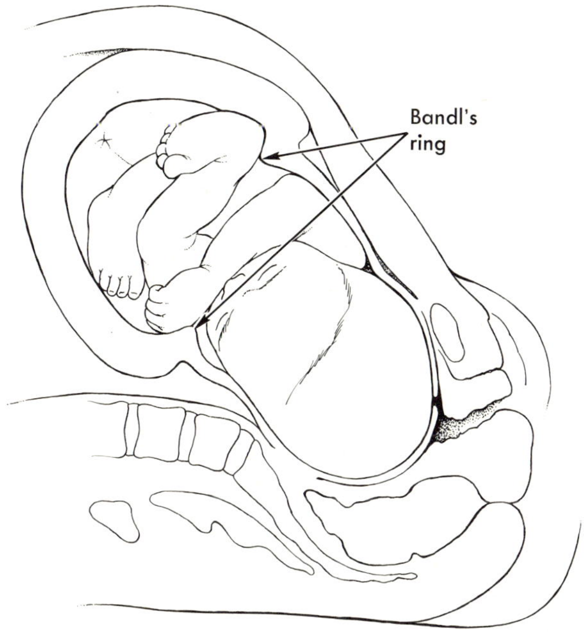

Fig. 20-1. Bandl's ring.

cervix is fully dilated, deep anesthesia will provide relaxation so that vaginal delivery may be accomplished.

Pathologic retraction ring

Bandl's ring (Fig. 20-1), a pathologic retraction ring, develops during obstructed normal labor. The ring forms at the junction of the active upper and passive lower uterine segments. Descent and expulsion of the infant are impeded, with the lower segment becoming thinner and longer and the upper segment shorter and thicker. Bandl's ring is a result of obstruction, and if immediate cesarean section is not done, the uterus may rupture. Cephalopelvic disproportion is a most common cause.

Dystocia of fetal origin

Dystocia of fetal origin is the result of excessive size, developmental abnormalities, and unusual positions in utero.

Excessive size. Overgrowth of the fetus may be a result of parental size, multiparity, or maternal diabetes. A large infant is suspected when the presenting part never enters the pelvic inlet with forceful contractions. X-ray pelvimetry is done whenever overgrowth is suspected. Often disproportion may be minimal and the head may descend into the true pelvis, yet the shoulders may be too broad and impede progress. The only treatment is surgical intervention.

Developmental abnormalities. Although developmental anomalies do not often cause dystocia, in some instances, such as hydrocephalus, enlargement of the body or abdomen, or monstrosities, labor may be faulty. With breech presentation, hydrocephalus may be difficult to diagnose but should be suspected. If the vertex is presenting, fluid can be withdrawn by puncturing the enlarged ventricle through a suture or fontanel with a spinal needle. This can be accomplished only with a cervix dilated 3 to 4 cm. The procedure decompresses the head so that labor can progress normally. Cesarean section is seldom done, unless decompression cannot be accomplished.

Transverse lie. With transverse lie, the baby's head lies in one flank of the mother and the buttocks in the other (Fig. 20-2). Transverse lie is frequently associated with a placenta that occupies the lower segment or with hydramnios. Diagnosis is made when the abdomen appears wide rather than long. On palpation the head can be felt on one side, the breech on the other, with no presenting part in the inlet. X-ray examination will usually confirm diagnosis.

Management may be individual depending upon fetal size and pelvic size. If transverse lie is diagnosed in late pregnancy, external version to either a breech or vertex position may be attempted. If this is unsuccessful, an x-ray or isotopic examination for placental site should be done.

Infant mortality rate is high with vaginal delivery since there is often prolapse of the umbilical cord or fetal parts with resulting maternal infection. Cesarean section is the method of choice for safe care of mother and baby.

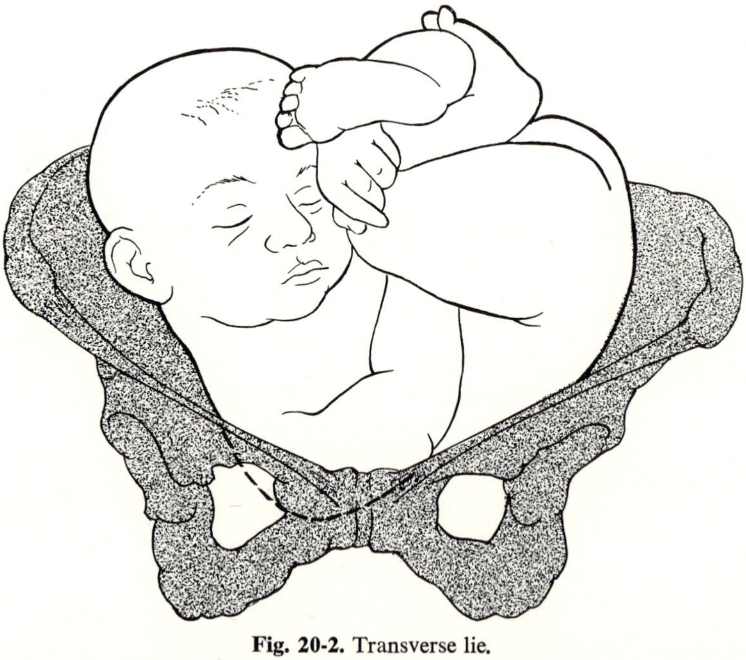

Fig. 20-2. Transverse lie.

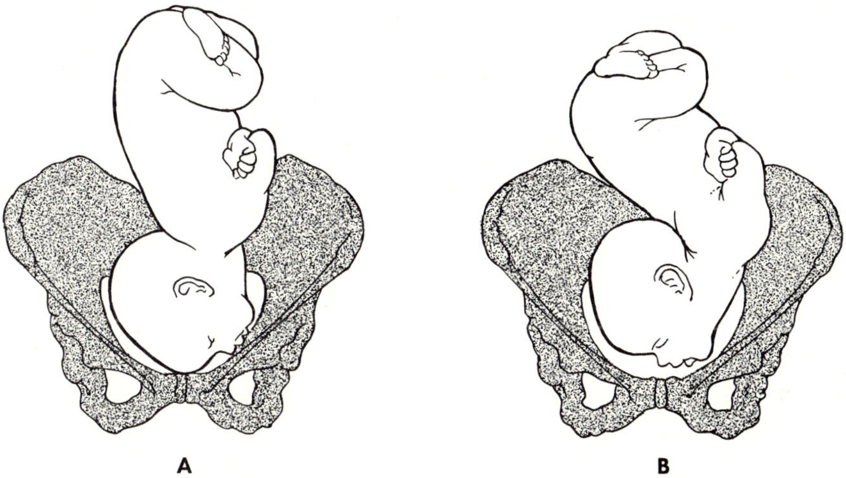

Fig. 20-3. A, Brow presentation. B, Face presentation.

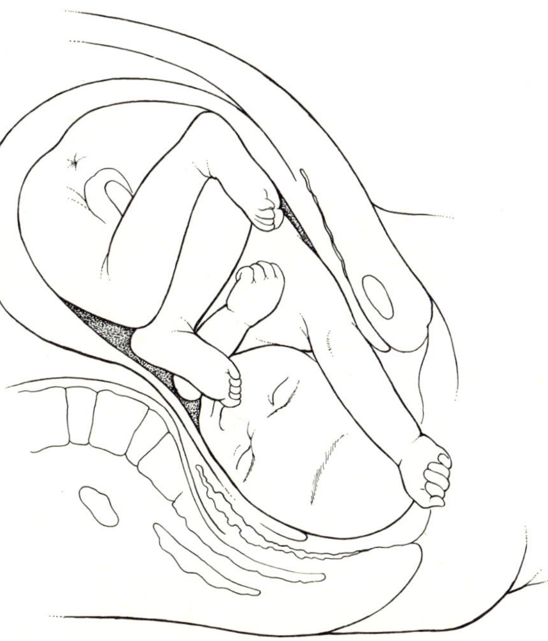

Fig. 20-4. Compound presentation.

Occiput posterior position. In one fourth of all vertex deliveries the occiput points toward the posterior quadrant of the mother's pelvis. As the head engages in the true pelvis, the occiput rotates anteriorly. In some women the baby's occiput remains posterior and causes pressure on the sacrum and coccyx, with resulting backache in the mother and prolongation of labor.

At times the head rotates and the occiput may be delivered anteriorly. However, often if the occiput remains posterior, the head may advance to a +2 station and then need to be rotated manually or with forceps. Cesarean section is never done for an occiput posterior position if the pelvis is normal.

Face and brow presentation. Deflexion of the head in varying degrees causes face or brow presentation (Fig. 20-3). Usually x-ray examination is done to determine the size of the pelvis, the size of the baby, and the amount of deflexion. Management depends upon these factors.

Compound presentation. Compound presentation occurs when one or more of the infant's extremities prolapse with the presenting head or breech (Fig. 20-4). It is more common in multigravidas or in premature infants. If an entire arm or leg has descended with the presenting part, the limb may have to be replaced by disengaging the presenting part vaginally.

Dystocia caused by contracted pelvis

A clinical estimation of the pelvis is made in all women at this initial prenatal visit. If the pelvis is suspected to be small or abnormal, an x-ray study is indicated when the mother is close to term. This shows the relationship of the size of the pelvis and the size of the fetus.

Indications for roentgen pelvimetry

Indications for roentgen pelvimetry are the following:

1. Dysfunctional labors considering oxytocin stimulation
2. Question of pelvic adequacy during early labor
3. During a trial of labor for contracted pelvis to determine whether stimulation with oxytocin or cesarean section is indicated
4. In breech or abnormal presentations

Trial of labor

A trial of labor may be afforded a mother in whom the physician feels that effectual labor may bring about vaginal delivery. The physician designates the number of hours the mother will be given in labor before a decision is made to proceed with operative intervention. A trial of labor is never used as an endurance test for mother and infant when dystocia is anticipated.

Many trials of labor terminate in successful vaginal delivery. It is a common belief by many physicians that once labor starts there is assurance that the baby is not premature, that the lower uterine segment is more easily delineated if cesarean section is indicated, and that there is less likelihood that the uterus may become atonic during surgical intervention. In known borderline pelves with disproportion, a 12-hour trial is given. If there is definite inlet disproportion, a 6-hour to 8-hour trial is allowed. With signs of maternal exhaustion or fetal distress, immediate surgical intervention is indicated.

Nursing care for prolonged labor

The nurse caring for the mother in prolonged labor needs to be alert to signs of maternal exhaustion and fetal distress. Signs of dehydration in the mother are elevation in body temperature, a fruity odor to the breath, general skin dryness, and a diminished urinary output with marked acetone reaction. Often glucose and oxytocin are ordered parenterally to strengthen uterine contractions and alleviate dehydration.

Long labors are frightening to mothers, and assurance given by the nurse affords support that is an adjunct to effective therapy. Comforting measures, such as a soothing sponge, a cool mouth rinse, or a back rub, are most welcomed. Provisions for a quiet environment augment the effect of sedation.

Following a difficult delivery ineffectual uterine contractions may result in postpartum hemorrhage. Vigilance in checking the fundus, pulse, and blood pressure is imperative in the early postpartum period. Often parenteral fluids are continued with added oxytocics to aid in keeping the uterus well contracted.

Signs and symptoms of fetal distress are a result of a depletion of oxygen to the infant, with ensuing hypoxia. Frequent checking and immediate reporting of any variations in rate, regularity, and strength of fetal heart tones are essential. As the baby is further depleted of oxygen, signs of fetal distress are excessive fetal movements and meconium staining of the amniotic fluid (with vertex presentation). Administering oxygen to the mother until the physician arrives will alleviate symptoms of hypoxia.

Equipment for aspiration and resuscitation of the newborn is essential in preparation for delivery. Intravenous equipment for administration of glucose or whole blood should be available for the mother.

Other causes of fetal distress are the following: (1) cord around the neck, which becomes tighter as the baby moves downward into the pelvis; (2) placental separation with oxygen depletion to the baby; (3) prolonged labor as just cited; (4) maternal diabetes; (5) toxemias of pregnancy; and (6) Rh sensitization.

PRECIPITATE LABOR

A labor of 2 hours or less is known as a precipitate labor. The hazards of a rapid labor and delivery affect mother and infant. Frequently precipitate labor occurs in multigravidas who give a history of a previous short labor. Contractions usually occur suddenly with increasing intensity and frequency, allowing for little relaxation in between. At the same time the infant becomes anoxic, since the intervillous blood flow is impaired, and rapid delivery may result in intracranial hemorrhage. Often delivery is unattended, and the mother may experience lacerations of the perineum, labia, urethra, and clitoris. Occasionally following delivery the fundus relaxes, and postpartum hemorrhage occurs.

Management with a history of previous precipitate labors warrants early admission. The onset of labor may be induced with amniotomy and the character of contractions closely observed. If contractions become tumultuous, some form of safe anesthesia may be administered to slow down labor. Controlling contractions will permit adequate oxygenation of the infant and will prevent maternal trauma.

LABOR INDUCTION

Induction of labor is a means of therapy for the welfare of mother and baby. Indications for elective induction are both medical and obstetric. The methods used are either medical in which the use of oxytocic drugs initiates uterine contractions or mechanical in which membranes are ruptured artificially. At times both methods are used. Indications for induction, contraindications for induction, and obstetric criteria for safe induction follow.

Indications for induction

1. *Medical*
   a. Diabetes
   b. Pyelonephritis
2. *Obstetric*
   a. Toxemia
   b. Sensitization to Rh or blood incompatibility
   c. Polyhydramnios
   d. Premature rupture of membranes at term without contractions
   e. Abruptio placentae

Contraindications for induction

1. Cephalopelvic disproportion
2. Malpresentation
3. Grand-multigravida
4. Previous cesarean section
5. History of uterine surgery in which danger of rupture of uterus exists
6. Reconstructive surgery of the uterus or cervix

Obstetric criteria for safe induction

1. No evidence of cephalopelvic disproportion
2. Cervix must be "ripe" (partially effaced) and 1.5 or 2 cm. dilated
3. Vertex presentation with engagement
4. No abnormally distended uterus

Elective induction of labor may be a matter of convenience for the mother and the physician in the multigravida at term. Induction is attempted only when the baby is at term, the pelvis is adequate, and the cervix is soft and partially dilated. Attempts without these prerequisites are usually unsuccessful.

Medical methods of induction

Posterior pituitary extracts such as oxytocin and sparteine sulfate (Tocosamine, 75 to 150 mg. I.M.) are being used in small doses to initiate labor contractions. An intravenous drip of 5 units of oxytocin to 1,000 ml. of 5% glucose in water is started at a rate of 5 to 10 drops per minute. If the patient is not sensitive to oxytocin and labor contractions do not become initiated, the rate of flow is increased to 20 drops per minute depending upon uterine response. If contractions become strong and last 2 minutes with no relaxation periods, the infusion is discontinued immediately.

In pregnancies beyond 20 weeks in which fetal death has occurred, labor may be induced by intra-amniotic instillation of normal saline or hypertonic glucose; 200 ml. of amniotic fluid is withdrawn, and 200 ml. of either normal saline or hypertonic glucose solution is injected into the amniotic sac, by means of an abdominal amniotomy. This is believed to cause necrosis of the placenta with beginning labor contractions. This method is at times unsuccessful, and hysterotomy may be performed.

Buccal oxytocin, tablets of which are inserted between the upper gum and lip for absorption by the mucous membranes, has been found effective and is being widely used. If labor is not initiated within 4 hours and no apparent change in cervical effacement and dilatation occurs, induction has been unsuccessful.

Sparteine sulfate (Tocosamine), 75 to 150 mg., is used and administered every hour for four doses. In some women cumulative effects may result in tetanic contractions or sensitivity, and the drug may produce marked depression with bradycardia. Buccal and intravenous injections of oxytocin have an advantage over sparteine since they may be terminated, whereas sparteine injections may not be.

Mechanical methods of induction

With the vertex well engaged and fixed in the true pelvis and the cervix somewhat effaced and dilated, artificial rupture of the membranes may initiate labor contractions promptly. Rupture or stripping of the membranes is contraindicated when the vertex is high, since sudden escape of amniotic fluid may prolapse the cord, cutting off oxygen supply to the baby. At times rupturing the membranes is done prior to medical induction.

Nursing care during induction

Preparation of the mother by explaining the planned treatment is essential to alleviate anxiety. Prior to artificial rupture of the membranes, the nurse checks fetal heart tones and administers perineal care to prevent introduction of organisms into the vagina. The mother is draped properly and supported since relaxation is essential during vaginal examination. Coaching the mother in breathing keeps her occupied during the examination and promotes relaxation. Immediately following examination the nurse checks fetal heart tones and observes the amount and color of the amniotic fluid. Any change in rate and regularity of fetal heart tones or discoloration of amniotic fluid warrants immediate attention. Oxygen may be given to the mother until the physician arrives. At times elevating the mother's hips above the shoulder level (Trendelenburg position) relieves umbilical cord compression with improvement in fetal heart tones.

Astute checking and timing of uterine contractions, vital signs, blood pressure, and fetal heart tones are done in most institutions by a doctor-nurse team for safety of the mother and the baby. Induction warrants availability of oxygen, resuscitative equipment, and delivery facilities if an emergency arises.

If labor progresses rapidly, sedation and halothane (Fluothane) anesthesia must be available. *The mother is never left unattended during induction of labor.* The doctor must be available during induction.

When oxytocin is used by drip method, checking the rate of flow is done frequently. In most institutions the doctor is responsible for adding the oxytocic to the intravenous fluid and increasing the rate of flow.

Prior to induction, blood typing and crossmatching are done, and availability of whole blood is essential should an emergency occur. Shaving the abdomen and spinal area is also done if emergency cesarean section is necessary.

Induction of labor is safe when preparation of the mother is adequate, when there are indications without contraindications, and when a doctor-nurse team is in constant attendance.

SELECTED REFERENCES

Allen, S.: Nurse attendance during labor, Amer. J. Nurs. **64:**70, July, 1964.

Eastman, N. J., and Hellman, L. M.: Williams obstetrics, ed. 13, Philadelphia, 1966, Appleton-Century & Appleton-Century-Crofts.

Fields, H., and others: Induction of labor, New York, 1965, The Macmillan Co.

Goodlin, R. C., and others: Therapeutic abortion with hypertonic intraamniotic saline, Obstet. Gynec., vol 34, no. 1, July, 1969.

Goodman, R. R.: Psychological support in labor: a supervisor's view, Hosp. Top. **45:**97, August, 1964.

Jordan, M. J.: Induction of labor, Hosp. Med. **1:**35, December, 1964.

Schaefer, G.: Induction of labor, Amer. J. Nurs. **61:**89, September, 1961.

Schiffer, M.: Induction of labor by intra-amniotic instillation of hypertonic solution for therapeutic abortion or intrauterine death, Obstet. Gynec., vol. 33, no. 5, May, 1969.

Van Praagh, I. G., and others: Primary cesarean section in the multipara, Obstet. Gynec., vol. 36, no. 6, December, 1968.

Questions for study

1. Define dystocia.
2. What are the frequent causes of dystocia?
3. Mrs. X., a gravida III para II, is admitted at 42 weeks gestation with ruptured membranes. Twenty-four hours later she is still not in labor. The doctor ordered 1,000 ml. of 5% glucose in water with 2 units of oxytocin to begin induction of labor. Should contractions not occur, 2 units of oxytocin were to be added to the infusion every half hour (no more than four added doses) until labor was established. Check with the resident before adding any additional oxytocin following the first dose.
   How would you prepare Mrs. X. for induction? How would you give Mrs. X. safe nursing care during oxytocin induction?
4. Mrs. C., a gravida I para 0, has been in labor for 12 hours. She has been fully dilated for 2 hours and is pushing with each contraction. A portion of the baby's head is visible, fetal heart tones are regular, good quality 146, and there is suddenly meconium-stained amniotic fluid. The doctor orders her taken to the

delivery room for elective low forceps application.

Why was operative intervention indicated for Mrs. C.? In lieu of forceps application, how would you plan for safe care of Mrs. C. and her baby following delivery?

5. Mrs. K., a gravida I para 0, is admitted to the labor and delivery unit in active labor at 37 weeks gestation. Her abdomen appears taut and as large as a full-term pregnancy. Fetal heart tones are not audible, yet Mrs. K. feels the baby moving. She is diagnosed as a possible polyhydramnios. After 3 hours of 3-minute to 4-minute contractions of moderate intensity lasting 30 to 40 seconds, membranes ruptured spontaneously. Following rupture of the membranes, contractions ceased. Fetal heart tones were now audible 140, regular and good quality.

   What is polyhydramnios?

   Write a nursing care plan for Mrs. K. considering the preceding history.
6. Name the indications and contraindications for labor induction.
7. What are the medical and mechanical methods used to induce labor?
8. What are the nurse's responsibilities in the care of the mother during induction of labor?
9. What are the signs and symptoms of maternal exhaustion and fetal distress?
10. What are the nursing responsibilities if maternal exhaustion or fetal distress occur?

CHAPTER 21

OPERATIVE OBSTETRICS

FORCEPS DELIVERY

The obstetric forceps (Fig. 21-1) is an instrument designed to facilitate delivery of the baby's head by traction or rotation. It is a surgical instrument that possesses great potential in saving the infant's life when used properly. The outcome of a forceps application depends not only upon the skill of the operator but also upon specific criteria that designate its judicious use.

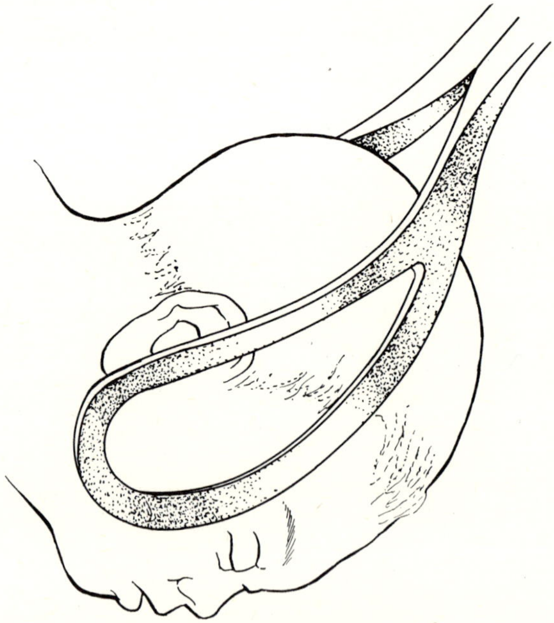

Fig. 21-1. Forceps application.

History

Instruments were used to assist in the delivery of infants prior to the sixteenth or seventeenth century with little respect for safety of the mother or the baby. Various instruments were used in ancient times when normal delivery was not possible. Most of these instruments, however, were tools of mutilation of the child, and they were used only in an attempt to save the life of the mother. Hindu writings 1,000 years before Christ refer to a knife and hook used for difficult labors.

The Chamberlen family over several generations (A.D. 1601-1818) are credited with devising an effective forceps for delivery of a living infant. It was during this period that the physician, rather than midwives, gained the privilege of delivering infants.

The Chamberlens contributed outstanding features of design in the obstetric forceps. Up to this period blades could not be disjointed, making application quite difficult. The Chamberlens introduced a disjointed blade, making possible introduction of one blade at a time. The blade was enlarged, fenestrated, and had an added pelvic curve to the already present cephalic curve.

In 1848 Sir James Simpson introduced an obstetric forceps that perfected the cephalic curve to follow the contours of the baby's head. Some thirty years later, Tarnier introduced a forceps whereby traction could be exerted along the pelvic axis.

Parts and design of the obstetric forceps

The parts of a forceps (Fig. 21-2) include the handle, lock, shank, and blade. All forceps have variations in details as to handle, type of lock, length and width of shank, fenestration of blades, and degree of cephalic and pelvic curves.

The most commonly used forceps are the following: (1) Simpson or Elliott, applied as low-outlet forceps when the head is visible; (2) Barton, used for rotation and traction of the occiput in transverse positions; (3) Kjelland, for rotation and traction of the head in transverse arrest, occiput posterior, and face presentation; and (4) Piper, for the aftercoming head in a breech delivery.

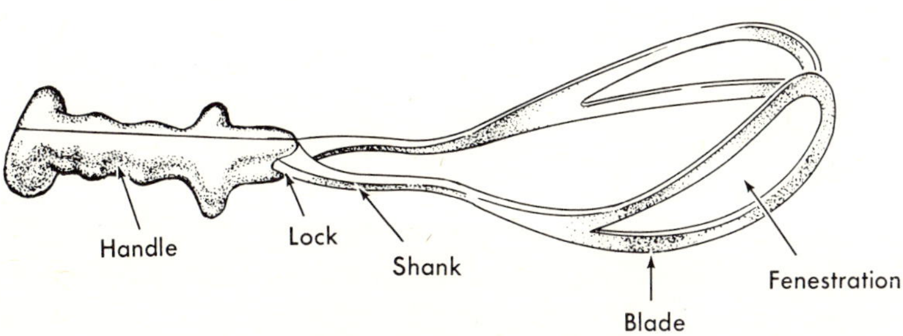

Fig. 21-2. Parts of forceps.

Indications for forceps delivery

Most forceps applications are performed to reduce the length of the second stage of labor, which eliminates undue stretching of the perineal muscles and reduces compression of the baby's head. Forceps are indicated should there be a slowing of fetal heart tones or the passage of meconium, signs of fetal distress. In the cardiac mother and with premature labor, forceps application conserves the mother's cardiac reserve and prevents undue trauma to the baby's skull. Maternal indications for forceps application are prolonged second stage with uterine inertia, inability of the mother to participate when caudal or saddle block anesthesia has been given, toxemias of pregnancy, active tuberculosis, pneumonia, poliomyelitis, and persistent malpositions of the occiput.

Classification of forceps delivery

Forceps are applied when the vertex is at various levels in the pelvis. The following classification is the one in current use:

1. *High forceps:* The biparietal diameter of the baby's head is in the inlet and barely above the ischial spines. Should the vertex be higher and unengaged, forceps application is hazardous. This type of high forceps application is contraindicated, and abdominosurgical intervention is the method of choice.
2. *Midforceps:* The bony part of the vertex is just below the ischial spines.
3. *Low midforceps:* The biparietal diameter is at or below the ischial spines, and the bony portion of the vertex is a fingerbreadth above the perineum between contractions.
4. *Low forceps:* The bony portion of the vertex is on the perineum and visible with contractions. The biparietal diameter is below the ischial spines with the anteroposterior diameter at the outlet.

Prerequisites to forceps application

Prior to the application of forceps, the following criteria are essential for safety of mother and baby: (1) indication of an adequate pelvis; (2) complete effacement and dilatation of the cervix; (3) rupture of the membranes; (4) position of the vertex correctly diagnosed; (5) vertex must be engaged; and (6) anesthesia is essential for perineal floor relaxation.

Nursing care in forceps delivery

The nurse's role in the delivery room prior to forceps application is one of frequent auscultation of fetal heart tones. Suction and resuscitation equipment must be in readiness should respiratory distress occur in the delivered infant.

Following delivery maternal dangers include injury, hemorrhage, and infection. Observing the lochia and checking vital signs are essential. Extensive injury to the soft tissues of the vagina, urethra, and clitoris or extension of the episiotomy may cause the mother much discomfort. A perineal heat lamp improves circulation to the area and is soothing and comforting. Asepsis at all times will lessen the possibility of infection. Attention to bladder function is an adjunct to astute observation.

The dangers to the infant include asphyxia, skull fractures and brain concussions, cephalohematoma, hemorrhage from rupture of the sinus at the base of the brain of the tentorium cerebelli, facial paralysis from nerve compression, deafness from injury to the auditory organs, Erb's paralysis, and susceptibility to pneumonia and atelectasis.

The nurse observes the infant for noticeable skull abrasions or protrusions, asymmetry of the face, or malposition of the scapula and arm. A newborn with brain damage is restless, has a shrill cry, a poor sucking reflex, and experiences tremors. Respiratory distress symptoms such as cyanosis, increased respiratory rate, sternal retraction, flaring of the nostrils, and grunting on expiration are not uncommon.

The infant with possible brain damage should be elevated in semi-Fowler's position to alleviate intracranial pressure. Oxygen is ordered and administered following adequate suctioning to provide an open airway. Feedings are omitted to conserve energy and improve respirations, and parenteral fluids are ordered. Careful observation and checking of vital signs every hour assure safe nursing care.

At times forceps marks are apparent following delivery. These usually disappear within 48 hours but may be of concern to parents. Abrasions with skin breakdown are kept clean to prevent infection.

The emotional status of the mother following a difficult delivery is of great concern in planning for care. Allowing the mother to talk about her delivery and keeping her informed of the baby's condition are essential for return to optimum health. The interruption of contact with the infant may be traumatic for the parents who anticipated a well infant. Preparing the mother before she visits the nursery is important if the baby is receiving oxygen and parenteral therapy. Although false hope cannot be given parents, any slight improvement will alleviate much anxiety. When improvement is not apparent, conveying concern and understandign for the parents' anxiety is supportive. Conveying that all is being done for the infant gives comfort and reassurance.

The added financial expense for extended hospitalization of the mother or the infant has a direct impact on each family member. The nurse provides continuity in care by referral to community agencies such as the social caseworker, homemaker service, and the public health nurse.

ABDOMINAL DELIVERY—CESAREAN SECTION

History

Cesarean section and abdominal hysterotomy are terms used for abdominal delivery through a surgical incision made into the uterus.

In ancient history this operation became a procedure under Roman law. The purpose greatly differed from the present-day indications, since during Roman days it was done to salvage a living baby if the mother died prior to delivery and also to provide a separate burial for the baby. The purpose for cesarean section in ancient times is still an indication for it today. Statistics show that the fetal mortality rate was high, and probably irreparable brain damage existed resulting from hypoxia in the infant.

The first cesarean section was performed on a living woman by Trautman and Wittenberg in 1610. The infant survived, but the mother died 3 weeks later with generalized sepsis. Within the next two centuries little progress was made, with an 85% mortality rate. The mortality rate existed since little was known of asepsis, anesthesia was nonexistent, failure to close the uterine wound resulted in complications, and often the surgery was done as a last resort following days of prolonged labor.

In 1876 Porro favored removal of the uterus and ovaries, leaving the cervix in situ with cesarean section. It was the hope that this procedure would reduce infection and hemorrhage.

In 1882 Saenger of Leipzig recommended suturing of the uterine wall with a double row of sutures to assure closure. Although American surgeons had attempted closure, the method that was used (silver wire sutures) proved unsuccessful.

During the nineteenth and early part of the twentieth centuries, two important contributions made the abdominal route less hazardous. Attempt to enter the uterus extraperitoneally and the entrance by incision into the lower uterine segment decrease the hazard of peritoneal infection.

In 1909 Latzko advocated an extraperitoneal cesarean section in which incision was made into one section of the lower uterine segment. In 1950 Waters performed an extraperitoneal cesarean section with an approach to the lower uterine segment and surgical treatment of the peritoneum overlying the bladder.

Incidence and indications

Advances in surgical techniques, improvement in anesthesia, availability of blood for transfusion, and the use of chemotherapy have greatly reduced the maternal mortality with abdominal delivery. Cesarean section is chosen as a method for delivery to avoid risk to the baby during labor. There is also a trend toward fewer difficult midforceps deliveries or internal podalic versions.

Indications for cesarean section include: (1) cephalopelvic disproportion, (2) placenta previa, (3) abruptio placentae, (4) uterine inertia, (5) toxemia, (6) fetal distress, (7) malpresentations, (8) Rh isoimmunization, (9) diabetes, (10) postmaturity (previous infant deaths in utero), (11) uterine growths blocking the vaginal canal, and (12) maternal risks such as cranial aneurysm or brain tumor.

Contraindications

Contraindications for cesarean section are (1) fetal death (with no other complications), (2) major fetal anomalies, (3) eclampsia, and (4) infections of the peritoneal cavity.

Types of cesarean sections

Low-segment cesarean section. Low-segment cesarean section (Fig. 21-3) is the most frequent type, in which the midline incision is made just below the umbilicus down to the symphysis on the skin, and a transverse incision is made just above the symphysis into the lower uterine segment. Incision into this lower por-

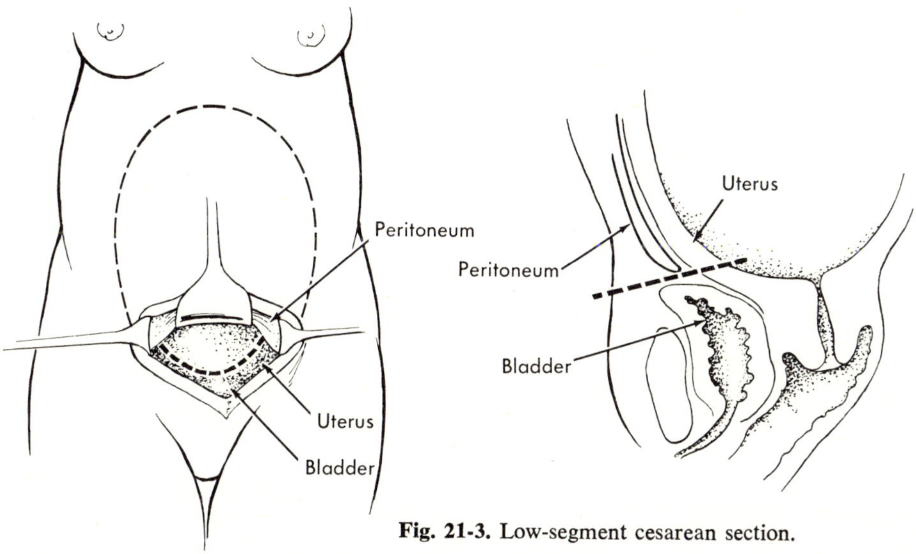

Fig. 21-3. Low-segment cesarean section.

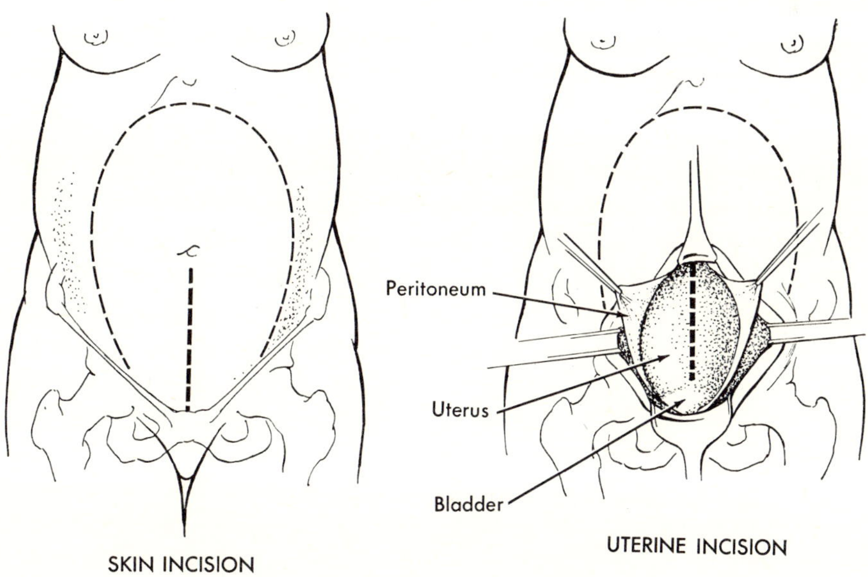

Fig. 21-4. Classical cesarean section.

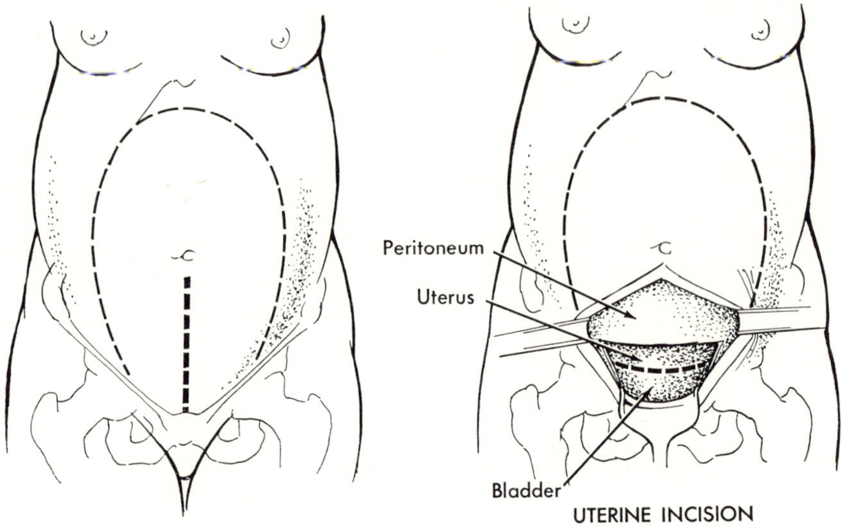

Fig. 21-5. Extraperitoneal cesarean section.

tion reduces the incidence of infection, blood loss, and the possibility of rupture of the scar since it is not the contractile portion.

Classical cesarean section. Classical cesarean section (Fig. 21-4) is performed with the same skin incision of the low transverse type. The incision into the uterus, however, is longitudinal, terminating just above the reflection of the bladder peritoneum. Classical cesarean section is indicated when placenta previa occurs or when adhesions from a previous section are present.

Extraperitoneal cesarean section. Extraperitoneal cesarean section (Fig. 21-5) is done by dissecting the bladder downward and exposing the portion of the uterus not covered by peritoneum. This type is indicated when there have been prolonged ruptured membranes or long labor. Since infection may be anticipated, effort is made to avoid entering the peritoneal cavity.

Nursing care in cesarean section

With cesarean section that is elective and anticipated, there is time to prepare the mother physically and emotionally. However, cesarean section is often an emergency measure to save the mother and the infant. Most mothers expect and anticipate vaginal delivery and normally have fears of the outcome. The prospect of a possible abdominal incision, which is a deviation from the normal birth route, brings added fears and anxieties. The body reacts in various ways to stress, the most common being an increase in epinephrine with added heart action. It is essential that nursing care be directed toward alleviation of fears and anxieties in emergencies. Spiritual attendance by a priest or clergyman gives added strength and support at this time. Letting the mother know that everything possible will be done for her safety and that of her infant gives reassurance. Preparation prior to introduction of treatment alleviates fear of the unknown.

Physical preparation preoperatively consists of shaving the spinal area, the abdomen (from beneath the breast line to the symphysis), and the vaginal and rectal areas. Shaving hair growth facilitates removal of surface bacteria. Catheterization is often ordered before surgery since the bladder is in close proximity to the uterus. The catheter is left in place to keep the bladder empty during surgery. Blood typing, Rh, and crossmatching with availability of blood are imperative should bleeding occur. Preoperative medications are ordered with due consideration to mother and infant, and the type of anesthesia is selected.

Postoperatively, checking vital signs and observing for incisional and vaginal bleeding are the nurse's primary responsibility. Ambulation is started early, and encouraging deep breathing and leg motion improves circulation. Warm fluids and soft foods are ordered within 24 to 36 hours to promote peristalsis and prevent abdominal distention. Parenteral fluids may be ordered for the first 24 hours following a long labor. Attention to bladder and bowel function for cesarean section does not differ from that for normal vaginal delivery. At times, especially in the extraperitoneal type of cesarean section, the catheter may be left in the bladder for a 48-hour to 72-hour period postoperatively. Sedation is ordered and given for comfort of the mother.

Cesarean section is not a contraindication for breast-feeding. The baby is put to breast as soon as the mother is comfortable and able to meet the infant's needs. Women who have had an abdominal delivery are usually discharged 8 to 10 days following surgery. The nurse helps the mother plan activities before discharge, and referral to community agencies ensures return to optimum health.

VACUUM EXTRACTOR

The vacuum extractor is a suction device used on the baby's head to facilitate delivery. Known devices of this type were used as early as 1706 by Yonge and as early as 1849 by Simpson. The present vacuum extractor was designed by Tage Malmström in 1954 and was further developed and used in 1957.

The vacuum extractor is composed of a traction cup of metal, a traction chain that is passed through a rubber suction tube terminated by a metal handle. The suction cups are manufactured in varying sizes of 30, 40, and 50 mm. The apparatus is attached to a glass container, fitted with a vacuum gauge and fine metal connectors. To each of the connectors is attached the rubber tube from the suction cup and the tube leading to the suction pump.

The metal suction cup is adjusted over the small fontanel (at the posterior occiput), and a vacuum is created. The physician then applies traction with each labor contraction.

Although vacuum extractions have been used over the centuries, they are not a universally accepted practice. Maternal risks include cervical tears, increased incidence of retained placenta, and postpartum hemorrhage. Infant risks include intracranial hemorrhage and brain damage in the years following birth.

SELECTED REFERENCES

Baird, Sir D.: Combined textbook of obstetrics and gynecology, London, 1962, E. & S. Livingstone, Ltd.

Bourne, A. W., and Williams, L. H.: Recent advances in obstetrics and gynecology, New York, 1963, The Blakiston Division, McGraw-Hill Book Co.

Eastman, N. J., and Hellman, L. M.: Williams obstetrics, ed. 13, New York, 1966, Appleton-Century & Appleton-Century-Crofts.

Fenton, A. N., and Steer, C. M.: Fetal distress, Amer. J. Obstet. Gynec. **83:**354, 1962.

Greenhill, J. P.: Obstetrics, ed. 13, Philadelphia, 1965, W. B. Saunders Co.

Kelly, J. V.: Instrument delivery and fetal heart rate, Amer. J. Obstet. Gynec. **87:** 529, 1963.

Laufe, L. E.: Obstetric forceps, New York, 1968, Harper & Row, Publishers.

Malmström, T.: The vacuum-extractor, Acta Obstet. Gynec. Scand. **43,** supp. 1:5, Jan. 5, 1954.

McLenahan, I. G.: Helping the mother who has no baby to take home, Amer. J. Nurs. **62:**70, April, 1962.

Reid, D. E.: A textbook of obstetrics, Philadelphia, 1962, W. B. Saunders Co.

Shaefer, G., Taggart, E., and Ivey, E.: The pregnant woman with tuberculosis, Amer. J. Nurs. **63:**68, August, 1963.

Questions for study

1. What are the indications for forceps application?
2. Define low, low-mid, mid, and high forceps delivery.
3. What are the nursing responsibilities during and following forceps application?
4. What are the indications for cesarean section?
5. What are the nursing responsibilities in caring for mothers preoperatively and postoperatively with abdominal delivery?
6. Mrs. G., a gravda III para II, has been admitted at 39 weeks for elective cesarean section. The preoperative order read:
   a. Soft diet tonight, nothing p.o. after midnight
   b. Abdominal, vaginal, and spinal preparation
   c. Insert Foley catheter, catheterize before going to O.R.
   d. Atropine, gr. 1/150, subcutaneously ½ hour prior to surgery
   e. Clerical attendance

   You are the nurse assigned Mrs. G.'s care preoperatively and postoperatively. Write a nursing care plan.

CHAPTER 22

MEDICAL AND SURGICAL DISEASES IN PREGNANCY

Medical diseases are responsible for a great majority of maternal and fetal deaths, but they have been lessened by the great strides in obstetric care. There are, however, an increasing number of women who attempt pregnancy with superimposed medical problems. Even with the new scientific knowledge, there remains evidence of an increase in the number of stillbirths and fetal deaths from prematurity associated with severe hypertensive disease and other infections and metabolic disorders.

The relationship of the increased incidence of congenital anomalies found in pregnancy complicated by medical disease is now of great concern. Premarital physical examination with due respect to family history is essential in preparation for marriage and childbearing. Genetic counseling services are in demand and available in varying parts of the United States. Genetic counselors enter into discussion with young people on issues such as: Will a pregnancy aggravate the medical problem? What effect will it have on the baby, and what considerations are to be given to planning of children for safety of mother and infant? Nurses in the health field provide young people with anticipatory guidance to maintain optimum health in families.

Disorders of the heart and blood vessels contribute to the largest proportion of maternal deaths. The normal physiologic changes during pregnancy that include an increase in interstitial fluid, an increase in blood volume, an increase in cardiac output, and the physiologic anemia of pregnancy are all a temporary burden to the cardiovascular system. It is evident that the mother with an existing medical problem who becomes pregnant needs zealous care and supervision.

HEART DISEASE

The highest incidence of heart disease is influenced by the frequency of rheumatic fever and syphilis in a geographic area. Less frequent are coronary heart disease, thyroid heart disease, arteriosclerotic heart disease, acute pericarditis, and rarely hypertension. Hypertension is more often associated with toxemia of pregnancy.

Approximately 1% of all pregnant women have organic heart disease. Of all women with heart disease, in 90% the history shows it to be of rheumatic origin, and in the remaining 10% the heart disease is attributed to congenital lesions and syphilis. The severity of heart disease during pregnancy may be related to its being the fourth cause of maternal deaths, preceded by hemorrhage, infection, and toxemia.

Hemodynamics during the maternity cycle

A full understanding of the hemodynamics of pregnancy is essential in the study of heart disease. Changes in the maternal reproductive organs during the first trimester require more oxygen to the rapidly growing fetus. The increased oxygen need is present whether the mother is at rest or at work 24 hours a day. The heart rate accelerates 10 beats per minute during the latter half of pregnancy, accounting for 14,000 extra heartbeats daily. The physiologic anemia of pregnancy warrants an increase in iron intake.

Blood volume and cardiac output are greatest at 24 to 32 weeks gestation or in the sixth, seventh, or eighth month. Danger of heart failure during this period would be preceded by dyspnea, hemoptysis, and cough. Since normally there is an increase in vital capacity during pregnancy, any sudden decrease would be suggestive of impending heart failure. Any severe anemia, toxemia, or upper respiratory infection at this time would precipitate failure.

After the twenty-seventh week, the cardiac output falls and at term reaches the level of that prior to gestation. Blood volume reaches its peak at 36 weeks and declines somewhat the last 4 weeks of pregnancy.

During labor oxygen consumption rises with each contraction. Heart rate accelerates with the beginning of each contraction and is considerably slowed at the height of contractions. During delivery tachycardia is common, and a decided bradycardia follows delivery.

During delivery and immediately postpartum the cardiac output is markedly increased. The blood volume increases 20% to 40% due to the contracting uterus and venous return from the lower extremities.

Functional and therapeutic classifications of patients with diseases of the heart*

Functional classification. The classification of patients according to their cardiac functional capacity gives only a part of the information needed to plan the management of the patient's activities. A recommendation or prescription

*Excerpted from Diseases of the heart and blood vessels—nomenclature and criteria for diagnosis, ed. 6, Boston, Little, Brown and Co.; copyright 1964 by the New York Heart Association, Inc., and available from the publisher, medical bookstores, and through local Heart Associations.

regarding physical activity should be based on information derived from many sources. The functional classification is an estimate of what the patient's heart will allow him to do and should not be influenced by the character of the structural lesions or by an opinion as to treatment or prognosis.

Class I: Patients with cardiac disease but without resulting limitations of physical activity. Ordinary physical activity does not cause undue fatigue, palpitation, dyspnea, or anginal pain.

Class II: Patients with cardiac disease resulting in slight limitation of physical activity. They are comfortable at rest. Ordinary physical activity results in fatigue, palpitation, dyspnea, or anginal pain.

Class III: Patients with cardiac disease resulting in marked limitation of physical activity. They are comfortable at rest. Less than ordinary physical activity causes fatigue, palpitation, dyspnea, or anginal pain.

Class IV: Patients with cardiac disease resulting in inability to carry on any physical activity without discomfort. Symptoms of cardiac insufficiency or of the anginal syndrome may be present even at rest. If any physical activity is undertaken, discomfort is increased.

Therapeutic classification. The therapeutic classification is intended as a guide to the management of the activities of cardiac patients. It gives a prescription for the amount of physical activity that is advised for those in each functional class. From a practical point of view, it should be translated into terms of daily physical activity, such as walking a certain number of yards, climbing a specified number of stairs, lifting a certain number of pounds, and standing for an unlimited or limited part of the working day. For children it is necessary to individualize with permissible play programs, specifying the type and duration of outdoor and indoor activity that may be performed.

Class A: Patients with cardiac disease whose physical activity need not be restricted in any way.

Class B: Patients with cardiac disease whose ordinary physical activity need not be restricted, but who should be advised against severe or competitive efforts.

Class C: Patients with cardiac disease whose ordinary physical activity should be moderately restricted, and whose more strenuous efforts should be discontinued.

Class D: Patients with cardiac disease whose ordinary physical activity should be markedly restricted.

Class E: Patients with cardiac disease who should be at complete rest, confined to bed or chair.

The functional capacity of the patient does not always determine the amount of physical activity that should be permitted. For example, although a child at the onset of active rheumatic carditis may not experience discomfort on playing baseball, rest in bed is imperative. Such a patient would be designated as Class I (Functional), E (Therapeutic). There is frequently a difference between the amount of activity that a patient can undertake in terms of his functional capacity and that he should attempt in order to prevent aggravation of his disease. The recommendation of physical activity is based not only upon the amount of effort possible without discomfort but also upon the nature and severity of the cardiac disease.

Management and treatment of heart disease

Management of the cardiac patient during pregnancy and good tenets of prenatal care are explicit in Gorenberg's* principles, which follow:

Rule 1. Extra bed rest
2. Weekly clinic visits for the cardiac who is 25 years of age or older
3. Immediate hospitalization for Class III and Class IV cardiacs and absolute bed rest until after delivery
4. Immediate hospitalization for the patient with a history of cardiac failure, with absolute bed rest until after delivery
5. Immediate hospitalization at the first suspicion of decreasing cardiac reserve
6. Cesarean section for obstetric indications only

The cardiac patient may experience heart failure at any time during pregnancy. Medical and obstetric health supervision includes a low-sodium dietary regime and prompt reporting of unusual fatigue, dyspnea, hemoptysis, or edema of the feet. On physical examination any excessive weight gain, arrhythmia, or heart rate of 90 to 100 per minute with mitral stenosis warrants immediate hospital admission and treatment.

Management during labor and delivery should foster minimal analgesia and anesthesia to protect the decreased cardiac reserve.

Forms of anesthesia such as saddle block, caudal, and presacral are safe providing hypotension and tachycardia do not occur. Inhalation anesthesia is contraindicated since respiratory embarrassment due to oxygen depletion is common, and vomiting (a sequela) increases heart action. During delivery Class III or Class IV cardiac patients are safer in Walcher's position than in lithotomy position. In Walcher's position the legs are not lifted beyond the horizontal and are held widely adducted by two assistants, giving ample room for delivery and repair. Sims' position may also be assumed. If acute congestive failure occurs, "bloodless phlebotomy" or the rotation of tourniquets on the extremities is used to reduce circulating blood volume. Pooling of blood in the extremities is dangerous in the cardiac mother and should be kept in mind at the time of delivery. Lowering the legs should be done slowly following delivery.

Intravenous injections of ergot have a tendency to raise venous pressure, resulting in high blood pressure, and are contraindicated. To keep the uterus contracted, oxytocin may be given intramuscularly or intravenously in a solution of 5% glucose in water. When parenteral therapy is instituted, the volume and rate of flow are significant since added heart action predisposes to pulmonary edema.

---

*Slowinski, E. J., D'Alessandro, G., and Stein, J.: Heart disease in pregnancy. A three-dimensional view, J. Med. Soc. New Jersey **61**:215, June, 1964.

Following delivery Fowler's position and administration of oxygen are often ordered. The previous methods of applying abdominal binders and sandbags to the fundus are contraindicated since they obstruct normal respirations and predispose to thrombophlebitis. Breast-feeding in severe cardiac disease is discouraged because of the increased fluid and metabolic demands and the increased incidence of mastitis.

The puerperium is managed with great care since 88% of all maternal deaths occur during this period. Vital capacity readings are done because a decrease and a sudden increase in venous pressure and cardiac output are indicative of impending heart failure. Bed rest and a low-sodium diet are maintained for a period of 2 weeks. Antibiotics are given for a period of 3 days to prevent infection. Digitalis preparations and diuretics are ordered to strengthen heart muscle and to increase circulation time to prevent complications such as heart failure and pulmonary edema.

Following discharge continued medical supervision of the mother is essential. Discussions on daily activities, diet, and planning of future pregnancies assure maintenance of optimum health for the cardiac mother.

Nursing care of the heart patient

During the maternity cycle there are major considerations in caring for the mother with moderate or severe heart disease.

Prenatal period. During pregnancy discussions related to foods low in salt content will clarify the dietary regime for the mother. Correction of any existing anemia is imperative. During the prenatal period stressing the importance of rest by early retirement, late rising, and rest periods during the day is the nurse's responsibility. Often, helping the mother plan specific times is difficult when other siblings need to be considered. Knowledge of community agencies that offer homemaker service is important to the nurse in helping families plan for limitation of activities.

Emotional stress causes tachycardia with an increase in cardiac output. Cooperation of family members in avoiding stress is an adjunct to adequate nursing care during pregnancy. Preparation for labor and delivery is of primary importance for the cardiac mother. She has many fears and anxieties concerning her ability to withstand the work during labor. The nurse is the person with whom the mother establishes close rapport, and free discussion and reassurance will alleviate added stress. The mother who is prepared approaches labor and delivery with less fear and will do better physically and emotionally.

Teaching the importance of reporting a common cold early will avoid respiratory difficulty and cardiac embarrassment. The importance of medical supervision by a cardiologist and an obstetrician is stressed to assure early recognition of heart failure and pulmonary edema. The beginning signs of heart failure are persistent audible rales at the lung bases, edema, tachycardia, cough, and hemoptysis.

Labor period. The cardiac mother is prepared for oncoming labor by early admission a week or two prior to term. The added rest before labor starts and getting to know staff personnel are of physical and psychologic importance. Barbiturates are often used to assure relaxation when there is evidence of apprehension.

During labor, vital signs, labor progress, and astute observations for signs of heart failure are the nurse's primary responsibility. Small doses of meperidine (Demerol) and barbiturates are given to assure alleviation of pain and to allay apprehension. If signs of cardiac embarrassment occur, small doses of morphine may also be ordered. Although this may stop labor entirely for a short time, it is justified to prevent cardiac collapse. *Scopolamine is contraindicated since it increases heart action.*

Maintaining the bed in semi-Fowler's position facilitates breathing. Coaching the mother promotes relaxation, augmenting labor progress. Keeping the mother informed and constant attendance by the nurse are essential for safe care. Oxygen equipment should be available on the labor unit for emergency purposes.

Delivery period. With full effacement and dilatation the second stage is managed with local pudendal block. Caudal anesthesia may be used safely if administered by a qualified anesthesiologist. With caudal anesthesia there may be a resulting hypotension; therefore, frequent checking of the blood pressure is important. In severe cardiac disease the mother is not moved but delivered under aseptic technique in the labor bed. Often elective low-outlet forceps are used to shorten the second stage. This practice avoids strenuous activity and increased heart action associated with pushing.

Since the mother is awake during delivery, the supportive role of the nurse is an important one. Continual coaching by the same person during delivery adds comfort and relieves apprehension.

Postpartal period. The nurse's responsibility augments following delivery since this is the most crucial period. Following delivery there is a 30% increase in cardiac output—it remains at a high level for 3 to 4 days. There may also be a delayed period of decompensation occurring as late as the fifth day due to diuresis. The nurse is responsible for careful observations of vital signs. Tachycardia and respiratory difficulty are reported promptly. Often the mother is kept sedated, and providing a quiet environment allows for added rest.

Pulmonary embolism is the greatest hazard following delivery, and often anticoagulants are started routinely if there is endocardial damage.

For congestive heart failure digitalis may be ordered to strengthen heart action. Intravenous solutions are rarely given since they increase the work load of the heart. If parenteral fluids are ordered, they should be administered slowly, and the mother should be observed carefully for signs of pulmonary edema.

Bed rest is maintained for at least 2 weeks depending upon the severity of heart disease. Ambulation is gradual, and care of the baby is assumed for short periods when the mother's condition permits. Although the cardiac mother is to be at complete rest, her concern for the new baby is paramount. Keeping the mother informed and feeding the infant at the bedside as the mother shows improvement alleviate added anxiety and encourage beginning mother-infant relationships. Breast-feeding is usually discouraged since it would interfere with the rest needed to prevent complications. Hormones to prevent lactation are contraindicated since they have a tendency to retain sodium.

Mitral valvotomy is usually performed in the nongravid state. Only with severe Class III or Class IV diseases of the heart, valvotomy may be indicated and done prior to 18 weeks gestation and prior to the increased blood volume and cardiac output periods. Following mitral valvotomy, 2 or 3 years is optimum time for a new pregnancy. Pregnancy should not be delayed for too many years, since this is palliative treatment, and deterioration of the heart valve may occur.

Referral to public health nursing service, homemaker service, or social service agencies for the deprived family assures continuity in care. Family planning becomes an integral part of care when the mother's cardiac status is Class III or Class IV. The nurse works closely with family, clergy, and social service agencies to provide comprehensive nursing care.

DISEASES OF BLOOD VESSELS

Arteries

Diseases of the arteries associated with pregnancy are Raynaud's disease and dissecting aneurysm of the aorta.

Raynaud's disease is characterized by attacks of peripheral cyanosis (hands more than feet) occurring sometime between puberty and the menopause. Raynaud's disease is seldom complicated during pregnancy.

Dissecting aneurysm of the aorta is uncommon in the young pregnant woman but is associated with pregnancy and the puerperium. The majority of symptoms occur in the last trimester of pregnancy with sudden and severe chest pain, cyanosis, dyspnea, and weakness with ensuing cardiac failure and uremia.

Veins

Varicose veins. Varicose veins are often seen during pregnancy. Aggravation occurs because of the retarded venous flow from the lower extremities due to pressure of the gravid uterus. Varicose veins occur either when there is a weakness in the venous musculature or when there is a lack of normal functioning of valves, or both. The increase in blood clotting power during pregnancy also predisposes to venous thrombosis should circulatory stasis occur.

Symptoms. Discomfort characterized by burning or pruritus of the skin area, fatigue, ache on standing, and occasional skin discoloration is common. As pregnancy progresses, the enlarging uterus increases peripheral vascular pressure with exacerbation of symptoms.

Treatment and nursing care. The objectives in treatment are as follows:

(1) to relieve symptoms, (2) to reduce the incidence of phlebothrombosis and thrombophlebitis with ensuing embolism, (3) to prevent further damage to vein walls, and (4) for cosmetic reasons.

The nurse is responsible for instruction in proper application of an Ace bandage to ensure venous return and for elevation of the extremities when feasible throughout the day. Often varicosities are found in the vulva area, and they produce much discomfort. Comfort may be provided if the mother wears a panty maternity support during pregnancy.

Proper positioning of the mother during delivery without undue pressure on the varicosities will reduce the incidence of complications with thromboembolic disease. Ace bandages are applied immediately following delivery, and ambulation is begun early.

Thromboembolic disease. Thromboembolic disease is of two types: *thrombophlebitis,* in which there is inflammation of the vein wall, and *phlebothrombosis,* in which there is a clot formation without vessel involvement. A clot formation soon adheres to the vessel wall, and the hazard of embolism with thrombophlebitis is great.

The incidence of thromboembolic disease in pregnancy has decreased over the years. The low incidence is related to less traumatic deliveries, control of pelvic sepsis with the advent of chemotherapy and antibiotics, and better care and supervision during the prenatal and postpartal periods.

Thromboembolic disease develops either in the deep pelvic veins, the femoral vessels, or both. Involvement of the femoral veins is referred to as phlegmasia alba dolens. Often it is a sequela of pelvic infection or a traumatic pelvic delivery, and it may occur as late as 7 to 10 days following delivery.

Symptoms. Diagnosis of thromboembolic disease is difficult in the early stages. Elevation of pulse rate and basal body temperature often occurs. At times fleeting chest pain may be the only indication. Local tenderness, increase in the size of calf muscles or in the area along the femoral veins, redness, heat, and pain on dorsiflexion of the foot (Homans' sign) are visible manifestations. A blood count reveals a leukocytosis. Danger signs of pulmonary embolus are hemoptysis, pleuritic pain, and positive findings on roentgen examination of the lungs.

Treatment. Management and treatment of thromboembolic disease during pregnancy are controversial between anticoagulant and surgical therapy. The majority favor anticoagulant therapy when emboli are present. Drugs, however, that depress prothrombin production are contraindicated during the antepartal period. The drugs will deplete the growing baby of prothrombin activity, with resulting intrauterine death due to placental bleeding.

Heparin intravenously or bishydroxycoumarin (Dicumarol) by mouth may be given. When heparin is given, the clotting time of the blood is followed carefully; when bishydroxycoumarin is given, the prothrombin time is checked. Heparin is usually given in doses of 50 mg. every 6 hours until the clotting time is approximately 20 minutes, and subsequent doses are ordered to maintain a delayed clotting time. If the clotting time becomes excessively prolonged, 50 mg. to 100 mg. of protamine sulfate is administered intravenously to correct the deficit. Bishydroxycoumarin is given by beginning with an initial 300-mg. dose, followed by 250 mg. 24 hours later. Then daily doses of 50 mg. to 100 mg. are continued in order to keep the prothrombin time within 10% to 30% of normal. Vitamin K in doses of 50 mg. to 70 mg. is kept on hand as an antidote. Although vitamin K may be given intravenously, its action is slow, and at times administration of whole blood may be necessary to reduce the prothrombin time quickly. Heparin is usually the drug of choice since it can be controlled more easily, is more effective within 48 hours, and is continued for at least 10 days.

Surgical treatment consists of incision into the vein and removal of the clot by suction and subsequent vein ligation. Thromboembolic disease complicated by pulmonary emboli necessitates ligation of the inferior vena cava.

Nursing care. The psychologic implications in caring for the woman with thromboembolic disease need consideration in planning nursing care. The fear associated with circulatory involvement is great, since the danger of blood clots is common knowledge to most patients. Strict bed rest and leg immobilization constrict activity. Daily prothrombin times are done to pursue safe therapy. The nurse needs to listen, convey understanding, and reassure the mother that she is being given all the necessary care. Thromboembolic disease during pregnancy brings added fears and anxieties of the unborn baby's welfare. The emotional components of care are just as important as the physical aspects.

Elevation of the affected leg with due respect to pressure areas assures safe care and provides comfort. The weight of the bedclothes may add to the discomfort, and a leg cradle is useful and beneficial. Any rubbing or washing of the affected area is containdicated so that an adherent clot will not be dislodged. Medications for pain relief are given. When anticoagulant therapy is given, vital signs are checked, and any elevation in pulse rate or drop in blood pressure is reported immediately to the physician. At times the Ace bandage may become unraveled or wrinkled, decreasing its effectiveness, and reapplication is necessary. In handling the affected limb the leg is raised from the ankle to avoid pressure on the calf. Any sudden, severe chest pain with labored breathing, indicative of pulmonary embolism, warrants immediate reporting to the physician. Oxygen equipment should be in readiness for an emergency. At times surgical intervention with ligation of the inferior vena cava is attempted with recurrent pulmonary infarction caused by embolism. The ovarian vessels may be involved as often as the uterine veins, and they are also ligated. Following surgery there may be a resulting edema of the lower extremities if collateral circulation is not adequate. Women with ligations have been known to have subsequent uneventful pregnancies.

DIABETES MELLITUS

Prior to the discovery of insulin in 1921, only a few diabetics became pregnant. Amenorrhea and infertility were common, and mild diabetics were prewarned of the hazards of pregnancy. Sterility before that time was probably related to restriction in diet to control diabetes, and to hypofunction or hyperfunction of the anterior pituitary gland. Today, with the advancement of scientific knowledge and the improvement of obstetric care, women with severe diabetes may successfully complete a pregnancy.

The advent of insulin therapy has increased the numbers of childhood diabetics reaching childbearing age. The frequency with which pregnancy is complicated by diabetes is variable since the incidence increases with age. In many women symptoms of diabetes occur more frequently in the fifties and during the menopause.

Heredity

Since diabetes is genetically transmitted, a history of one or both parents with the disease may suggest a prediabetic state. Young people with diabetes have question as to the proportion of offspring genetically liable to diabetes. Generally diabetes is inherited as a recessive trait; however, in some families it is a dominant one. In a recessive trait, when only one parent has diabetes, approximately one fourth of the children may inherit the disease. When one parent has the disease and the other has a diabetic background, one half of the children may inherit the disease. Studies from family histories show that diabetes is twice as prevalent among children of diabetics who have diabetic parents as among those who do not have an affected parent.

Incidence

The incidence of diabetes ranges from 0.25% to 1% of all pregnancies. Of the total 1%, 30% have the disease prior to 40 years of age. A history of repeated stillbirths, fetal deaths, or excessively large babies weighing over 4,000 grams is suggestive of possible latent or prediabetes.

The severity of diabetes depends upon age, duration of the disease, and amount of renal and vascular damage. With adequate prenatal care and control of diabetes, maternal deaths are rare. Prognosis for the infant is contingent with the length of time the mother has had diabetes, since vascular and renal damage will ultimately affect the fetus.

Classification of diabetes during pregnancy

A classification of diabetes proposed by Priscilla White considers the age of onset of the diabetes, its duration, and the presence or absence of vascular or renal changes. The classification is as follows:

Group A: Diabetes on the basis of glucose tolerance test; dietary regulation only; no insulin requirement

Group B: Onset of diabetes after age 20, duration less than 10 years; no associated vascular disease

Group C: Onset of diabetes between the ages of 10 and 19, with a duration of 10 to 19 years; no vascular disease

Group D: Onset of diabetes under age 10, or duration of 20 years or more; vascular disease becoming established—retina or leg vessels (excluding pelvic arteriosclerosis)

Group E: Pelvic arteriosclerosis by roentgen-ray examination

Group F: Vascular nephritis

Group G: Multiple obstetric failures

Groups A and B may be expected to have an uneventful pregnancy with no difficulty. In contrast, Groups C, D, E, and F will frequently have maternal and fetal complications.

Physiology of pregnancy related to diabetes mellitus

The physiologic changes occurring in the various systems during pregnancy make diabetes difficult to control. Vomiting during the first trimester greatly decreases the carbohydrate intake, resulting in dangers of acidosis. The increased activity of the anterior pituitary gland decreases the tolerance for sugar, and larger quantities of insulin are required. During pregnancy the elevated basal metabolism and the decrease in the carbon dioxide combining power increase the tendency toward acidosis.

It is common to find glucose or lactose in the urine. Early in pregnancy sugar may be found in the urine since there is a lowered renal threshold. The presence of lactose in the urine in the latter part of pregnancy may be due to changes in preparation for lactation. During labor the muscular activity of the uterus depletes the glycogen reserve; therefore carbohydrate with insulin coverage is essential. Hypoglycemia during the puerperium is common as involution and lactation occur.

Regardless of these physiologic changes during pregnancy, any excretion of sugar is followed by fasting blood sugars and glucose tolerance tests. Oral glucose tolerance tests during pregnancy are not accurate since there is a known decrease in gastric motility and a delayed absorption of sugar from the intestinal tract. Interest is now centered on the intravenous glucose tolerance test (I.V.G. T.T.) for detection of early diabetes during pregnancy. For the test, women are given 2 ml. of a 10% glucose solution per 3 kg. of ideal body weight in a fasting state. Blood samples are then drawn at ½, 1, 2, and 3 hours after administration of the glucose. Women with suspected diabetes have a 2-hour postprandial blood sugar done, and then, if indicated, an I.V.G.T.T. in the third trimester.

The vast changes occurring in the maternal organism make diabetes difficult to control during pregnancy. Women with diabetes have a greater tendency toward toxemia and hydramnios. With these complications, there is a greater incidence of premature labor, stillbirth, congenital malformations, and neonatal deaths due to hypoxia and hypoglycemia.

Babies of diabetic mothers are larger than usual in 75% of cases, and their size may cause difficult labor and delivery. The increased birth weight is due to acceleration in growth of the true skeleton, excessive fat, and increased water retention in the subcutaneous tissue. However, in the mother with juvenile diabetes, the baby may not grow so rapidly, and the birth weight may be less than normal. This is important in determining when to terminate pregnancy.

The newborn is usually sluggish at birth, has poor temperature control, and has difficulty establishing respirations for proper lung oxygenation. Often the infant has ingested excessive amounts of amniotic fluid, and stomach aspiration is routinely a good practice. Since the baby is quite edematous at birth, a weight loss of as much as a pound may occur within a few days. Signs of hypoglycemia in the newborn are lethargy, poor sucking reflex, cyanosis, or twitching. Feedings of glucose water are started early when the infant's condition permits. Should the sucking reflex be poor, glucose is given parenterally to prevent hypoglycemia.

Management and nursing care in diabetes

The primary objectives of antepartal care of the diabetic pregnant woman are the prevention of acidosis and toxemia. Acidosis and toxemia are maternal complications that pose grave hazards for the unborn baby, predisposing to death in utero.

Prenatal examination includes urinalysis for protein and ophthalmoscopic examination to determine renal-vascular damage. If albumin is present, renal function is determined by urine concentration ability by further testing. A diet low in salt but adequate in protein and calories is prescribed. Insulin coverage is adjusted to prevent marked glycosuria and acetonuria. Fasting blood sugar levels of 140 to 150 mg. per 100 ml. and mildly positive sugar reactions are harmless during pregnancy. If vomiting makes the diabetes difficult to control, temporary hospitalization is indicated.

The internist and the obstetrician work as a team to control the diabetes. Weekly visits are necessary to check weight gain carefully. Excessive retention of fluids is treated with diuretics. Once the diagnosis is established, hospital admission for careful evaluation of the diabetic status is essential. It is often necessary to readmit women for a period of a few days every other month to keep the diabetes under control. The danger period of diabetes during pregnancy includes the last 7 weeks, beginning with the thirty-fourth week to term. It is during this period that 10% to 15% of fetal deaths occur. The majority of obstetricians recommend admission to the hospital 4 weeks prior to term. The purpose for early admission is twofold: (1) stabilization of the diabetes in preparation for delivery and (2) evaluation of the possibility of early delivery by induction or cesarean section.

Blood sugar levels are used to determine diet and insulin dosage. Priscilla White recommends a dietary regime of 30 to 40 Cal. per kilogram, 150 to 250 gm. of carbohydrate, 2 gm. of protein per kilogram, and fat to complete the caloric requirement. An average diet would include: 60 gm. of protein, 150 to 180 gm. of carbohydrate, and 80 to 90 gm. of fat with an added 15 to 20 gm. of carbohydrate at bedtime. White specifies that a liberal intake of carbohydrate prevents ketosis.

During the first trimester when nausea and vomiting may occur, diabetes is difficult to control and acidosis is a common occurrence. During the last trimester acute observations are made for beginning signs of toxemia and for variations in glucose tolerance. Any sudden changes in insulin requirements, where an increased amount is needed, may result in hypoglycemia. It is recommended that some spilling of sugar is safer than consistent negative readings. During labor it is a common practice to administer 10 gm. of glucose parenterally every hour since glucose is being utilized at this time. Diabetes is *most* difficult to control in the early puerperium. Marked fluctuations of blood sugar are common at this time due to the following: (1) endocrine and metabolic changes with the termination of pregnancy, (2) conversion of blood glucose to lactose in preparation for lactation, (3) sudden withdrawal of the fetal pancreas, and (4) the occurrence of an infection. Fluctuations in sugar tolerance are also common during the first week postpartum. Antibiotics are ordered at the first indication of puerperal infection. Although fluctuations in sugar tolerance are common during the first week postpartum, the diabetic status returns to its prepregnant state following this period.

The nurse's role in caring for the diabetic pregnant woman includes guidance in relation to diet, urinalysis, exercise, and personal hygiene. Planning a list of exchange foods will facilitate following a diet since food cravings are common. Teaching the technique of testing urine and interpreting signs and symptoms of hypoglycemia and acidosis is essential for safety of mother and baby. Hypoglycemic reactions include a feeling of inner nervousness and apprehension, blurred or double vision, tingling sensations, and a staggering gait. When untreated, symptoms progress to twitching, convulsions, and unconsciousness. Acidosis is preceded by a significantly large amount of sugar and acetone in the urine. Symptoms include increased thirst and urination, hunger, weakness, easy fatigue, loss of weight, and genital pruritus. When these symptoms are untreated, loss of appetite, nausea, vomiting, headache, rapid deep breathing, impaired vision, and finally unconsciousness occur. Awareness of these symptoms is essential for prompt reporting to the physician. Infections, fever, colds, accidents, and emotional upsets increase the amount of insulin required.

Care of the teeth, bowel regularity, and adequate rest and sleep are essential for maintenance of health. Skin care includes daily bathing and gentle drying to prevent skin breakdown. Loose garments alleviate constriction of blood vessels and prevent blood stasis in the lower extremities.

The patient must be taught the following for maintenance and control of diabetes during pregnancy: (1) the importance of regular visits to the internist and the obstetrician; (2) adhering to a schedule of diet, urine testing, and medication; (3) taking adequate exercise daily without undue overexertion; (4) maintaining an adequate regime for sleep and rest; (5) avoiding emotional stress whenever possible; and (6) always carrying an identification card saying, "I am a diabetic and I have been taking ______________________" (indicate dosage of insulin or dosage of antidiabetic oral drug).

Referral to public health nursing service is an adjunct to continuity in care.

DISORDERS OF THE RESPIRATORY SYSTEM

Acute infectious diseases of the lung during pregnancy are less serious since the advent of chemotherapy. The dangers of uncontrolled upper respiratory infections are fetal death in utero and premature labor, a result of high fever with toxicity. The control of chronic pulmonary lesions through the advancement in medical and surgical therapy permits more women to undertake pregnancy.

Chronic pulmonary disorders may be categorized into three groups. The first group includes infectious conditions, the most common being tuberculosis and bronchiectasis. The second group includes those conditions such as pulmonary fibrosis, in which there is interference with alveolar capillary oxygen exchange. The third group includes those diseases that alter the capacity of the thoracic cage through chest deformities such as kyphoscoliosis.

Tuberculosis

Incidence. Tuberculosis in pregnant women has not shared the decline in prevalence that has occurred in the general population. A 2% to 3% rate of tuberculosis has been found in roentgenographic examination of pregnant women, with approximately one third of these women having active tuberculosis. The value of prenatal chest roentgenograms is obvious. Fetal and gonadal irradiation is minimal with the improvement in roentgen-ray equipment.

Since the advent of chemotherapy, the prognosis of tuberculosis during pregnancy is good. There is general agreement that maternal tuberculosis rarely affects the baby. In instances in which the baby is affected, there has been a penetration by the tubercle bacillus into the placenta. It is also believed that pregnancy exerts little or no influence on the incidence and course of pulmonary tuberculosis. This belief is based on the assumption that during pregnancy and puerperium the woman receives close health supervision and therapy.

Management. Hospital care and total bed rest are not required by the majority of women, but therapy of this kind is reserved for the gravidas with advanced disease and positive sputum tests. Most women remain at home to rest and receive chemotherapeutic drugs such as streptomycin and isoniazid together, or either of these in combination with para-aminosalicylic acid. It was believed that streptomycin had an effect on the vestibular and auditory apparatus in the fetus—however, such evidence is not conclusive.

Thoracic surgery such as pneumolysis or thoracoplasty may be performed in the early months of pregnancy, when indicated. Data indicate that 10% to 15% of pregnant women with tuberculosis react unfavorably in the early puerperium, with exacerbation of the tuberculosis process. When this occurs, pneumothorax and pneumoperitoneum have been recommended within the first 24 hours following delivery and periodically thereafter. The newborn is protected by the use of BCG vaccine. Prior to delivery consent of the parents is obtained for tuberculin testing, BCG vaccination of the infant, and breaking contact between the mother and the infant.

BCG vaccination, however, is only one step in the prevention of tuberculosis. Vaccination is accomplished by injecting a very small amount of nonvirulent bovine tubercle bacilli, which produces a small pustule similar to that of smallpox vaccination. The pustule appears in 3 to 5 weeks and disappears within a month. At times there may be enlargement of the lymph nodes in the axilla, and the lesion may take 6 to 8 weeks to heal.

Vaccination of the infant is done on the second day after birth providing he is normal and weighs more than 5 pounds. Eight weeks later, a tuberculin test is done on the infant. The Vollmer patch test is used for a positive reaction; the Mantoux test is used for a negative reaction. With a positive reading the child is returned to his mother if her condition permits. The infant with a negative tuberculin test is revaccinated 10 to 12 weeks following BCG vaccination, isolation is continued, and tuberculin testing is repeated. Tuberculin testing and roentgenographic examination of the infant's chest are continued and repeated every 6 months.

Bronchiectasis

Bronchiectasis, a severe necrotic type of bronchitis, occurs early in life. It results in chronic respiratory difficulty with secondary emphysema. Symptoms include intermittent low-grade fever, cough, and occasionally foul sputum.

The course of bronchiectasis is not altered during pregnancy nor is pregnancy affected by the lung changes. The treatment is the same as in the nonpregnant state: postural drainage and antibiotic therapy to prevent further infection. When lobectomy has been performed, pregnancy is uneventful.

Pulmonary fibrosis and allied conditions

Viral and bacterial infections may result in a chronic respiratory condition involving the lung parenchyma, causing pulmonary fibrosis. With fibrosis, there is interference with oxygen diffusion because of an impaired alveolar septum, with a resulting reduction in arterial oxygen saturation. There is also enlargement of the thoracic cage and diminution of motion, which embarrass respirations. These patients are relieved of respiratory discomfort by assuming a supine position.

Management has included ACTH and cortisone therapy. ACTH and cortisone therapy are seldom used during the first trimester unless they are urgently needed, since studies show a higher incidence of harm done to the developing fetus during this early stage of pregnancy. When given in the second or third trimester for prolonged periods, serum electrolytes are checked frequently. Cortisone may induce hyperglycemia and metabolic acidosis, which may affect the fetus. The course of the disease is not accelerated by pregnancy, and pregnancy is rarely contraindicated.

Kyphoscoliosis

Marked distortions of the chest are a result of changes in the cervical and thoracic vertebrae caused by rickets, tuberculosis of the spine, or poliomyelitis. These produce a reduction in the lung volume by decreasing the capacity of the thorax as a result of interference with normal mobility.

Although kyphoscoliosis presents no special problem during pregnancy, cardiac and respiratory evaluation is pursued. Vital capacity determinations reveal the approximate index of functioning pulmonary parenchyma. Other tests are used to determine functional residual capacity.

The course of pregnancy with kyphoscoliosis will depend upon whether cardiac hypertrophy and dilatation are present, and to a lesser extent on the degree to which pulmonary volume is reduced.

• • •

In summary, the respiratory changes associated with pregnancy do not impose any burden on the woman with pulmonary involvement.

Nursing care in respiratory distress

The role of the nurse is one of prevention by careful health supervision through referral to public health agencies. The primary objective of maintaining optimum health during pregnancy is prevention of infection through health teaching. Stressing the importance of having all family members seen by a physician yearly will ensure early treatment and cure.

If tuberculosis is diagnosed, the nurse as a member of the health team teaches the etiology, prevention, and control to all family members. Follow-through on all contacts assures adequate public health measures. With children of school age, the school nurse becomes an integral part of the health team. When prolonged hospital care is needed for the mother, community agencies such as social welfare and homemaker service will relieve stress by keeping the family together.

DISORDERS OF THE URINARY SYSTEM

Incidence. The increase in frequency of infections of the urinary system is attributed to the physiologic changes during pregnancy. Ureteral dilatation, kinking, and displacement are changes occurring due to the rotation and enlargement of the uterus. These factors predispose to urinary stasis with resulting bacterial invasion. Calculi and congenital anomalies of the urinary tract are also etiologic factors.

The most common infections during pregnancy are acute and chronic pyelonephritis, and only these will be treated in this text.

Acute and chronic pyelonephritis

Acute pyelonephritis is a diffuse inflammatory process of the interstitial connective tissue of the kidney, the nephron only being involved with extensive infection.

Pathology. Pathology reveals leukocytes and bacteria in the connective tissue or lymphatics surrounding the glomeruli. The tubules may contain purulent material, and occasionally but rarely there may be scattered multiple abscesses in the cortex and the medulla. Blood vessels may be damaged in areas where there is marked inflammation with deposition of fibrin upon the lumen of involved arterioles. With chronic pyelonephritis in addition to inflammatory changes, the renal cortex becomes narrow from scar tissue formation.

With acute pyelonephritis, healing without scarring or kidney dysfunction is the usual outcome. However, with repeated recurrent attacks the disease may become chronic, resulting in progressive renal impairment with death from hypertensive disease and renal failure.

In 75% of women the *Escherichia coli* are the invading organisms in acute pyelonephritis. Occasionally the staphylococcus and the streptococcus are responsible organisms.

Signs and symptoms. In the majority of women acute pyelonephritis appears in the latter part of pregnancy, particularly in the last trimester. Systemic reactions are more profound when *Escherichia coli* is the responsible organism.

Urinary frequency and urgency with or without dysuria are common symptoms in mild forms. In severe infections, chills, fever, and severe backache with tenderness over the kidney region are characteristic symptoms. On examination there is a moderate rise in nonprotein nitrogen, some decrease in phenolsulfonphthalein excretion, and a delay in dye excretion on pyelography. With severe and prolonged toxicity, there may be a resulting fall in hemoglobin levels.

Management. Management of women with pyelonephritis of pregnancy depends upon the degree of severity of signs and symptoms. Women with severe toxicity require prompt hospitalization, while women with milder forms can be treated on an outpatient regime.

With severe toxicity, urine is obtained for culture, and blood is drawn for a blood culture, for nonprotein nitrogen determination, and studies of the peripheral blood. Roentgenographic examination is done to rule out the presence of calculi or kidney enlargement. Acute infections are treated with broad-spectrum antibiotics, forcing fluids by mouth or parenterally when vomiting occurs. Checking the intake and output is a good indication of kidney function.

When alleviation of signs and symptoms fails, urinary blocking may be due to kinking of the ureter. An intravenous pyelogram in 3 or 4 months will rule out pathology.

Problems related to the chronicity of pyelonephritis include the recurrence of the condition in future pregnancies and the long-range effects on the cardiovascular system with repeated attacks. Although pyelonephritis is not a cause of toxemia of pregnancy, nor is the incidence of toxemia greater with the condition, it is a cause of hypertension in pregnant women. Severe hypertension in approximately 15% to 20% of individuals is a direct result of chronic pyelonephritis. When not treated promptly, mild acute pyelonephritis results in permanent renal damage and vascular disease.

Nursing care. The nurse, caring for the mother on an outpatient regime, plans with her the maintenance of an adequate diet, chemotherapy, and proper rest to alleviate symptoms. Teaching and stressing the importance of frequent health visits and reporting signs of frequency, dysuria, and tenderness or pain in the kidney region assure prompt treatment. The importance of forcing fluids is essential with chemotherapy.

Long-range goals include medical examinations a few months following delivery. Discussion on family planning will avoid the added risk of recurrence with an early unexpected pregnancy before the urinary tract is free of infection and the mother's optimum health has been restored.

For the hospitalized mother with severe pyelonephritis, nursing measures include bed rest, forcing fluids, and checking intake and output. Adequate urinary drainage is accomplished with the mother in Sims' position, which relieves the pressure of the enlarged uterus on the ureters. If a catheter is ordered, checking the flow and maintaining a closed system prevent added infection. Since premature labor may occur, observing for signs of labor is essential. If the mother has recurrent attacks, the importance of periodic urologic examinations should be stressed following delivery.

VIRUSES DURING PREGNANCY

Rubella

Rubella in the first trimester is known to cause congenital eye defects in the infant. Often the infant is born prematurely and does poorly in the neonatal period. Exposing young girls to rubella produces a permanent immunity and has been advocated. However, care must be taken because some of these young girls may have mothers in the childbearing age whom they may be exposing to rubella.

Varicella

Varicella (chickenpox) occurs only rarely in pregnant women. When it does it is usually serious in the mother, and the infant can be infected in utero.

Scarlet fever

The only treatment for scarlet fever is early administration of penicillin. However, abortion is usually the sequela.

Mumps

Mumps during pregnancy produces a 15% incidence of abortion and fetal death and a much higher incidence of congenital anomalies.

HERPES GESTATIONIS

Herpes gestationis is a rare form of dermatitis herpetiformis that appears during the third month of pregnancy. It subsides spontaneously following delivery. Symptoms are pruritus, burning, and pain. The lesions are papules, vesicles, or bullae arranged symmetrically over the groin, buttocks, trunk, or thighs. Hydrocortisone or adrenocorticotropic hormone is effective in treatment. Analgesics are sometimes given if severe pain occurs.

SELECTED REFERENCES

American Heart Association: Heart disease and pregnancy, New York, 1963, The Association.

Anderson, B.: Diabetes mellitus—the crisis arising in pregnancy, Abbottempo **2:**4, June, 1964.

Baker, D., and others: Comparison of standard oral and rapid intravenous glucose tests in pregnancy, Obstet. Gynec., vol. 31, no. 4, April, 1968.

Burwell, C.: Heart disease and pregnancy, Boston, 1958, Little, Brown and Co.

Chesterman, H.: The public health nurse and family planning, Nurs. Outlook **12:**32, September, 1964.

Croasman, R.: Pregnancy and diabetes: nursing care, Amer. J. Nurs. **58:**101, January, 1958.

Eastman, N. J., and Hellman, L. M.: Williams obstetrics, ed. 13, New York, 1966, Appleton-Century & Appleton-Century-Crofts.

Garnet, J., and others: One hour intravenous glucose tolerance test, Obstet. Gynec., vol. 32, no. 2, August, 1968.

Garnet, J. D.: Pregnancy in women with diabetes, Amer. J. Nurs. **69:**1900, September, 1969.

Gelber, I.: Family planning in a growing world, Amer. J. Nurs. **64:**98, August, 1964.

Goodrich, F.: The problem of anxiety in obstetrics, Child and Family **4:**62, Winter, 1965.

Guttmacher, A.: Planning your family, New York, 1964, The Macmillan Co.

Hamilton, Sister M.: The obstetrical patient—family member, Catholic Nurse **13:**56, September, 1964.

Handjani, A.: Grand-multiparity and rheumatic heart disease, Obstet. Gynec., vol. 32, no. 2, August, 1968.

Haynes, M.: Teaching continuity of care, Amer. J. Nurs. **62:**84, May, 1962.

Heap, B.: Sodium restricted diets, Amer. J. Nurs. **60:**206, February, 1960.

Hughes, E. C.: Diabetes and pregnancy, Postgrad. Med. **42:**487, 1967.

Kelly, D. N.: Change is the rhythm, Catholic Nurse **13:**18, December, 1964.

Kelly, G. A.: Birth control and Catholics, New York, 1964, Doubleday & Co., Inc.

Latham, H. C.: Thrombophlebitis, Amer. J. Nurs. **63:**122, September, 1963.

Le Mat, A. F.: The public health nurse in a maternity service, Nurs. Outlook **12:**58, October, 1964.

Martin, M. M.: New trends in diabetes detection, Amer. J. Nurs. **63:**101, August, 1963.

Mendelson, C. L.: Cardiac disease in pregnancy, Philadelphia, 1960, F. A. Davis Co.

Minkler, D.: Public policy in family planning, Nurs. Outlook **12:**28, September, 1964.

Morlock, M.: The broadened horizons of homemaker services, Children **11:**152, July-August, 1964.

Morris, E.: How does a nurse teach nutrition to patients? Amer. J. Nurs. **60:**67, January, 1960.

Peel, Sir J.: Progress in the knowledge and management of the pregnant diabetic patient, Amer. J. Obstet. Gynec. **83:**847, 1962.

Reid, D. E.: A textbook of obstetrics, Philadelphia, 1962, W. B. Saunders Co.

Robinson, A.: The principle, not the method, Nurs. Outlook **12:**27, September, 1964.

Rodman, M.: Drugs used in heart disease, RN **27:**37, May, 1964.

Schenker, J. G., and Polishuk, W. Z.: Pregnancy following mitral valvotomy, Obstet. Gynec., vol. 32, no. 2, August, 1968.

Schlesinger, B.: The Canadian conference on the family, J. Marriage & Family **27**:81, February, 1965.

Shaefer, G., Taggart, E., and Ivey, E. D.: The pregnant woman with tuberculosis, Amer. J. Nurs. **63**:68, August, 1963.

Shyne, A. W., Le Mat, A. F., and Kogan, L. S.: Evaluating public health service to the maternity patient and her family, Nurs. Outlook **11**:56, January, 1963.

Slowinski, E. J., D'Alessandro, G., and Stein, J.: Heart disease in pregnancy. A three-dimensional view, J. Med. Soc. New Jersey **61**:215, June, 1964.

Taylor, H. P., Lammert, A. C., and Zeit, P. R.: Current medical therapy in obstetrics, Amer. J. Nurs. **62**:86, August, 1962.

Veray, F., and Cibes-Hernandez, J. J.: Heart disease and pregnancy, Obstet. Gynec., vol. 32, no. 3, September, 1968.

Welton, T. B.: Rhythm birth control, New York, 1963, Grosset & Dunlap, Inc.

Questions for study

1. What are the normal physiologic changes during pregnancy that need be considered in the care of the cardiac mother?
2. Define the criteria for classifying heart disease as set down by the American Heart Association.
3. How is the cardiac mother managed during the prenatal, intrapartal, and postpartal periods?
4. What are the nursing responsibilities of the cardiac mother during the maternity cycle?
5. What are the inherent dangers of varicose veins during pregnancy?
6. Define thrombophlebitis and phlebothrombosis. Discuss the management and treatment.
7. What are the nursing implications for thromboembolic disease during pregnancy?
8. Relate the physiologic changes during pregnancy that would make diabetes difficult to control.
9. What are the primary objectives in caring for the diabetic pregnant mother during the prenatal, intrapartal, and postpartal periods?
10. What are the nursing responsibilities during pregnancy, labor, delivery, and the postpartal periods?
11. List the objectives in caring for the pregnant mother with tuberculosis.
12. What are the nurse's responsibilities in caring for the mother with a urinary tract infection?
13. Mr. and Mrs. C. have been married 6 years and are white Americans of middle-class income. They live in a well-furnished 5-room house they recently purchased. Mr. C. is 26 years old, and Mrs. C. is 24 years old.

 Mrs. C. has had diabetes since she was 12 years of age. The onset of the disease was dramatic, and she was immediately put on insulin and a diabetic diet.

 Since their marriage Mr. and Mrs. C. have been anxious to have a baby—yet pregnancy had never occurred. Mrs. C. had now missed two periods and suspected she was pregnant. She visited her obstetrician who confirmed the diagnosis.

 At two different times during her pregnancy she had been admitted for re-evaluation of her diabetic status. On each occasion she verbalized concern about her own well-being and that of the baby. She had been visiting her internist once a week and her obstetrician once a month.

 At 38 weeks gestation Mrs. C. was admitted for evaluation and for induction. On admission this information was found on her chart:

Weight	120 lb. prior to pregnancy 148 lb. at present
Blood pressure	140/90
Sugar	2+
Acetone	Negative
Albumin	Trace
Blood sugar	200 mg./100 ml.
Cholesterol	270 mg./100 ml.
CO_2 combining power	Stat.
Hemoglobin	13 gm.
B.U.N.	Stat.

 Three days following admission Mrs. C. was started on an infusion of 1,000 ml. 5% glucose in water with 10 units of Syntocinon at 12 drops per minute. Labor progressed quickly, and in 4 hours Mrs. C. was 2½ fingers dilated, fully effaced, and frustrated in coping with uterine contractions. She was given 50 mg. of meperidine and 50 mg. of promethazine I.M. stat. Within another 3 hours she was fully dilated. Following an 8-hour labor under epidural block anesthesia, she delivered spontaneously a living baby boy weighing 4,200 grams. Although exhausted, she was very much elated when she saw her baby.

The baby needed to be aspirated and resuscitated, and the Apgar score was 7 in one minute, 9 in 5 minutes. The baby was taken to the premature nursery, placed in an Isolette, and given glucose water within 2 hours. His blood sugar and serum calcium levels remained within normal limits.

Mrs. C. was hospitalized for 2 weeks and was well controlled upon discharge. Referral was made to the local public health office for follow-up care.

Suggested reflections on the preceding study

a. How would you plan nursing care for this family in light of the information you have? Prenatally, during labor and delivery, and during the puerperium?
b. Following your reading, interpret the findings upon admission of Mrs. C.
c. What are some of the teaching plans for continued health maintenance of Mrs. C. and her baby?
d. What are your plans in caring for Mrs. C. and the baby following delivery?

Directions

14. Using the following case as a frame of reference, apply the information you have gained from your readings that will enable you to:
    a. Identify areas of physiologic and emotional stress that are specifically related to the cardiac patient in the pregnancy cycle.
    b. Identify what you see as the responsibility of the nurse to this type of patient in the various phases described.
    c. Relate this information to designing and adjusting nursing care plans for this type of patient as she progresses through the pregnancy cycle.

Phase I:

Mrs. C. is a 29-year-old primigravida of Greek extraction who has been married for 5 years. Her husband is 31; he is employed as a bookkeeper at a moderate salary. They live in a 4-room apartment in the upstairs of a two-family house. She is not employed at this time.

Because of a history of a heart murmur and a siege of subacute bacterial endocarditis, which responded to treatment, she was referred by a family physician to a cardiology clinic for evaluation when she suspected she was about 7 weeks pregnant. Examination revealed a systolic murmur, long thrill over the pericardium, enlarged heart, predominantly right-sided, blood pressure, 125/70. Tentative diagnoses were made—the latter two would probably be ruled out:

a. Ventricular septal defect
b. Atrial septal defect
c. Rheumatic heart disease with mitral insufficiency

The patient was to be followed in the special obstetric-cardiac clinic. She was classified as having congenital heart disease, compensated-functional Class II and therapeutic classification of Class C (New York Heart Association).

Phase II:

The patient continued to do well until she reached 22 weeks gestation, when she became short of breath and had an irregular pulse, 120/minute. She was digitalized, and her condition improved.

Phase III:

At 30 weeks gestation, she was admitted to the hospital in heart failure, pulse rate was 100, there was vein distention in the neck but no peripheral edema. Her hemoglobin at this time was 11.3 gm., hematocrit, 32%. She responded well to the medical treatment. Four days after admission her weight went from 117 to 112. Five weeks later she was discharged to continue bed rest at home.

Phase IV:

In the thirty-ninth week of pregnancy her membranes ruptured spontaneously, and she was readmitted to the hospital. When her contractions became weak, she was given oxytocin in an intravenous drip. After a total labor of 10 hours, 28 minutes, she was delivered of a boy, 6 lb., 9 oz., by midforceps and an episiotomy under pudendal block anesthesia.

Phase V:

Postpartally, she was placed on a conventional unit. She complained of fullness in her chest the next day, but this disappeared by the following day. She held and fed the infant at regular times. She was discharged 10 days later with the plan of returning in 2 or 3 months for diagnostic cardiac procedures.

15. Mrs. J., a 25-year-old primigravida of Puerto Rican extraction, had been married for 3 years. She and her husband had just come to the United States and settled in a 3-room, 4-story walk-up apartment in a low-income housing project.

    When seen in the clinic at 12 weeks gestation, Mrs. J. gave a history of rheumatic fever at the age of 7 with two recurrent episodes of streptococcal throat infections at 9 and 12 years of age. At that time, she was told she had developed rheumatic heart disease with mitral insufficiency. She was referred to the cardiac clinic, and evaluation revealed an enlarged heart, predominantly right-sided, blood pressure 128/74, and she was classified as a compensated functional Class II cardiac.

    a. What determines the classification of a patient with cardiac disease? What is the underlying disease process in rheumatic heart disease?
    b. During pregnancy what measures would be essential for safe care of Mrs. J. and her baby?
    c. What members of the health team might be involved in her care?
    d. During which trimester would close observation and visits be imperative? Why?
    e. What signs would indicate a worsening of her cardiac condition?
    f. Mrs. J. has ben put on a 1,500 calorie low-sodium diet and asks you about what she could eat. How would you help her?
    g. How would labor and delivery differ with Mrs. J. as compared to a normal primigravida with no complications superimposed on pregnancy?
    h. What kinds of drugs used in obstetrics would be definitely contraindicated for Mrs. J.? Why?
    i. How would the care of Mrs. J. and her baby differ from the normal postpartum mother and baby?
    j. What are some of the long-range goals in caring for this family that are nursing responsibilities?

16. Mrs. Bell is a 19-year-old primigravida, who was first seen in the clinic with a history of amenorrhea for a period of 3 months. While giving her history, she mentioned being in bed with a fever for many weeks when she was 11 years old. She was told that she had "growing pains," but since this time has been well. In fact, she said she had not mentioned the illness to her husband. A diagnosis of pregnancy of 3 months was made. On the basis of a murmur picked up on physical examination plus the medical history, rheumatic heart disease was noted. Initial laboratory work showed the following:

Hemoglobin	10.6
Sedimentation rate	Normal limits
Urinalysis	Sugar, negative Albumin, negative

    a. What do we know about "growing pains"?
    b. What significance do you think the diagnosis of rheumatic heart disease has for this family?
    c. On the basis of this visit, what would be your immediate concerns?

    You first meet Mrs. Bell when she is 24 weeks pregnant, and her husband accompanies her to the clinic. He stops you and says his wife woke up in the night with shortness of breath and some coughing. You speak to Mrs. Bell and note that she does appear slightly dyspneic and that her legs appear edematous. The doctor sees her and orders immediate hospitalization on the basis of incipient heart failure.

    Her orders read:

    Strict bed rest
    Vital signs q, 4 h.

Diet, high protein, 1 gm. Na.
Mercuhydrin, 1 ml. I.M. stat.
Intake and output

a. What is the underlying disease process?
b. Why is hospitalization needed at this time?
c. What might this mean to the wife? the husband?
d. How do the orders relate to the disease process? Are there any others you might anticipate?
e. How might we use the health team?

After two weeks of bed rest followed by progressive ambulation, Mrs. Bell is allowed to go home. She does well at home and is readmitted at 38 weeks. Ten days later she complains of low intermittent back pain. The doctor comes and verifies that labor is progressing. You go with Mrs. Bell to the labor room. During labor she receives 50 mg. of meperidine and is taken to the delivery room when fully dilated. She is delivered of a living baby girl by low forceps. You care for her during the postpartal period. On the fifth day the father takes the baby home. Mrs. Bell remains 10 more days and goes home on the fifteenth postpartal day.

a. What might Mrs. Bell's regime be at home, in the hospital prior to delivery, during the four stages of labor?
b. What implications does Mrs. Bell's continued hospitalization have for the attainment of new roles?
c. What future needs can you anticipate?

CHAPTER 23

COMPLICATIONS OF THE NEWBORN

Prior to birth the infant lives in an environment completely protected and nourished by the maternal organism. The majority of infants begin their extra-uterine existence without any great difficulty. However, in reality, the rapid change from placental to pulmonary respirations that occurs at birth is one of the most dramatic of cardiovascular pulmonary phenomena occurring in one's lifetime. The success of this transition is related to the events that occur during prenatal life and to the course of labor and delivery. Prenatal factors causing respiratory distress in the neonate are *a*sphyxia, *p*rematurity, *n*arcosis, *e*ncephalo-spinal injury, *i*nfection, and *c*ongenital anomalies. The first letters of these causative factors spell out *apneic*. Asphyxia may occur as a result of etiologic factors related to their site of origin, which may be maternal, placental, and fetal. Complications that produce hypoxia or acidosis within the mother or that decrease maternal blood flow to the placenta are causes of asphyxia. Placental causes of asphyxia are placenta previa, abruptio placentae, placental infarction, or reduced diffusion of oxygen through the placenta. Fetal complications include fetal anemia, umbilical cord occlusions, and fetal shock.

NEONATAL RESPIRATORY DISTRESS

Asphyxia neonatorum

Normally the newborn infant cries immediately after birth, and respirations become rhythmic within the first minute. The newborn is pale or cyanotic at birth but rapidly develops a pink color as soon as respirations are well established. Two methods in current use for evaluating the newborn are the Apgar (page 138) and the Silverman-Anderson (page 190) scoring systems.

When respirations are not well established within one minute, the condition is known as *asphyxia neonatorum*. With this complication the infant may show signs of brief periods of apnea or total apnea. Mild cases are characterized by persistent cyanosis of the entire body; the muscle tone is good, and the infant will resist the examiner who attempts to open the mouth. This condition is known as *asphyxia livida*. With severe symptoms the infant has a marked pallor, general muscle limpness, and there is no resistance to the examiner. This is known as *asphyxia pallida*.

The three main causes of asphyxia neonatorum are either one or a combination of the following: (1) anoxia (oxygen deprivation), (2) cerebral damage, and (3) narcosis.

Anoxia

Prior to birth the infant is oxygenated by the placenta, and any interference with this exchange produces either death in utero or asphyxia at birth. The contractions of labor that are lengthy and strong may cut off placental exchange. Any mechanical or accidental interference with the umbilical cord, such as pressure, knotting, or malformation, deprives the infant. Placental detachment as in placenta previa or abruptio placentae produces varying degrees of asphyxia.

Cerebral injury

Disturbed respirations at birth commonly follow difficult deliveries. Often the head is so compressed that pressure on the blood vessels causes hemorrhage and damage to the respiratory center. Difficult forceps application with extraction, breech presentation, or an unusually large infant and small pelvis cause cerebral injury. A sudden precipitate delivery or a long labor and difficult delivery without the use of instruments may also produce brain damage.

Narcosis

The mother who is heavily sedated often has an infant with delayed respiratory effort at birth. Often it is the time sedation is given prior to delivery that causes narcosis. If anesthesia is administered at the same time sedation is at its peak, asphyxia of the newborn occurs.

Prevention of neonatal respiratory distress

It is evident that preventive treatment encompasses early and adequate prenatal medical supervision. Early prenatal care will aid in the prevention and management of toxemia, pelvic disproportion, premature birth, and other abnormalities.

The nurse's role is one of teaching mothers good nutrition and hygiene. The physiology of labor and delivery should be discussed so that there is less fear and anxiety during labor, eliminating the use of large doses of sedation and anesthesia. The nurse who cares for the mother in labor checks the fetal heart frequently and reports immediately signs of fetal distress so that prompt treatment is given.

Many of the preventive measures are a direct responsibility of the obstetrician as he provides prenatal care and manages the labor and delivery.

Treatment of neonatal respiratory distress

The nurse on the labor and delivery unit is responsible for having available oxygen and resuscitative equipment for the infant at all times. Often it is the anesthetist who assumes the responsibility of aspiration and resuscitation of the newborn, but the nurse must also be cognizant of the needs of the infant. Any help the nurse gives the anesthetist at this time will prove valuable to the baby in distress.

Care of the infant with asphyxia neonatorum demands early and prompt treatment if the infant does not assume rhythmic respirations within one minute following birth. Since shock is present the infant should be handled *gently,* kept *warm,* and positioned properly in order to *clear the airway* of mucus. The infant's head should be lower than his buttocks, and his chin should be held backward to straighten the trachea.

To promote drainage of mucus, the infant may be held upside down by the ankles with one hand. The forefinger is held between the ankles, and the other hand supports the infant's head or milks the trachea. If this method is not sufficient, a bulb syringe or a tracheal catheter may be used. The bulb of the syringe is compressed prior to inserting the tip into the baby's mouth and nose, and the pressure on the bulb is released gently after insertion. Secretions that have been suctioned into the syringe are then discarded, and the procedure is repeated. If a catheter is used, it is inserted as far as the pharynx and gently rotated so as not to injure the mucous membranes in the mouth. The catheter is inserted about one fourth of an inch beyond the opening of the nares to suction both nostrils. The safest suctioning apparatus is the De Lee mucus trap (Fig. 13-2), in which the operator uses his own mouth to suction and clear the infant's airway gently. A simple method is to position the infant's head downward and to milk the trachea so that the mucus may be aspirated when it appears at the pharynx. Once the airway is rid of mucus, oxygen may be administered at controlled concentrations by mechanical devices.

When mechanical devices are not available, an old method of resuscitation is mouth-to-mouth insufflation. The physician or prepared nurse places a few pieces of gauze over the infant's mouth, and with the head well extended the operator puts his mouth over the infant's nose and mouth (Fig. 23-1). He then gently exhales into the infant's mouth and at the same time slightly compresses the chest following each insufflation. The operator never uses force by blowing air into the infant's lung, since this would cause pulmonary alveolar damage.

The primary objective of resuscitation is to establish adequate pulmonary respiration. Prompt and effective resuscitation prevents permanent brain damage and death. The method used for resuscitation depends upon the physical signs of depression at the time of delivery. The Apgar score and the heart rate are the best present-day guides to resuscitation need.

The moderately depressed infant with a heart rate of over 100 per minute with weak respirations or cry (immediate Apgar 3 to 6) is treated with 100%

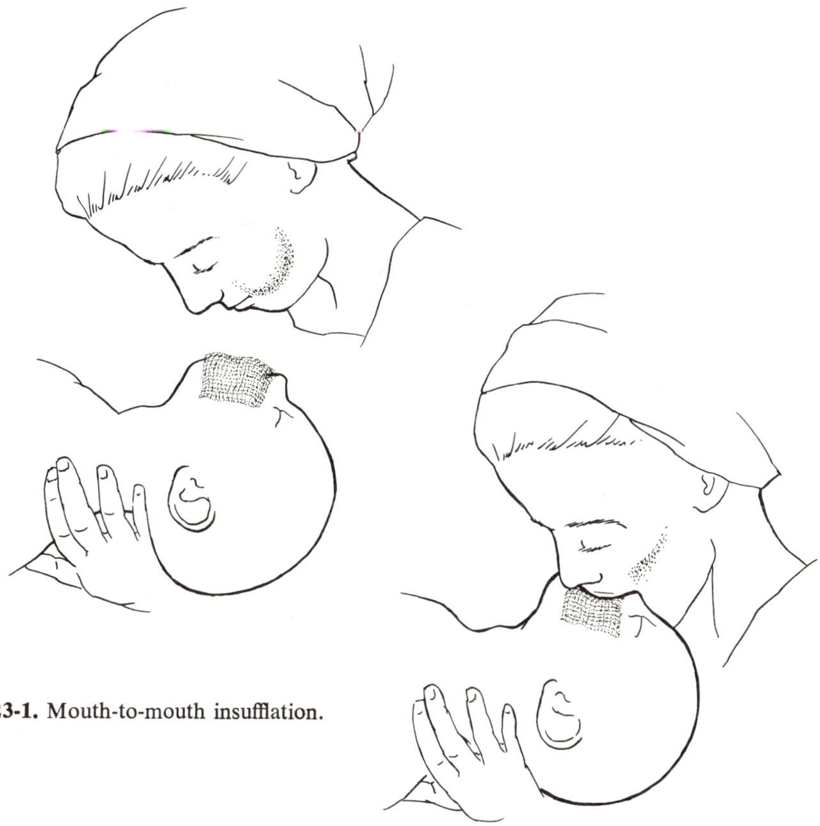

Fig. 23-1. Mouth-to-mouth insufflation.

oxygen blown over the face. A brisk slap on the soles of the feet (with the legs raised and the infant lying flat) is the only safe and effective tactile stimulation that may initiate respirations. If respirations are not initiated and the heart rate decreases despite these measures, intermittent positive pressure breathing with oxygen is applied. Prior to any positive pressure application, the larynx should be directly visualized for the presence of fluid since the fluid may be forced into the trachea. Because positive pressure may rupture the lung in the newborn, pressure should not exceed 35 ml. of water for a duration of 1 to 2 seconds. When moderate chest movements occur, with an increase in heart rate and improvement in color, treatment is usually discontinued.

The markedly depressed infant is limp, has a heart rate that is less than 100, and is usually apneic (Apgar 0 to 3). These infants require immediate tracheal intubation, suctioning, and careful gentle mouth-to-tube insufflation. This is accomplished safely by using the cheek muscles to expel the oxygen the operator has in his mouth. Mouth-to-tube breathing is continued until spontaneous respirations are established.

With cardiac arrest, intubation and external cardiac massage are recom-

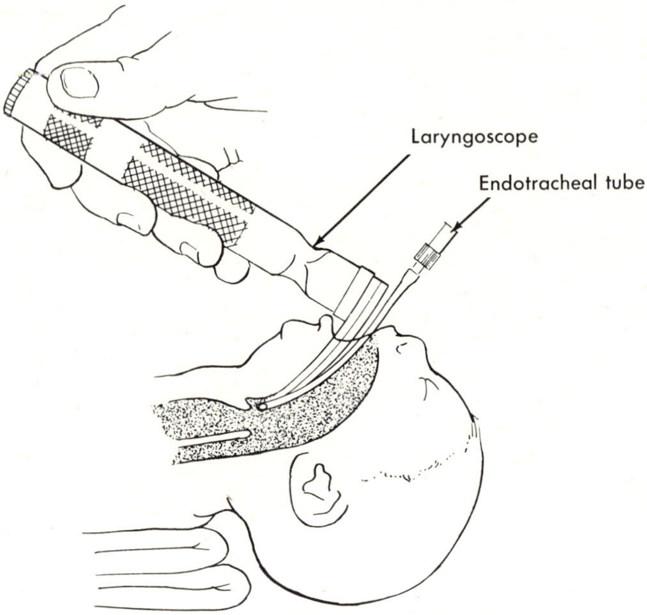

Fig. 23-2. Intubation with a laryngoscope.

mended. Cardiac massage is accomplished by two-finger compression at the middle third of the sternum. While insufflation is being carried out, external massage is discontinued. Effectiveness of heart emptying during massage is determined by palpating the femoral pulse. Direct intracardial injection of 0.05 to 0.1 mg. of epinephrine may be helpful to reestablish spontaneous cardiac activity.

Stimulant drugs such as nikethamide (Coramine) and pentylenetetrazol (Metrazol) are hazardous and may cause further respiratory depression. Drugs are seldom given as stimulants unless respiratory distress is attributed to maternal narcosis. In such instances, particularly when opiates are given the mother, levallorphan (Lorfan, 0.25 mg.) or nalorphine (Nalline, 0.1 mg. per kilogram of body weight) is given directly into the umbilical vein. Unless these drugs are given for opiate narcosis, they may cause further respiratory depression.

Persistent metabolic acidosis is treated with intravenous therapy (Usher treatment). Risks of this treatment require careful and repeated evaluation of blood acid-base levels. Glucose and sodium bicarbonate are given. Dosage and rates of administration are regulated carefully to the size, weight, and condition of the infant.

Newer theories in relation to neonatal respiratory distress

Placental transfusion in which there is delayed cord ligation is believed to increase the neonate's blood volume by as much as 50% to 60%. This increase in blood volume is beneficial to the infant. It is now believed, however, that most of this blood enters the newborn at the onset of respirations. With this knowledge, the onset of respirations with respect to the time of cord ligation is a better index of placental transfusion.

However, not all infants would benefit from additional placental blood. In some infants increased blood volume predisposes to hyperbilirubinemia (contraindicated in Rh sensitivity factor), and the effects on pulmonary function need further study.

Prompt initiation of treatment has also been found to be more beneficial to the depressed infant. Hyperbaric oxygen is of little therapeutic use at present. Hypothermia as a resuscitative measure is still disputable. Deep hypothermia, which formerly was believed to reduce oxygen consumption by the newborn, is now believed to increase oxygen consumption. At present it is a method not being used but still being studied.

ATELECTASIS

At birth the newborn begins his own respiratory efforts, and in a few days the lungs are completely expanded. At times, because of pulmonary immaturity, inadequate respiratory effort due to weak muscles, oversedation, damage to the respiratory center, or inhalation of mucus or amniotic fluid, the lungs will expand only partially. This condition is known as *atelectasis*. Atelectasis means incomplete expansion of a lung or a portion of a lung. Premature infants frequently develop atelectasis.

Symptoms of atelectasis include cyanosis (since the blood does not receive an adequate oxygen supply), rapid and irregular respirations, flaring nostrils, and visible intercostal and suprasternal retraction on inspiration with an audible grunt on expiration.

Treatment consists of maintaining a patent airway, continuous administration of oxygen, high humidity (to liquefy secretions), and changes in position. The nurse who frequently stimulates these infants encourages deeper respirations with resulting lung expansion. Occasionally whiffs of carbon dioxide under pressure are ordered. Antibiotics are frequently given to prevent infection.

PULMONARY HYALINE MEMBRANE SYNDROME (HYALINE MEMBRANE DISEASE)

Hyaline membrane disease is manifested by an accumulation of a protein material, a sticky exudate that fills the alveoli, preventing lung aeration. Symptoms of respiratory distress are cyanosis, dyspnea, and sternal retraction. In the majority of infants these symptoms are apparent a few hours after birth and not immediately at the time of birth.

Premature infants and those delivered by cesarean section frequently develop hyaline membrane disease. Although the nurse is astute in observing all infants, she should be particularly careful in observing premature and cesarean section infants. Reporting symptoms early will assure prompt treatment.

Treatment consists of placing the infant in an Isolette with oxygen and high humidity. Maintaining an open airway is imperative. Antimicrobial drugs are given to prevent infection. When respirations are embarrassed, parenteral fluids are administered. Often with cesarean section infants, the stomach contents are aspirated at birth as a prophylactic measure.

BIRTH INJURIES

Caput succedaneum

Prolonged pressure of the occiput against the cervix during a long and difficult labor causes edema of the soft scalp tissues. The molding is a result of pressure of the infant's head on the cervix.

Although caput succedaneum is commonly seen in the newborn infant, for parents it is frightening. The first mother-infant contact deserves an explanation to alleviate anxiety. Letting parents know that it is a temporary swelling and that it will subside in a few days eliminates undue worry.

Cephalohematoma

A cephalohematoma is also characterized by edema of the scalp, a result of effusion of blood between the bone and the periosteum. It is seldom visible at birth but may be noticed a day or two following delivery. As blood exudes between the bone and the periosteum, the area swells gradually and increases in size. After a few days reabsorption occurs, and the hematoma disappears. Often cephalohematomas are a result of a forceps delivery or follow a breech presentation when fundal pressure is used to deliver the head.

Intracranial hemorrhage

Cerebral hemorrhage or brain hemorrhage is a serious complication of the newborn. It is the result of tearing of the tentorium cerebelli with bleeding into the cerebellum, the pons, and the medulla oblongata. It is obvious that damage to these areas concerned with respiration often proves fatal to the infant.

Intracranial hemorrhage occurs most often with prolonged labors, difficult forceps deliveries, versions and breech extractions, and in precipitate deliveries. With prolonged labors, the constant pounding of the head against the cervix and the perineum causes marked molding and overriding of sutures, injuring the tentorium and causing rupture of blood vessels.

Symptoms. Symptoms of brain damage or cerebral hemorrhage are the nurse's responsibility since she observes the newborn infant closely. The development of symptoms may be sudden or gradual depending upon the severity of hemorrhage. At times the infant appears normal at birth and develops symptoms several hours or several days later.

Abnormal respirations, cyanosis, a sharp, shrill, or weak cry, flaccidity, spasticity, restlessness, wakefulness, convulsions, and poor sucking reflex are signs and symptoms of varying degrees of brain damage.

Treatment. Prevention of intracranial hemorrhage is a responsibility of the physician as he supervises and intervenes during labor and delivery.

Treatment is effective providing severe damage has not occurred. Since the infant often has respiratory difficulty, an Isolette with oxygen and humidity provides warmth and allows for adequate observation of respiratory effort. The head of the infant is raised above the hips to decrease intracranial pressure. Trendelenburg position is contraindicated with cerebral hemorrhage.

Vitamins C and K may be used to control the hemorrhage, and antibiotics are given to prevent infection. Since the sucking reflex is often impaired and there would be too much effort used during feeding, gavage is frequently carried out.

Support of the parents in times of stress is the nurse's greatest responsibility. Although she does not give false hope, she conveys that all is being done to help the infant. Discussing with parents how the infant is faring day by day is safer than talking of what will happen at a future time. Parents need to know, they want the truth, and they are strong enough to accept it during times of stress if the nurse shows understanding, kindness, and sincerity.

Facial paralysis

Facial asymmetry is caused by injury to the facial nerves during a difficult forceps delivery. It is often more noticeable when the infant cries, is temporary, and disappears in a few hours or days. Explanation is imperative prior to mother-infant contact. Often the baby has difficulty in sucking, and mothers need to be supported during feeding periods.

Arm paralysis (Erb-Duchenne paralysis, brachial palsy)

Paralysis of the arm is commonly referred to as Erb's palsy. It is a result of pulling of the shoulder away from the head during a difficult forceps delivery or breech extraction. The pull on the nerve fibers that run from the neck through the shoulder and down the arm, known as the brachial plexus, causes them to become excessively stretched. Since the muscles of the upper arm are involved, the arm is held at the side with elbow extended and hand rotated inward. When mild stretching occurs, healing is rapid. With severe stretching, the nerves are severed from their sheaths, and healing takes several months. If healing does not take place, surgical intervention is indicated. To relieve tension on the brachial plexus a splint or cast may be applied. Gentle massage and motion of the arm are necessary to prevent contractures. Teaching the mother will provide continuity in care following discharge. Referral to public health nursing service when indicated will provide added support.

Dislocations and fractures

During the initial appraisal of infants, the nurse feels for crepitation of bone, immobility, and variations in normal range of motion. Fractures usually involve the jaw, clavicle, or long bones. These are a result of difficult breech extraction or a difficult delivery.

Fractures of the newborn heal rapidly with simple immobilization of the part in proper alignment. Swaddling, positioning, splints, and slings are useful. Handling of the infant often becomes cumbersome and difficult for parents. Allowing the mother to care for the infant at the hospital will prepare her for discharge. Referral to a public health agency will provide continuity in care.

Infections

Scrupulous cleanliness and medical asepsis are a practice in all nursery units. Since the newborn is vulnerable to infection, any sign of beginning infection warrants immediate separation from other healthy infants.

Thrush. Thrush is a mouth infection caused by *Candida albicans* (Chapter 25). The organism is transmitted either by the mother as the infant passes through the birth canal, by trauma and uncleanliness of the mother's breasts or uncleanliness of bottles and nipples in artificial feeding, or by a break in hand washing technique. It is common in premature infants, weak infants, or ill infants. Thrush is characterized by white patches on the tongue, palate, or sides of the inner cheek surfaces. Any attempt to wipe away the white patches will cause bleeding. Often the infant refuses to nurse or suck because it is painful.

Treatment for thrush consists of painting the mouth areas with a 1% gentian violet solution or oral administration of nystatin (Mycostatin). A specific for *Candida albicans,* nystatin is given in dosages of 1 to 4 ml. (200,000 units per milliliter) by medicine dropper three to four times a day. Nystatin is absorbed poorly by the gastrointestinal tract and is excreted in the feces.

The equipment for breast care of mothers and bottles and nipples of infants with thrush are kept separately, washed thoroughly, and boiled before they are put into general use with other equipment. Infants with thrush are isolated from other newborns since thrush is transmissible.

Impetigo. Impetigo is a skin eruption of infectious origin. It is characterized by small eruptions that are semiglobular vesicles or pustules. The bacterium found in the vesicle is either staphylococcal or streptococcal in nature.

The blebs are generally found where the infant's skin surfaces meet, such as the undersurface of the neck, in the axilla, groin, and face. Once the blebs break, the purulent matter reinfects another skin area and spreads rapidly. Prevention of impetigo is accomplished by proper hand washing techniques of all nursery personnel. Rarely does impetigo occur when nursery technique is meticulous.

Treatment consists of immediate separation of the infant from other infants and local treatment of the lesions. Baths using hexachlorophene (pHisoHex) are given daily, and the blebs are broken and exposed to dry heat. Local application of gentian violet, alcohol, bacitracin, or neomycin ointment may be ordered. Antibiotics by intramuscular injections may be required for severe infections.

To prevent the infant from scratching the blebs with chances of reinfection and spread, keeping the infant's shirt sleeves over the hands loosely to allow for adequate hand movement may be necessary. Should restraints be necessary in severe eruptions, periods of untying the restraints with the nurse in attendance will allow the infant freedom, which is essential for normal growth and development. The infant needs to be held for feedings since this builds a beginning sense of trust and security.

Ophthalmia neonatorum. Through state legislation requiring prophylactic treatment with silver nitrate of all infants' eyes at birth, ophthalmia neonatorum has been prevented. It is caused by the *Neisseria gonorrhoeae* (Chapter 25), which may be found in the mother's genital tract at the time of delivery or may be transmitted by infected hands and articles on a maternity unit.

The condition is caused by the gonococcus and is characterized by a profuse, purulent discharge in the eyes. It is the nurse's responsibility to report promptly, isolate, and take a culture of the purulent material to confirm the diagnosis. Ophthalmia neonatorum differs from a silver nitrate reaction in that both eyes are involved, the lids become reddened and swollen, the discharge is thick and greenish yellow, and the eyes are difficult to open. As the infection progresses, corneal opacity and conjunctival ulceration occur, with subsequent blindness.

Prompt treatment with intramuscular injections of penicillin is imperative to prevent eye damage. The infection subsides within 24 to 36 hours with antibiotic therapy. All materials and equipment used on the eyes are handled with care since they are highly infectious. Boiling all equipment and strict hand washing techniques are imperative. Since the gonococcus has an affinity for the eyes, nurses caring for the infant must be careful not to transmit infection.

Staphylococcal infection. Epidemiologic studies have revealed that many normal infants harbor staphylococcus organisms in the nasopharynx. Because of the numbers of infants in newborn nurseries, resulting in crowding of cribs, and numbers of personnel caring for newborns, the outbreak of staphylococcal infection is not uncommon. Many hospital personnel are carriers of staphylococcus coagulase-positive organisms, which are highly resistant to antibiotics.

The skin lesions are similar to those of impetigo, and the organism may cause pneumonia, conjunctivitis, septicemia, omphalitis, or other forms of mild infections. The transfer of organisms becomes a vicious circle, from infant to infant, from infant to mother, and from mother and infant to other family members and the community.

Prevention includes meticulous technique in nurseries, hand washing, medical asepsis, and isolation of all suspects. Treatment is accomplished by giving antimicrobial drugs parenterally.

It is now becoming common practice to limit the number in each nursery to approximately eight infants. Once the eight infants are together in a central nursery, they are not transferred to any other nursery. The eight infants remain together until the time of dismissal from the hospital. By following this practice only seven other infants are exposed if an infection occurs. When all infants from one nursery have been dismissed, it is cleaned thoroughly and a new set of infants is admitted.

Epidemic diarrhea of the newborn. Diarrhea in the newborn is a serious infection, and there is a high infant mortality rate. The onset is sudden with frequent watery, yellow-green stools that are expelled with force. The infant becomes markedly dehydrated and acidotic with a rapid drastic weight loss. As the infant becomes severely dehydrated, the fontanels become sunken, the skin becomes dry, the respirations become rapid and markedly labored, and the infant appears ill.

The organism commonly found in the stool is *Escherichia coli*. It may be transmitted through faulty technique or by the adult carrier caring for the newborn. Personnel with diarrhea should be taught to report infections and refrain from caring for the newborn until they are cured.

Treatment consists of oral administration of neomycin (Mycifradin) and colistimethate sodium (Coly-Mycin). These drugs are often used prophylactically for exposed infants. Penicillin and streptomycin are also given to prevent occurrence of other infections. Dehydration is treated by replacement fluid therapy of 5% glucose in water or Lytren (commercially prepared electrolyte) given orally in small amounts.

All infants with diarrhea are immediately isolated, and new babies are not admitted to the nursery of exposed babies. Prophylactic treatment of all exposed babies is carried out with careful observation for symptoms of beginning infection. Public health follow-up is mandatory. If an outbreak occurs following discharge, readmission to the pediatric unit is advised. All infants treated prophylactically are followed by public health nursing service for 2 weeks following discharge. Nurseries are completely emptied following diarrhea epidemics, are repainted, and are used only after meticulous and scrupulous cleansing.

Syphilis. Prevention of congenital syphilis in the newborn is accomplished by adequate medical supervision of the mother during pregnancy. The mother admitted into the labor and delivery unit sans prenatal care warrants immediate Wassermann or cord blood testing at the time of delivery.

Lesions of the newborn infected by the spirochete are maculopapular and appear on the palms of the hands and soles of the feet. With time, desquamation of these areas occurs. Other signs are restlessness, rhinitis (snuffles), and a hoarse cry. The liver and spleen are enlarged, the lymph nodes are palpable, and the ends of the long bones are enlarged on roentgenographic examination.

Penicillin or a broad-spectrum antibiotic is used in treatment. Infants are usually followed for a 1-year to 2-year period following therapy. Mothers who are treated early during pregnancy have babies showing no signs of infection. (See discussion of syphilis in Chapter 25.)

SELECTED REFERENCES

Barnes, A. C.: Intrauterine development, Philadelphia, 1968, Lea & Febiger.

Bellam, G.: The first year of life, Amer. J. Nurs. **69**:1244, June, 1969.

Berrien, A.: Evaluating the newborn, Nurs. Outlook **9**:93, February, 1961.

Canice, Sister Mary: Rotation plan in the nurseries, Amer. J. Nurs. **61**:96, November, 1961.

Chernick, V.: Respiratory emergencies in the infant, Hosp. Med. **5**:18, February, 1969.

Gordon, R. D.: An infant with a visually disabled mother, Amer. J. Nurs. **68**:1943, September, 1968.

Harper, P. A.: Preventive pediatrics—child health and development, New York, 1962, Appleton-Century & Appleton-Century-Crofts.

Hervada, A. R.: Nursery evaluation of the newborn, Amer. J. Nurs. **67**:1669, August, 1967.

Mortimer, E. A., Jr., Fischer, P., Jenkins, N., and McGirr, O.: Staphylococcus in the nursery, Amer. J. Nurs. **61**:56, October, 1961.

New chest-massage method found safe for infants, RN **27**:28, May, 1964.

Oshin, E. S.: Sudden death in the crib, RN **25**:58, January, 1962.

Pavenstedt, E.: To help infants weather disorganized family life, Amer. J. Nurs. **69**: 1668, August, 1969.

Pidgeon, V.: The infant with congenital heart disease, Amer. J. Nurs. **67**:290, February, 1967.

Ravenholt, R. T., and Nixon, M.: The telephone in epidemiology of staphylococcal disease, Amer. J. Nurs. **61**:60, August, 1961.

Shaffer, A.: Diseases of the newborn, Philadelphia, 1963, W. B. Saunders Co.

Spotting the baby with a brain involvement, RN **24**:59, July, 1961.

Von Schilling, G.: The birth of a defective child, Nurs. Forum **7**:424, 1968.

Why the rise in birth-in-transit deliveries? RN **27**:48, September, 1964.

Questions for study

1. List the three main causes of complications in the newborn infant.
2. What preventive measures are a responsibility of the nurse and the physician?
3. What role does the nurse play in detecting complications? List some significant observations.
4. What are nursing responsibilities in caring for the ill infant?

CHAPTER 24

CONGENITAL MALFORMATIONS

HISTORY OF BIRTH DEFECTS

Birth defects or congenital malformations have been recorded, and these records are available going back thousands of years. The birth of abnormal children interested primitive man more than the reproductive process. Prior to hieroglyphics, wood and stone carvings of double-headed human beings and Siamese twins are a contribution of the Stone Age civilization. Legends have been passed down through generations by the Australian aborigines of attached twin girls and of minor malformations.

As legends were passed on, many of the factual stories became wondrous tales and fables of cyclopean people with one eye in the middle of the forehead, double-headed deities with many arms, etc. As time went on, the ancient Babylonians engraved clay tablets depicting deformities of the ears, nose, mouth, the sex organs, and various forms of twinning. These are displayed in museums in London. Legends and records of deformed children spread from Babylonia to many countries in Europe and America. The term *monster* is derived from the Latin *monstrare* meaning to show. Often the term *monstrosity* is used. Romans believed that birth defects were predictions for the future.

Belief in maternal impressions originated with finding a way to explain the cause for birth defects. The idea that mental impressions on the pregnant woman affected the baby was a belief of many peoples with no geographic and cultural connections. This belief spread widely to the Near East, Far East, Africa, and South America. One hears of maternal impressions such as that the mother frightened by a mouse will have an infant with the imprint of a mouse on its body—these are still superstitions of today. During the Middle Ages, maternal impressions did not produce guilt feelings since they could not be better explained due to lack of knowledge concerning the reproductive process.

Greek mythology suggested that perhaps crosses of human beings and animals were responsible for monstrous births. However, as Mosaic and Christian laws became a practice, condemnation of relations between man and animals became widespread. During the fifteenth and sixteenth centuries strong beliefs in demons, witches, etc. spread through Europe, and birth anomalies were thought to be a result of sorcery.

The most outstanding contribution to birth defects was made by William Harvey in 1651. Harvey, the discoverer of blood circulation, described a cleft lip as an abnormal continuation of normal embryologic development. His concept that congenital malformations are manifestations of arrested embryonic development resulted in a rational analysis of birth defects.

The nineteenth century opened new fields of research with the science of genetics and embryology. Although much of the new knowledge gives answers to the why and how of birth defects, the where, who, and when still need much research.

DEFINITION OF BIRTH DEFECT

A birth defect is "a structural or metabolic disorder present at birth genetically determined as a result of environmental interference during embryonic or fetal life. Birth injuries are not included."*

INCIDENCE OF BIRTH DEFECTS

Over half a million (one infant in 16 of all live births) have defects evident at birth or during the first year of life. One family in every ten has a defective child—43% are apparent at birth, and 57% are discovered later in life. Birth defects are numerous and range from the commonly known cleft lip and clubbed foot to heart and circulatory system, skeletal, gastrointestinal, central nervous system, and metabolic disorders.

Statistics of birth defects are difficult to obtain since they are frequently not reported or are unnoticed. Often babies that die before birth due to faulty development are not included. Birth defects affect both sexes and all races; however, certain defects are more common in some groups than in others. For instance, extra fingers occur more often in Negroes and Orientals than in Caucasians, malformations of the lips and mouth are more prevalent among Orientals and Caucasians than among Negroes, hip dislocations are more frequent in girls, and pyloric stenosis is more frequent in boys. Maternal age is also a factor—the mother younger than 18 or older than 40 runs a greater risk of having a child with a birth defect.

PREVENTION OF BIRTH DEFECTS

Prevention of birth defects starts early in the life of parents, perhaps from the time of their birth. The couple in optimum health comes to marriage as potential parents of healthy children. Professional counseling services afford parents the opportunity to discuss family heredity patterns and the risk and dangers of marry-

*The National Foundation, March of Dimes, New York, N. Y.

ing a close relative. Research and new methods of testing parents as hereditary carriers may prevent damage to the infant since treatment is instituted promptly at birth, for example, for galactosemia and phenylketonuria. Today prenatal care services are making great strides since there are adequate health histories, blood typing, and genetic counseling.

In 1958, the National Foundation, March of Dimes ventured into the research and study of birth defects. Their objectives are threefold:

1. Treatment centers have been established in large teaching hospitals and medical centers to study and treat children born with defects. Each center teaches the paramedical team (doctors, medical students, nurses, therapists, and other personnel), and new knowledge is disseminated rapidly to other centers.

2. Scientific researchers are studying hereditary and environmental factors affecting the developing embryo.

3. Educational material is being circulated to alert and familiarize the public with birth defects and with the treatment and research for the future. Educational programs are also provided for members of the health professions concerned with problems of birth defects.

The advance in medical science and research, new legislation, and public awareness are changing attitudes toward the child who is different. Prevention, early detection, and treatment will decrease the numbers of children with permanent disabilities and mental retardation.

ETIOLOGY OF BIRTH DEFECTS

Birth defects are classified into three categories: genetic, environmental, and a combination of both.

Genetic factors

Genetic factors are directly related to the chemical makeup in the original maturated ovum and sperm. Within each cell is stored a unique chemical substance known as DNA (deoxyribonucleic acid). The genes are found in larger units known as chromosomes located in the nucleus of each germ cell. Normal human cells contain 46 paired chromosomes. Once the ovum and sperm maturate there is a reduction of chromosomes to 23. With fertilization, the fusion of a mature ovum and sperm restores the original 46 chromosomes, and new life begins. In this process of cell division, aberrations or errors occur, producing a defective baby. The chromosomes often divide unpaired, with an end result of too many, too few, or separation or splitting of chromosomes. Aberrations in chromosomes are responsible for major birth defects such as Down's syndrome (mongolism) and abnormal sex characteristics. Errors in metabolism or hereditary defects are caused by a defective single gene (not a whole chromosome) or two abnormal genes. The two most common metabolic errors are galactosemia and phenylketonuria.

A pure genetic defect will always appear in each of a pair of identical twins. Both have the same chromosomal complement, and both display the defect, which means that the fetal environment is unable to overcome the genetic abnormality. The defect is then classified as "pure genetic." At present there is only one pure genetic defect, Down's syndrome. However, with a defect such as cleft lip or cleft palate, when only one of the identical twins has the defect, there is only a 30% chance that the other will inherit it. This means that there has been some other factor in the environment of one twin (since each has a unique environment) that enabled him to compensate for the inherited tendency in 70% of the cases.

The placenta therefore serves as a protective barrier since some materials, due to molecular size, for example, heparin, cannot cross the placenta. Since the placenta transports materials from the maternal bloodstream to the fetal bloodstream, small amounts of soluble substances pass the placenta readily from mother to baby, never reaching high levels. In some instances maternal levels may have to reach a certain level before there is "spillover" to the fetus, and in other instances, for example, vitamin C, material passes readily to the infant and yet cannot return from the baby to the mother.

Environmental factors

Virus infections, drugs, and radiation contribute to birth defects. The most common virus, rubella, contracted in the first trimester, causes abnormalities of hearing, vision, the heart, and mental retardation. A recently found parasitic salivary gland virus has no effect on the mother, yet it may produce serious congenital anomalies in the newborn. Certain tranquilizers, hormones, anticancer drugs, and radiation to the abdominal pelvic organs often cause severe damage to the developing baby in utero. Diet and general health of the mother provide a healthy environment.

Environmental factors affect the growing baby during the first trimester of pregnancy. The effect on the baby depends upon the stage of development at the time of exposure.

Two sociologic principles in relation to drugs and their chemical effects on the fetus are that the majority of times pregnancy is unplanned and often prenatal care starts after the second missed period. Therefore, the responsibility of a growing fetus also rests with the internist treating the nonpregnant woman.

Drugs and their effects on the fetus are outlined as follows:

Gamete effects

Alcohol

Cadmium (Capsebon): Found in increased amounts in the kidney of hypertensive women

Busulfan (Myleran): A male contraceptive that acts directly on gamete-producing tissue

The embryo and organogenesis

Salicylates: Picked up readily by blastocyte, slow in excretion

Thalidomide: Phocomelia (missing limbs)

- 4-Aminopteroyl glutamic acid (Aminopterin): Abortifacient, 100% effective, given a week following implantation
- Progestins: Masculinization of female
- Corticosteroids: Cleft palate

Fetal growth

- Oxytetracycline (Terramycin): Stunts fetal growth, deciduous teeth affected
- Propylthiouracil: Congenital goiter
- Orinase: Hypertrophy of fetal pancreatic islets
- Tolbutamides: Disturbs acid-base balance in mother and fetus
- Chloroquine (Aralen): Lesions of the eighth nerve and retinopathy
- Vitamin K and sulfisoxazole (Gantrisin): Neonatal hyperbilirubinemia (excessive vitamin K, sulfisoxazole last month of pregnancy)
- Quinine: Eighth nerve, thrombocytopenia
- Reserpine: Stuffy nose in baby, cyanosis, intercostal retraction, muscle flaccidity, and hypothermia
- Morphine: Withdrawal shortly after birth
- Mothballs: Carbon monoxide
- Bishydroxycoumarin (Dicumarol): Retroplacental hemorrhage (heparin is safe since it does not cross placenta)
- Novobiocin (Albamycin, Cathomycin): Jaundice in neonate

Fetal drug exposure during labor and delivery (narcotics, analgesics, and anesthesia)

- Barbiturates: Cross placenta within 2 to 3 minutes, equalized level between mother and baby
- Meperidine (Demerol): Nondepressant for fetus, safest drug choice in labor
- Muscle relaxants: Do not pass placenta in significant amounts and are safe
- Regional anesthesia: Epidural, caudal, saddle block, paracervical, and pudendal without fetal effect unless there is prolonged hypotension
- Paracervical block: Mild to moderate degrees of fetal bradycardia

BIRTH DEFECTS AFFECTING THE DIGESTIVE SYSTEM

Cleft lip and cleft palate

Genetic and environmental factors are responsible in cleft lip and cleft palate. During the fourth to eighth weeks of embryonic life the face takes form. Fusion of the lip occurs at 6 weeks, fusion of the palate occurs at 8 weeks. These deformities result from failure of the soft and bony tissues to fuse, and they may be unilateral or bilateral. At times only the lip is involved, or the cleavage may extend into the upper jaw or nasal cavity. The anomaly occurs in 1 out of every 1,000 births and is therefore the most frequent birth defect. In some instances there are hereditary tendencies; in others there is no known etiology. In cleft palate either the soft palate or the hard and soft palates may be cleaved.

Cleft lip is more common in Caucasians, affects more boys, and the incidence is higher in Japanese and lower in Negroes. Cleft palate is more common in Caucasians, affects more girls, and the incidence is higher in Japanese and lower in Negroes.

Cleft lip and cleft palate pose problems in feeding the newborn since the lips and the palate aid in the sucking and swallowing processes. Feeding is accomplished best by placing the infant in an upright position and directing the feeding against the side of the mouth. When it is possible to feed the infant by nipple, this is a means of strengthening and developing the muscles used for speech. Various nipples designed for these defects are available. Often just a large soft nipple with enlarged holes serves the same purpose. Should this method fail, a medicine dropper, Brecht feeder (bulb syringe with nipple attached to the end), or a spoon may be used successfully. The feeding should be given slowly and carefully to prevent milk aspiration into the lungs. Occasionally these infants swallow much air and need to be bubbled often. The mother needs much support, encouragement, and help before she becomes comfortable assuming the responsibility of feeding her infant. The mother who is determined and wishes to breast-feed may manually express or pump the breasts to keep a milk supply going until repair is completed. The milk obtained can be given to the infant by whatever method is feasible.

Repair of a cleft lip is planned rather early and is usually complete by 2 months of age. Cleft palates are usually repaired by 18 to 24 months of age. Surgical repairs of cleft lip and cleft palate involve a team of doctors that includes a pediatrician, an orthodontist, a dentist, a prosthodontist, a plastic surgeon, a speech therapist, and a public health nurse. At times, for particular individual needs, the services of a psychologist, psychiatrist, or social worker may be needed.

Galactosemia and phenylketonuria

Galactosemia and phenylketonuria are metabolic defects in which there is a deficiency of essential enzymes with an accumulation of toxic materials altering body chemistry. The toxic material may affect a vital body organ or is excreted in the urine, facilitating early recognition. It is becoming a universal practice in prevention that all newborns have blood drawn early after birth to detect enzymatic disturbances.

Phenylketonuria (phenylpyruvic oligophrenia) is inherited by a single recessive gene. There is a deficiency of phenylalanine hydroxylase, a liver enzyme that normally converts phenylalanine to tyrosine.

Five percent of the protein factor of all foods contains phenylalanine. Some infants cannot metabolize the excess phenylalanine ingested. The excess builds up in the baby's tissue and is excreted through the urine and through the skin by perspiration. If the infant is untreated, the toxic effects of the enzyme on the central nervous system cause mental retardation. Prior to birth there is no evidence of the enzyme defect since the placental circulation removes excessive phenylalanine. By the time the infant is a month or more of age, positive urine tests are found. Therefore early urine testing is not an accurate diagnostic measure.

The increased numbers of metabolites result in mental retardation, deficient pigmentation with a high frequency of infants with blond hair and bluc cycs, infants with agitated behavior, hyperactivity, and occasionally epilepsy and eczema.

The treatment consists of a diet low in phenylalanine. Commercial products such as Lofenalac (a special food mixed with water) are tolerated well by young infants. Synthetic products of casein hydrolysate are passed through charcoal to remove phenylalanine and tyrosine. To this end product are added tyrosine, tryptophan, methionine, a specific amount of milk and cream, sucrose, and inorganic salts and vitamins. Usually the diet is a restricted one for life. Teaching the parents and allowing them to discuss the problem will afford support. Referral to public health nursing service for continuity in care is essential.

Early detection and *treatment* prevent mental retardation. The most recent blood test using the Guthrie method is done before the newborn infant is discharged and is repeated in 4 weeks. The infant's heel is pricked, and a few drops of blood are obtained on filter paper. The urine test is simple but can be done only after the infant is 3 weeks old. A few drops of ferric chloride are added to a urine-saturated diaper, and a green reaction is positive for PKU.

Galactosemia is not as common as PKU and is known to occur in more than one sibling in a family. Galactosemia is a result of toxic effects due to depression of glucose concentration in the blood following regular ingestion of galactose. Infants begin to vomit and have loose stools a few days after human milk or cow's milk formula has been ingested. The liver becomes enlarged, the infant becomes jaundiced and fails to gain weight, and spells of weakness and unconsciousness may be noted. Cataracts may appear as early as the second week, and mental retardation is apparent in a few months. Diagnosis is made through glucose-galactose relationships in the blood and gross increases of amino acids in the urine. Treatment consists of absolute exclusion of any galactose-containing food in the diet as soon as diagnosis is established. There may be improvement in galactose tolerance as the child grows older, and then relaxation in diet is done cautiously.

Short frenum

The frenum is a vertical piece of mucous membrane that binds the tongue to the floor of the mouth. In most normal infants it is short, not too elastic, but allows the tongue to protrude to the bottom lip. Occasionally a considerably short and rigid frenum may prevent the tongue from curling around the nipple, thus interfering with sucking. Some physicians believe in snipping the margin of the mucous membrane, while others feel that the frenum will lengthen with time.

Atresia of the esophagus

This defect occurs during embryonic development and is characterized by the end of the esophagus terminating in a blind pouch rather than a continuous tube to the stomach. Occasionally a fistula occurs into the trachea at the bifurcation of the esophagus and the trachea. Diagnosis is made when there is excessive salivation with drooling, coughing, gagging, dyspnea, and cyanosis during feedings. For further confirmation of the diagnosis, a catheter is passed through the mouth or nose and often meets resistance or firm obstruction. The nurse who reports these symptoms promptly assures the infant immediate surgical intervention and prevents occurrence of bronchitis or aspirative pneumonia. For safety the infant's head is elevated to prevent aspiration into the trachea via the fistula. Following surgery, nasopharyngeal suction should be available. Infants are kept in a heated, humidified Isolette to liquefy the tenacious mucus. If labored breathing or cyanosis occurs, immediate nasopharyngeal and mouth suction is indicated. Parenteral fluids and antibiotics are given when indicated. Oral feeding is resumed when the infant's condition permits, with due respect to the extent of repair.

Obstructions of the duodenum and the small intestine

Vomiting that occurs during or after the first feeding is indicative of obstruction. The vomiting may or may not be bile-stained, and no meconium is eliminated. When the obstruction is in the lower bowel, there is marked abdominal distention. Immediate roentgenographic examination confirms the diagnosis, and surgery is done 12 hours following birth for survival of the infant. Postoperatively, fluids are administered by hypodermoclysis to maintain body temperature and as nourishment. Feedings are resumed at approximately 5 to 7 days following surgery when peristalsis is reestablished. If distention occurs, nasoduodenal suction and oxygen may be indicated.

Intussusception or a telescoping of the bowel is the most frequent type of obstruction. Symptoms include intermittent abdominal pain, vomiting, and bloody mucoid stool. Preoperatively insertion of an indwelling nasogastric polyethylene tube and lavage are done. Fluids are given parenterally, and feeding is resumed about the third or fourth postoperative day. Antibiotics to prevent infection and vitamin C to promote healing are commonly ordered postoperatively.

Imperforate anus

Improper formation of the anus during embryonic development of the alimentary tract may be partial or complete. Diagnosis is made when the nurse attempts to take a rectal temperature reading or when the infant is unable to pass meconium and is found crying and straining in an effort to evacuate the bowel. Abdominal distention is frequently found. Surgical intervention is essential for survival of the infant. The extent of the anomaly determines the surgical method of correction. In some infants incision of the membrane covering the rectum is indicated, and when there is extensive involvement a colostomy is performed.

BIRTH DEFECTS AFFECTING THE CIRCULATORY SYSTEM

Hemolytic disease of the newborn

Hemolytic anemia of the newborn is a congenital blood-destroying disease occurring prior to or shortly following birth. Erythroblastosis (destruction of red blood cells) occurs whenever there are differences in ABO blood groupings and in the Rh blood systems of parents.

Since blood groupings and Rh factors are genetically inherited, erythroblastosis is characterized by agglutination of red cells and by jaundice as bilirubin accumulates and then stains brain tissue, resulting in kernicterus (brain damage) or death of the infant.

Rh incompatibility. The Rh factor is absent in Rh-negative individuals and is present in Rh-positive individuals. Approximately 15% of all Caucasians are Rh negative, and 85% are Rh positive. It is obvious then that the chances of two Rh-negative persons marrying are small—therefore, 4 out of every 5 marriages have an Rh-negative female and an Rh-positive male. The over-all incidence of Rh-positive babies from these marriages is 65%. Fortunately not all these babies develop hemolytic disease; the reasons are not yet completely understood. Rh incompatibilities are found in approximately one out of every 250 pregnancies.

Etiology. Difficulty arises when there is a tranfer of incompatible blood from the fetal to the maternal circulation (Fig. 24-1). For instance, when the mother is Rh-negative and the father is Rh-positive, the baby may inherit either the negative or the positive factor. If the negative factor is in his genetic makeup there is

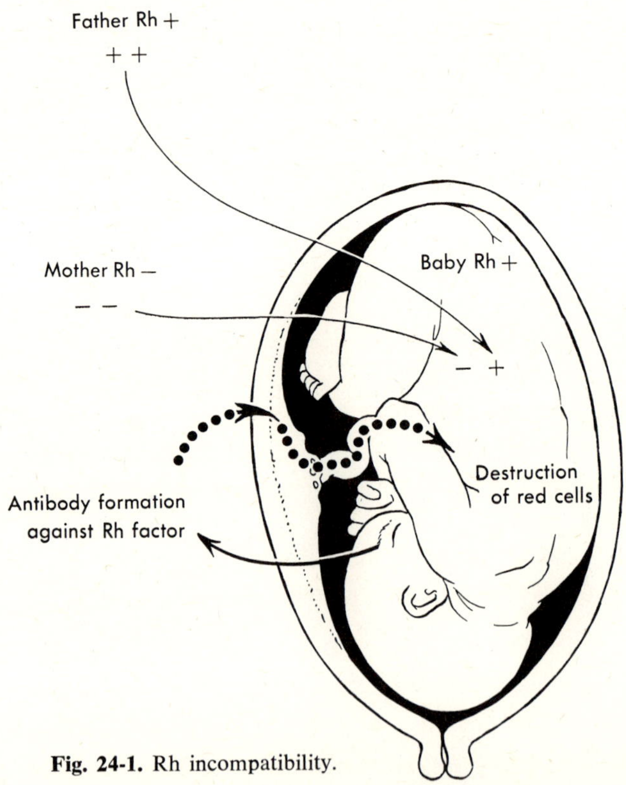

Fig. 24-1. Rh incompatibility.

no problem, but when the positive factor is inherited there is a 50% chance of sensitization. Sensitization occurs when the Rh-positive red cells escape the fetal circulation through the placental barrier and find entrance into the maternal circulation. To ward off Rh-positive antigens, the maternal circulation produces antibodies that return to the fetal circulation, causing red cell agglutination. The greater the number of antibodies formed, the greater the destruction of red cells.

Occurrence of sensitization is determined by the following: (1) antibodies already present in the mother's bloodstream from previous blood transfusions, (2) the possibility that although the father is positive he may have a paired chromosome in which a negative sperm penetrated the ovum, (3) there may be a strong placental barrier that prevents seepage of fetal blood into the maternal circulation, thus preventing sensitization, or (4) the fetal antigen may enter the maternal circulation and yet not produce antibody formation.

Symptoms. In 15% to 20% of Rh-positive infants born of Rh-negative mothers there may be no sign of illness. The babies who are sensitized show symptoms of jaundice, anemia, and edema in varying degrees.

Mild forms of sensitization are apparent when jaundice occurs within the first 24 to 36 hours following birth. The liver and spleen become enlarged and are palpable. About the fourth day after birth the jaundice and hepatosplenomegaly subside, leaving a moderate noticeable pallor that persists for a few weeks. Breast-feeding is not contraindicated in hemolytic disease of the newborn. Studies have revealed that antibodies transmitted through breast milk are destroyed in the stomach and will not produce further sensitization.

When the disease is severe, jaundice appears at birth or within a few hours. The jaundice becomes a deep greenish yellow hue by the third or fourth day, and the body, particularly the extremities, becomes puffy with pitting edema. The liver and spleen are markedly enlarged, and the infant appears critically ill. The heart enlarges, respirations become rapid and labored, and bloody material, suggestive of heart failure or pulmonary hemorrhage, exudes from the mouth. Feedings are taken poorly, and vomiting occurs. Tremors and convulsions are an indication of kernicterus.

Treatment. Observation for signs of hemolytic disease at birth is a responsibility of the nurse when the disorder is suspected. Prompt reporting of early jaundice affords immediate treatment. When Rh incompatibility is suspected, a specimen of the cord blood is taken in the delivery room for Coombs' test, Rh determination, blood group, red blood count, hemoglobin, and serum bilirubin. A positive direct Coombs test reveals the presence of maternal antibodies attached to the red blood cells of the baby. A negative direct Coombs test indicates the absence of maternal antibodies in the baby's blood system.

The results of the blood findings and the severity of symptoms are a determinant in treatment. In live infants prior to severe erythroblastosis and fetal hydrops, exchange transfusion accomplished early saves the infant's life. Normal cord bilirubin concentration is 2.5 mg. per 100 ml. or less. Bilirubin concentrations of 4 mg. or more require immediate transfusion. The high serum bilirubin level is caused by the inability of the liver to handle the numbers of erythrocytes being destroyed. If the increased bilirubin level continues, severe jaundice and staining of the brain cells result in irreparable damage.

Exchange transfusion is accomplished by insertion of a polyethylene tubing through the umbilical or saphenous vein. Rh-negative blood is introduced in small amounts (approximately 10 ml. to 20 ml. at a time). The procedure consists of first withdrawing a small amount of the infant's blood and then injecting a small amount of Rh-negative blood. The procedure takes a few hours. During exchange transfusion the blood is given at room temperature, and oxygen is given the infant to replenish the demand as body metabolism is lowered. Following transfusion repeated bilirubins, red blood counts, and hemoglobins are done to determine the need for repeated transfusion. Although the infant's blood is exchanged to remove maternal antibodies, the infant still remains Rh positive as new red cells are manufactured.

Researchers have devised newer methods in detecting sensitization of the baby in utero through *amniotic fluid evaluation* and *intrauterine transfusion.* Both methods will decrease the perinatal mortality from erythroblastosis fetalis. Amniocentesis is the removal of amniotic fluid through the abdominal route. The bilirubin level is determined by chemical and spectrophotometric evaluation of the amniotic fluid. Determining the bilirubin level provides an accurate picture of the amount of sensitization in the fetus. Often amniocentesis is performed when there is an increase in the maternal antibody titer.

Prior to amniocentesis a radiograph is done in which a radiopaque material is injected into the amniotic sac to outline the fetus. Fluid for analysis is removed either posterior to the neck of the fetus or in the area in which small parts are palpable and visible on the radiograph. While the procedure is in process, the fetal head is held stationary to ensure withdrawal of amniotic fluid and prevent traversing the placenta. If the fetus is stuck by the needle, marked fetal movements occur. If the mother is close to term, a radioactive material introduced into the bladder facilitates visualization prior to amniocentesis.

The nurse who prepares the mother adequately for this treatment alleviates some anxiety. Emptying the bladder and checking fetal heart tones prior to amniocentesis are imperative. The abdomen is prepared with an antiseptic solution. With the mother in a prone position, a spinal needle (No. 22) is inserted to aspirate amniotic fluid. If blood is found during aspiration, a stain technique determines whether it is fetal or maternal blood. If the stain indicates that placental circulation has been entered, checking for a rise in titer in 2 weeks is essential. Amniocentesis is performed from 29 to 32 weeks gestation and is often repeated in 2 weeks. Amounts of 40 ml. of amniotic fluid are removed if pregnancy is beyond 30 weeks, and less is removed prior to 30 weeks gestation. The results of amniocentesis, however, are not without risk of maternal infection, fetal injury, premature labor, and introduction of fetal cells into the maternal circulation, should the placenta be punctured. Amniocentesis is a valuable test in determining the time for preterm induction.

Intrauterine transfusion, in which the fetus is transfused with whole blood in utero, is being attempted in selected women. The first successful transfusion in utero was reported by Dr. A. W. Liley, of Auckland, New Zealand, in October, 1963. During amniocentesis the fetus swallows the radiopaque material, facilitating visibility of the gastrointestinal tract. A special Tuohy needle is passed through the maternal abdominal wall into the uterus and through the abdominal wall of the fetus. Rh-negative blood is then introduced into the fetal peritoneal cavity, which is later absorbed into the peripheral circulation. Roentgenograms are taken during intrauterine transfusion to establish accuracy in placement of the needle before transfusion is attempted. A catheter is then introduced so that the needle can be removed for safety should the fetus or the mother move. Blood consisting of packed red cells (plasma removed) is given at room temperature. For prophylactic measures, a million units of aqueous penicillin G is also given. Infants of 30 weeks gestation are given 100 to 150 ml. (10 ml. at a time), and those under 30 weeks gestation are given smaller amounts.

Estrogen studies are done occasionally since decreased production is indicative of fetal death. With fetal hydrops the placenta is excessively larger, which relieves depletion of oxygen to the fetus.

Amnioscopy is a new diagnostic method to detect fetal distress in late pregnancy. The examination is performed on an outpatient basis. The endoscope (amnioscope) is introduced through the cervix, and visualization of amniotic fluid is possible. Discoloration by meconium or bile pigments and lack of amniotic fluid are indicative of danger. Amnioscopy is done when amniotomy is not feasible. Indications are postmaturity and toxemia of pregnancy.

Preparation of the parents is paramount—treatment and the risks involved are discussed. Prior to the treatment the mother is given 100 mg. of meperidine hydrochloride (Demerol) for its analgesic effect. Following any of these treatments the nurse instructs the mother to report signs of labor immediately. False hope is never given parents when signs of severe incompatibility are evident.

RhoGAM (Fig. 24-2), a specially prepared gamma globulin derived from the plasma of persons previously immunized to the Rh_o (d) antigen, was approved by the Federal Drug Administration on May 1, 1968.* A dose of the antibody is administered after each Rh-incompatible pregnancy. These antibodies provide protection against foreign Rh-positive red cells that may enter the mother's bloodstream after delivery. An injection of RhoGAM prevents the mother's body from producing permanent antibodies. Any immunized Rh-negative mother who delivers an Rh-positive baby (or following a miscarriage) may be given an intramuscular injection of RhoGAM (1 ml. = 300 μg of anti-Rh_oantibody) within 72 hours after delivery. Additional injections are needed following each delivery.

*Marketed by Ortho Diagnostics, Raritan, N. J.

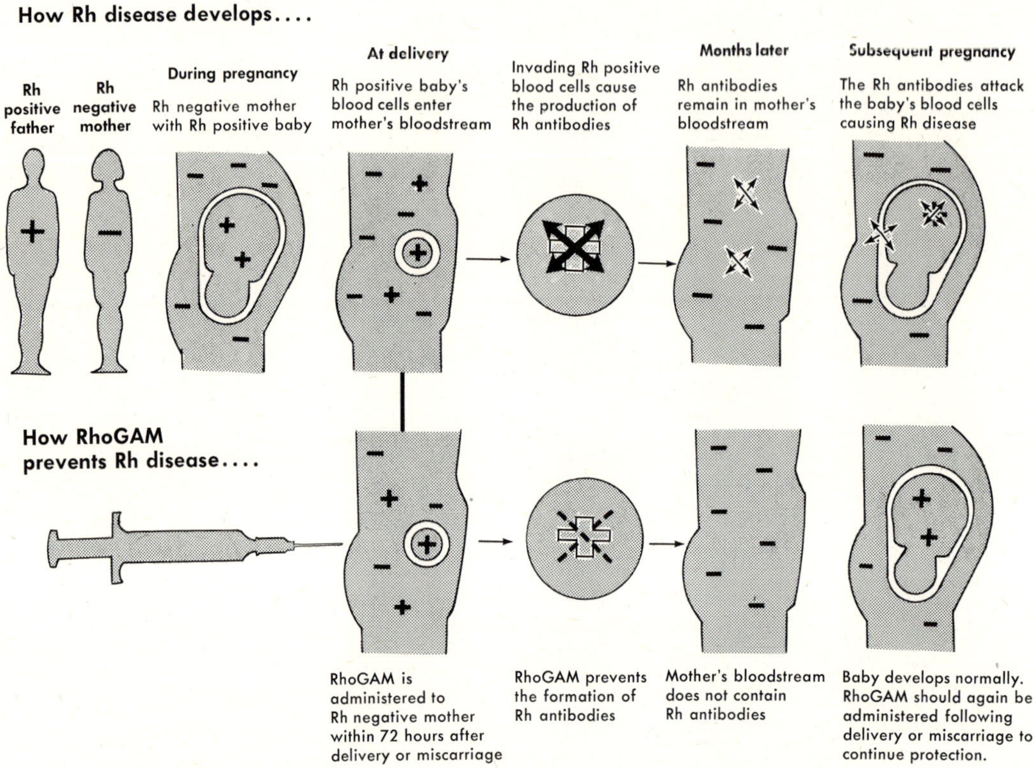

Fig. 24-2. How Rh disease develops. (From Ortho Diagnostics, Raritan, N. J.)

Adverse effects of RhoGAM are temporary soreness at the injection site or a slight elevation in basal body temperature.

ABO incompatibility. In this disease sensitization occurs when the mother is type O and the father is type A or B. Since A and B genes are dominant over O, the baby inherits type A or B. The mother's blood contains anti-A and anti-B agglutinins, and these may cross the placental barrier, attacking the red blood cells of the infant, with resulting hemolysis, anemia, and jaundice.

In ABO incompatibility, the disease is rarely as severe as in the Rh factor, and the Coombs' test is usually negative or slightly positive. Exchange transfusions are done with appropriate Rh type and with the mother's grouping of O blood. Bilirubin of below 20 mg. per 100 ml. of blood assures survival of the infant.

Patent ductus arteriosus

During fetal life there exists an abnormal opening between the pulmonary artery and the aorta since the placenta assumes the respiratory function. Normally at birth, closure of the ductus arteriosus occurs as respirations become established. Failure of closure results in dyspnea and retardation in growth. Surgical correction of this defect has now been perfected.

Tetralogy of Fallot

This congenital defect is manifested by four deviations: (1) a narrowing of the pulmonary artery, (2) a defect in the ventricular septum, (3) the aorta in dextroposition, and (4) a hypertrophy in the right ventricle.

Common symptoms are cyanosis at the nail beds, lips, and buccal mucosa and changes in the sclera. Later symptoms are dyspnea and clubbing of the fingers. Tetralogy of Fallot is usually diagnosed later and not at birth.

Surgical correction is palliative in relieving work load of the heart. The Blalock-Taussig operation bypasses the pulmonary stenosis by anastomosing the subclavian to the pulmonary artery side by side at a point beyond the stricture. Advances in open heart surgery are encouraging for the child born with tetralogy of Fallot.

BIRTH DEFECTS AFFECTING THE MUSCULOSKELETAL SYSTEM

Clubbed foot

Foot deformities are either positional or due to improper muscular and skeletal development. Positional deformities (due to position of feet in cramped intrauterine environment) are easily correctable. The nurse may instruct the mother to exercise the foot by proper rotation and alignment prior to each feeding. Exercises stretch the tightened muscles when there is minimal involvement.

For marked clubbing, plaster of Paris casts are applied and reapplied weekly since the infant outgrows the cast so rapidly. Nursing care includes instruction of the mother to observe the toes and upper leg for signs of edema or cyanosis, which indicate interference with circulation. At times a Denis Browne splint is ordered to be left in place during the infant's sleeping hours. With this type splint, the shoes are reversed so that the right shoe is put on the left foot to assure proper alignment. Referral to public health nursing service and to the Crippled Children's Bureau will assure correction and help for the infant's parents.

Congenital dislocation of the hip

This deformity occurs when the head of the femur does not fit or rotate properly within the acetabulum. The nurse who appraises the infant at birth should immediately report any difficulty in abducting the legs away from the midline with flexed knees. Another method is flexing both knees, and, with both feet flat on a hard surface, observation is made of the height of both knees. With congenital hip dislocation, one knee is lower than the other. Early detection with prompt treatment assures better results.

Treatment consists of keeping the legs abducted until a cast is applied. This may be accomplished by applying four diapers, the bulk of which provides abduction. Nursing care following cast application includes padding the cast edges to prevent skin irritation and soiling with urine and stool, observing the skin areas with attention to cleanliness, dryness, massage to prevent skin breakdown, frequent changes in position, and observing for impairment in circulation by edema or skin color changes.

BIRTH DEFECTS AFFECTING THE CENTRAL NERVOUS SYSTEM

Spina bifida

Spina bifida is a congenital anomaly in which the spinous processes of the laminae fail to unite during embryonic development. It is often complicated by a protrusion of meninges and spinal fluid, known as *meningocele,* or by protrusion of the spinal cord, known as *meningomyelocele.* The anomaly occurs anywhere in the spinal column; however, the lumbar and sacral areas are most common. With spinal cord involvement, paralysis is also present—the extent depends upon the amount of nerve damage.

Nursing care of the infant with spina bifida consists of proper positioning and cleanliness of the area since breakdown to tissue results in meningitis. Incontinent infants in whom paralysis has occurred need special attention to cleanliness and dryness of skin areas to prevent decubiti. Surgical intervention is attempted following thorough evaluation.

Hydrocephalus

Hydrocephalus is a result of increased amounts of cerebrospinal fluid in the ventricles due to obstruction, overproduction, or improper absorption of spinal fluid. Often spina bifida is complicated by hydrocephalus.

The nurse may detect hydrocephalus by an increased circumference of the infant's head, marked separation of the suture lines in the scalp, bulging fontanels, a high-pitched cry, vomiting, and later exophthalmia. The neurologic signs are indicative of increased intracranial pressure.

A surgical procedure now being widely used is a shunt operation in which the cerebrospinal fluid is directed from the ventricle into the jugular vein and right heart for elimination. This procedure is accomplished by inserting a Spitz Holter valve. Should spina bifida and hydrocephalus occur together, the shunt is done first since this alleviates pressure at the spinal opening. The valve is inserted so that it is visible through the skin behind the ear and may be pumped by digital pressure should blockage occur. Prior to surgery, however, all infants are evaluated carefully, and kidney and urinary tract function must be ascertained. There is a tendency toward multiple anomalies rather than one; therefore, thorough evaluation studies are imperative for infant survival.

BIRTH DEFECTS AFFECTING THE URINARY SYSTEM

Hypospadias and epispadias

Hypospadias is a congenital malformation in which the urethra terminates proximal to the usual site at the undersurface of the penis. With epispadias the opening is on the dorsal surface of the penis. Plastic surgery is usually attempted at the time of puberty when full growth of the reproductive organs has occurred. Until plastic surgery is accomplished, urinary flow may be impaired. Failure to correct this anomaly may produce infertility problems in later life.

Exstrophy of the bladder

Exposure of the bladder occurs during embryonic development with failure in uniting of the abdominal recti muscles. The amount of separation of the recti muscles is a determinant to the degree of bladder exposure. Plastic surgery is the only remedy to correct this deformity.

CHROMOSOMAL ABERRATIONS

There are approximately fifty chromosomal aberrations. The most common are Down's syndrome (mongolism) and two sex-linked aberrations known as Turner's syndrome (female gonad) and Klinefelter's syndrome (male gonad).

Down's syndrome results from an extra chromosome in pair 21. The infants are detected when the nurse observes the following characteristics: extra epicanthal folds of the eyelids, large fat pads at the nape of the neck, wide separation between the thumb and the index finger, flat surface at the top of the ears, protruding tongue, and poor muscle tone. These babies have feeding problems since they suck poorly. They are susceptible to upper respiratory infections and in later life demonstrate intellectual impairment in varying degrees. The incidence of Down's syndrome is higher in infants born to mothers in the latent childbearing periods.

Turner's syndrome (female gonad aberration) and Klinefelter's syndrome (male gonad aberration) occur when there is a missing sex chromosome—instead of XX in the female there is XO, and instead of XY in the male there is XO. These infants are hermaphrodites and may possess reproductive organs of both sexes. Diagnosis is made by examination of the external genitalia. Any apparent anomaly warrants further study. Chromosomal sex determinations are done by staining smears from the buccal mucosa. Often urethroscopy will reveal male or female internal reproductive organs. Roentgenographic visualization may be accomplished by injecting dye through a urogenital sinus. If doubt still exists as to sexuality, laparotomy is performed. Proper treatment is instituted following careful evaluation. In all instances when sex is doubtful, sex assignment is based not only upon chromosomal pattern and gonadal morphology but also upon the structure of the external genitalia.

PHOCOMELIA

Phocomelia is a congenital anomaly in which the infant is born with improper development of body limbs. In December, 1961, a large number of babies in Germany and Australia were born with these defects. Investigation proved that a sedative known as thalidomide had been taken by the mothers of these infants in early pregnancy. Although its use spread in Europe, the drug was not approved by the Food and Drug Administration for distribution in the United States.

Nurses need to be aware of instructing young women of childbearing age to refrain from injudicious use of drugs for minor complaints. Often the young woman of childbearing age is hardly positive of pregnancy until she has missed two menstrual periods. Perhaps reeducation of young women in high school will prevent injudicious use of common drugs for headache and irritability.

Strides are being made to supply deformed infants with prostheses rather early. Parents should be instructed to seek help and guidance early for more effective rehabilitation of the child. It is the nurse's responsibility to refer parents to community rehabilitative services. Small temporary prostheses are applied as early as 3 months of age so that the infant becomes accustomed to the device as being a part of self.

Nurses working with parents in the prenatal period will eliminate many of these anomalies with adequate teaching and medical supervision.

SUPPORT OF FAMILY OF INFANT WITH BIRTH DEFECT

The impact of a birth defect on the whole family lies ultimately in the strength and support given the parents by the paramedical team at the time of birth. Most parents expect a normal infant since the baby is a replica or extension of two healthy people. It is apparent that the first question often asked is, "Is the baby all right?" "All right" covers a multitude of intricate, fascinating mechanisms within our body structure to the point of perfection, making this question quite difficult to answer. Many times the "all right" means, "Is the baby all there?" referring to what can be seen with the naked eye. Therefore, this very first question asked in the delivery room need make one aware of the importance of careful and thorough appraisal of the newborn infant, since parents are entitled to be told.

Should the answer be in the negative, what do we say? When is the proper time? How do we know how much stress the mother can accept at this time? How does one proceed to say, "No, everything is not all right." What makes this so difficult an interaction for the paramedical personnel? What are the expectations of each in this two-way conversation? We would like to say, "Yes, your baby is perfectly all right," yet we cannot. What is the answer to, "Why did this happen to us?" "Will it happen again with a subsequent pregnancy?"

In times of stress, the person who knows the parents well and has established rapport may be better able to handle the situation. Acceptance of the immediate anguish, rejection, and feelings of guilt is essential in support by the nursing personnel and the physician. Time is very often necessary before acceptance and hope can be anticipated. Although frankness and the truth may add to the immediate despair, this is far better than giving false hope. At times we underestimate the stamina, fortitude, and faith of parents and learn they can accept and cope with more than we give them credit for.

Some parents will withdraw and become silent, finding it too difficult to talk. Creating opportunities for discussion by feeling at ease and remaining with the mother during feedings is one way the nurse can help her ventilate and feel free to ask questions. Preparation of the parents before showing them a baby with marked anomalies may greatly lessen the blow since often the defect is visualized to be far worse. The mother may need time to accept feeding the baby with a bilateral cleft lip. Perhaps feeding the baby in her presence will instill confidence and facilitate her moving toward accepting the responsibility. Visible defects especially are difficult for the whole family to accept.

When physical defects are complicated with mental defects, the problem becomes even greater for families to accept. The child then does not fit into normal family patterns; he needs and demands more time from the mother, resulting in family strains. The problem then of deciding upon institutionalization and how this will affect the family becomes of great concern. Economic factors also come into play and are burdensome for many families.

It is well for nurses to talk with each other as they plan to help parents in stress situations. Often the nurse has a difficult time caring for the infant with an anomaly and needs support herself before she can give support to the parents. Family members or a close relative or spiritual leader can be supportive and helpful during times of stress. It is well for the nurse to remember Caplan's* statement: "It is remarkable to see the power that ordinary people have to adapt to reality, however unpleasant. They have a great deal more strength than we often give them credit for. Unassisted in a time of crisis this strength may fail them. But if we recognize it, and build it up, we can help each other through times of trouble."

*Caplan, G.: Principles of preventive psychiatry, New York, 1964, Basic Books, Inc., Publishers.

SELECTED REFERENCES

Anderson, G. V.: Hazardous drugs in pregnancy, Amer. J. Obstet. Gynec. **93:**553, 1965.

Apgar, V.: Drugs in pregnancy, Amer. J. Nurs. **65:**104, March, 1965. (Reprinted from J.A.M.A. **190:**840, 1964.)

Barnes, A. C.: The clinical approach to the prevention of congenital anomalies, Amer. J. Obstet. Gynec. **90:**1242, 1964.

Bierman, J. M., Siegel, E., French, F. E., and others: The community impact of handicaps of prenatal or natal origin, Public Health Rep. **78:**839, 1963.

Bowes, W. A., Jr., Drose, V. E., and Bruns, P. D.: Amniocentesis and intrauterine fetal transfusion in erythroblastosis, Amer. J. Obstet. Gynec. **93:**822, 1965.

Brill, A. B., and Forgotson, E. H.: Radiation and congenital malformations, Amer. J. Obstet. Gynec. **90:**1149, 1964.

Brooks, M. B., Beal, L. L., Ogg, H. L., and Blakesler, B.: The child with deformed or missing limbs, his problems and prostheses, Amer. J. Nurs. **62:**88, November, 1962.

Bruce, S.: Reactions of nurses and mothers to stillbirths, Nurs. Outlook **10:**81, February, 1962.

Burks, J. L., Davis, M. E., and Bakken, A. H.: Autosomal trisomy, Obstet. Gynec. **25:**611, 1965.

Caplan, G.: The mental hygiene role of the nurse in maternal and child care, Nurs. Outlook **2:**14, January, 1954.

Cleft lip and cleft palate, Ross Laboratories, Nursing Education Service, No. 11, Columbus, Ohio, 1962.

Committee on handicapped child: Statement on treatment of phenylketonuria, Pediatrics **25:**501, 1965.

Congenital malformations, the problem and the task, National Foundation **9:**340, June, 1961.

Connor, A.: Improved accuracy of prediction of severity of hemolytic disease of the newborn, Obstet. Gynec., vol. 33, no. 1, January, 1969.

Davidson-Buchanan, D. J.: Erythroblastosis neonatorum, Amer. J. Nurs. **64:**110, April, 1964.

Diagnosis of hidden congenital anomalies, National Foundation **9:**588, October, 1961.

Dougherty, L.: The interactions between blood types and disease, Nurs. Forum **3:** 46, 1964.

Fishbein, M.: Birth defects, Philadelphia, 1963, J. B. Lippincott Co.

Freda, V. J.: The Rh problem in obstetrics and a new concept of its management using amniocentesis and spectrophotometric scanning of amniotic fluid, Amer. J. Obstet. Gynec. **92:**341, 1965.

Freda, V. J., and Robertson, J. G.: Amniotic fluid analysis in Rh iso-immunization, Amer. J. Nurs. **65:**64, August, 1965.

Glynn, E. M.: Nursing support during intrauterine transfusion, Amer. J. Nurs. **65:** 72, August, 1965.

Groves, R., and Schloesser, P. J.: A state program to control phenylketonuria, Amer. J. Nurs. **64:**74, August, 1964.

Guthrie, R., and Stewart, W.: Phenylketonuria, Children's Bureau Publication, No. 41, Washington, D. C., 1964, U. S. Government Printing Office.

Harper, P. A.: Preventive pediatrics—child health and development, New York, 1962, Appleton-Century & Appleton-Century-Crofts.

Hewitt, D.: A study of temporal variations in the risk of fetal malformations and death, Amer. J. Public Health **52:**1676, 1962.

Isler, C.: Treatment and care of the child with a congenital hip dislocation, RN **25:** 50, September, 1962.

James, W. H.: Teratogenetic properties of thalidomide, Brit. Med. J. **5469:**1064, 1965.

Jens, A.: Coping with Dietl's crisis, Amer. J. Nurs. **64:**108, January, 1964.

Kang, E. S.: The genetic basis of some abnormalities in children, Children **13:**60, March-April, 1966.

Krugman, S.: Rubella, new light on an old disease, J. Pediat. **67:**159, 1965.

La Du, B. N.: Inborn errors of metabolism, Amer. J. Obstet. Gynec. **90:**1024, 1964.

McDermott, M. M.: The child with cleft lip and palate: the pediatric ward, Amer. J. Nurs. **65:**122, April, 1965.

McLenahan, I. G.: No baby to take home, Amer. J. Nurs. **62:**70, April, 1962.

Mellin, G. W.: Drugs in the first trimester of pregnancy and the fetal life of homo sapiens, Amer. J. Obstet. Gynec. **90:**1169, 1964.

Murphy, P.: The simple soul, Catholic Nurse **12:**46, June, 1964.

Owens, C.: Parents' reactions to defective babies, Amer. J. Nurs. **64:**83, 1964.

Papadatos, C., and Paschos, A.: Single umbilical artery and congenital malformations, Obstet. Gynec. **26:**367, 1965.

Pollack, W., and others: Results of clinical trials of Rho-GAM in women, Transfusion, May-June, 1968.

Queenan, J. T., and Adams, D. W.: Amniocentesis for prenatal diagnosis of erythroblastosis fetalis, Obstet. Gynec. **25:**302, 1965.

Queenan, J. T., and Douglas, G. R.: Intrauterine transfusion: a preliminary report, Obstet. Gynec. **25:**308, 1965.

Ripley, I. L.: The child with cleft lip and palate through his years of growth, Amer. J. Nurs. **65:**124, April, 1965.

Saling, E.: Formation and circulation of amniotic fluid, Year Book of obstetrics and gynecology, Chicago, Ill., 1965-1966, Year Book Medical Publishers, Inc.

Schid, S.: Parents of children with phenylketonuria, Children **11:**92, May-June, 1964.

Shaeffer, A. J.: Diseases of the newborn, Philadelphia, 1963, W. B. Saunders Co.

Shapiro, S., Ross, L. J., and Levin, H. S.: Relationship of selected prenatal factors to pregnancy outcome and congenital anomalies, Amer. J. Public Health **55:**268, 1965.

Sussman, L. N., and others: The prophylaxis of Rh hemolytic disease with Rh immunoglobulin, Amer. J. Clin. Path., vol. 50, no. 3, September, 1968.

Symposium on congenital defects, Amer. J. Obstet. Gynec. **90:**983, 1964.

Tartakow, I. J.: The teratogenicity of maternal rubella, J. Pediat. **66:**380, 1965.

The National Foundation, March of Dimes, 200 2nd Ave., New York, N. Y.

U. S. Children's Bureau: Galactosemia: a selected bibliography, Washington, D. C., 1963, U. S. Government Printing Office.

U. S. Children's Bureau: The clinical team looks at phenylketonuria, Washington,

D. C., 1964, U. S. Government Printing Office.

Winick, M.: Birth defects: what is being done about them? Nurs. Outlook **14**:43, January, 1966.

Questions for study

1. Define a birth defect.
2. What are some preventive measures in curtailing birth defects?
3. List the major causes of birth defects.
4. Describe common birth defects affecting the body systems. What treatment and nursing care are indicated?
5. What is the nurse's role in supporting the parents of children born with birth defects?
6. What facilities are available in your community for children born with congenital defects?
7. What current research is being done by the National Foundation?
8. Make a survey of educational materials on birth defects.

UNIT IV

INTERPREGNANCY PERIOD

Few things are more important to a community than the health of its women. If strong is the frame of the mother, says a proverb, the son will give laws to the people. And in nations where all men give laws, all men need mothers of strong frame.

T. W. Higginson

CHAPTER 25

INFECTIONS OF THE FEMALE ORGANS OF REPRODUCTION

A routine yearly gynecologic examination of all women over 30 years of age for maintenance of optimum health cannot be overemphasized. Since the reproductive system is so closely related to the female function of sexual competency and childbearing, there is often much fear, anxiety, and reluctance in seeking health supervision. It is evident that nurses teaching this aspect of health need to be sensitive to the gamut of feelings associated with examination of the female genital organs.

The most common microorganisms invading the reproductive system are the fungus, protozoa, streptococcus, gonococcus, and spirochete (Table 6 and Fig. 25-1). Invasion is primarily via the vaginal canal, and it may spread to the uterus, fallopian tubes, Bartholin's glands, peritoneum, adjacent organs, and blood system. Primary local invasion of the tissues results in varied signs and symptoms differentiated by the specific bacteria present.

FUNGAL INFECTION

A yeastlike fungus *(Candida* [*Monilia*] *albicans)* is a common cause of vaginitis in women. Since the fungus needs a wet, dark environment for growth, the vaginal canal is ideal. Invasion produces pruritus, redness, and a thick, cheesy discharge. Fungi thrive on carbohydrate, and it is common to find diabetic and pregnant women prone to *Candida albicans*. Secondary infection may be found in the infant's mouth and is known as thrush (small white patches on the mucosa), sometimes transmitted during delivery.

Treatment. The infection may be treated with local application of a 5% aqueous solution of gentian violet three times weekly along with nightly insertion of Propion Gel. Gentian violet tampons (5 mg.) are more practical during menstruation, since they eliminate messiness. With the woman in a dorsal recumbent position, the gel is inserted with an applicator, preferably at bedtime. Instructions

Table 6. Infections of the reproductive system

Organism	*Diagnosis*	*Organ affected*	*Disease entity*	*Treatment*
Fungus, yeast	Cervical smear	Vaginal canal	*Candida albicans*	1. Local application of 5% aqueous solution gentian violet or tampon 2. Propion Gel 3. Mycostatin—broad-spectrum antibiotic
Protozoa, parasite	Cervical smear	Vaginal canal	*Trichomonas vaginalis*	1. Acid douches (vinegar) 2. Local application of medications that provide sugars 3. Antiprotozoal drugs (Flagyl)
Streptococcus	Blood count, high WBC; elevated basal temperature; elevated pulse	Blood system, uterus, ovaries, tubes, peritoneal cavity	Pelvic inflammatory disease	1. Bed rest 2. Sedation 3. Antibiotics 4. Intravenous therapy
Gonococcus, *Neisseria gonorrhoeae*	Cervical smear and culture; gram-negative stain	Vagina, fallopian tubes, Skene's glands, urethra	Gonorrhea	Penicillin therapy
Spirochete, *Treponema pallidum*	Blood serology; Kahn or Wassermann	Vulva, labia, vagina, cervix	Syphilis	Penicillin therapy

on directing the applicator downward and backward into the vaginal canal will provide effectual application. A vulva pad will provide comfort as body heat absorbs the medication. Nystatin (Mycostatin), a broad-spectrum antibiotic given orally, has proved effective in the treatment of fungal infections.

PROTOZOAL INFECTION

The protozoon, a parasite *(Trichomonas vaginalis),* is commonly found and thrives well in an alkaline environment. The vaginal canal normally has an acid environment; therefore any change in pH will favor invasion by protozoa.

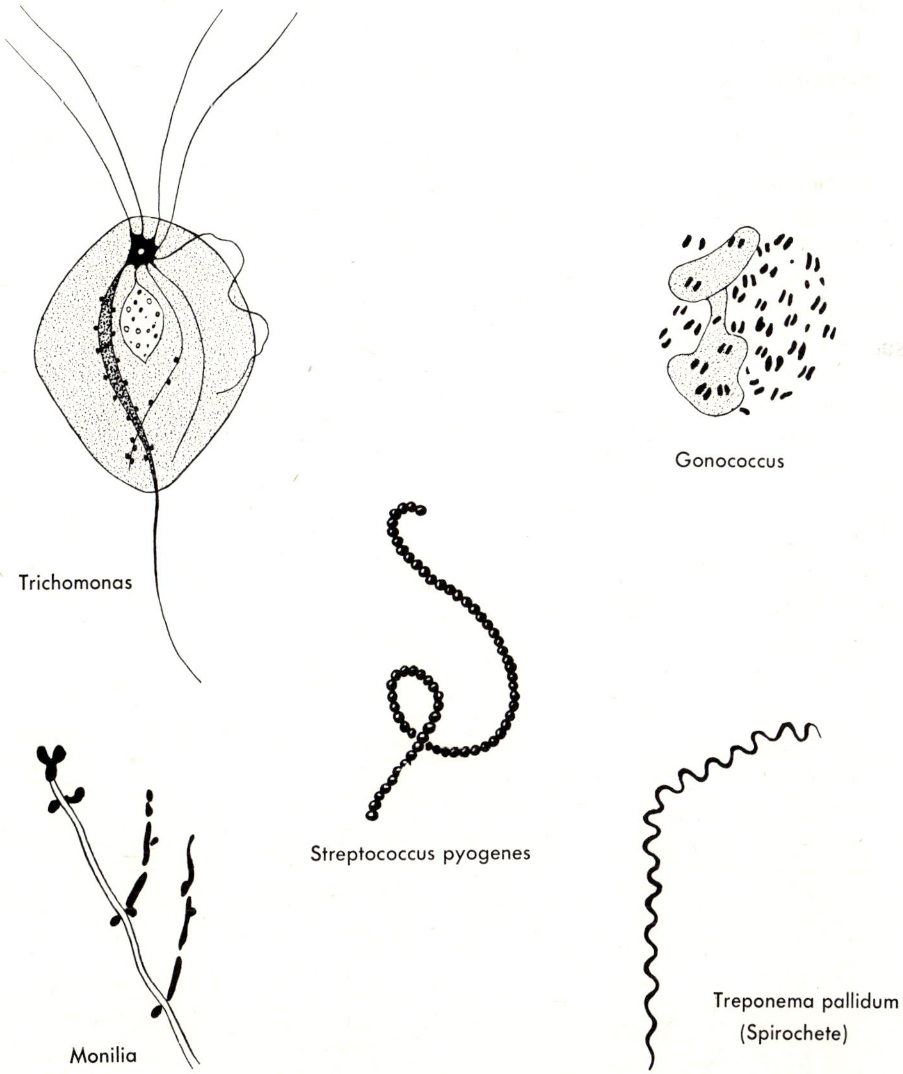

Fig. 25-1. Bacteria of the reproductive system.

Signs and symptoms. The common complaint is increased vaginal discharge, pruritus, and burning. The protozoa invade the vaginal tissue, causing redness, and often small hemorrhagic areas are visible on examination. During pregnancy invasion is common, and the organism is resistant to treatment.

Treatment and nursing care. The treatment for trichomoniasis requires decreasing the vaginal pH. Vaginal douches with vinegar (4 tbsp. to 2,000 ml. water), along with local application of medications containing sugars, restore the normal Döderlein's bacilli. When douches are ordered during pregnancy, the mother should be instructed to lie in the bathtub and to insert the nozzle just beyond the introitus, using a low-gravity flow. Douche equipment in which manual pressure is used should be discouraged since there is danger of air embolism. Flagyl (mctronidazole) is a new antiprotozoal medication now being ordered, and husband and wife are included in the therapy. Flagyl is contraindicated during pregnancy, since it crosses the placental barrier.

STREPTOCOCCAL INFECTION

The streptococcus invades the pelvic cavity through a breakdown in tissue. Accessible entrance into the bloodstream and lymphatics causes rapid invasion of the uterine lining, fallopian tubes, ovaries, and organs in the peritoneal cavity.

Streptococcal infection is likely following pregnancy, induced abortions, or intrauterine manipulation. Invasion of bacteria may occur when there has been a prolonged labor with general weakness, dehydration, and lack of resistance. A difficult delivery in which there is trauma to the tissues or excessive blood loss with retained placenta or membranes may also be a predisposing factor.

Prevention. Since it is evident that the streptococcus gains entrance through tissue breakdown, maintenance of strict aseptic technique during the maternity cycle is imperative. The importance of frequent gynecologic examinations to ensure a healthy status cannot be overstressed. Good nutrition and maintenance of optimum health are essential.

Signs and symptoms. The signs and symptoms of pelvic infection differ with the extent of tissue invasion. Common symptoms are elevated basal temperature, elevated pulse rate, and elevated white blood count. If there is peritoneal invasion, abdominal pain, distention, nausea, and vomiting may occur.

Treatment and nursing care. Bed rest, alleviation of pain with sedation, intravenous fluids, and antibiotics specific for the streptococcus are effectual. If the mother is on a postpartal unit, isolation to prevent spread of infection to other puerperal women is indicated. When abscess formation occurs with localization to a particular organ, surgical intervention is attempted following the acute inflammatory stage.

Nursing care in any staphylococcal infection includes prevention of the spread of the staphylococcal organism. The patient should be taught to dispose of dressings carefully because the organism is present in drainage following incision. Hand washing and keeping linens separate for washing are imperative.

GONOCOCCAL INFECTION

The gonococcus, a gram-negative diplococci, is the most common organism spread through sexual contact. Gonorrhea occurring during pregnancy may involve Skene's glands, Bartholin's glands, and the cervix. Infection sans pregnancy may also involve the urethra, fallopian tubes, and peritoneal cavity through the blood and lymph systems.

Signs and symptoms. Leukorrhea that is profuse and purulent, causing irritation, redness, edema, and pruritus, is the usual complaint. With involvement of the urethra, burning on urination is common. When untreated, purulent leukorrhea causes an overgrowth of epithelial tissue of the vulva and anus. At times the growth of tissue disappears with treatment, and at other times surgical removal is indicated when there is obstruction of the birth canal.

Treatment. Penicillin, 300,000 units given intramuscularly for 3 days, is therapeutic. When there is involvement of the urinary system, sulfa therapy is also indicated. Infected Bartholin's glands may subside with treatment or the infection may localize, causing a reddened, painful, inflamed edematous area on either side of the labia. Occasionally spontaneous drainage brings relief. At times the localized infection is treated by antibiotic therapy followed by surgical incision and drainage.

Involvement of the fallopian tubes is common with untreated gonorrhea. Prolonged damage to the muscular and peritoneal lining results in cicatrization and narrowing of the tubal lumen, causing menstrual disturbances and sterility. The gonococcus may also involve the knee, ankle, and wrist joints either during primary infection or as a latent manifestation. One single dose of kanamycin (Kantrex) given intramuscularly is now effective in the treatment of gonorrhea.

SPIROCHETAL INFECTION (SYPHILIS)

The spirochete *(Treponema pallidum)* is a corkscrew-shaped microorganism that invades the blood system and tissues through sexual contact. The infection progresses in stages from a primary sore or hard chancre to a generalized skin rash and gumma formation at the site of initial invasion.

Stages of syphilis

Primary stage. After 7 weeks of exposure, the primary chancre is a hard, indurated, painless ulcer found in the reproductive tract. The most common site is on the vulva and includes the cervix and the vaginal canal. This primary lesion often goes unnoticed when located in the vaginal canal. At times headache, malaise, and slight elevation in temperature may be noted.

Secondary stage. A characteristic maculopapular rash accompanied by malaise and headache is evident in the second stage. Swelling of the inguinal lymph nodes is common. At times hypertrophic growths are seen on the vulva and are known as condylomata lata. Occasionally surgical removal is necessary.

Tertiary stage. The lesion in the third stage of syphilis appears in the reproductive tract, usually on the vulva, and is known as a gumma. It is at first a "weeping" lesion containing active spirochetes. Eventually the lesion becomes a firm, indurated area.

Treatment. Treatment consists of penicillin given in massive doses. Primary, secondary, early latent, and late latent syphilis can be treated adequately with a single-dose deep intramuscular injection of 2,400,000 units of benzathine penicillin G. Patient discomfort is decreased by dividing the dose into 1,200,000 units given in each buttock. Vigorous shaking of the vial to ensure good suspension and warming to room temperature before injection are suggested.

Epidemiologic (prophylactic) treatment to prevent development of syphilis is recommended strongly for all persons who show no clinical manifestations but who are identified as sex contacts to primary or secondary syphilis. The treatment suggested is 2,400,000 units of penicillin G.

Patients with syphilis who are known to be sensitive to penicillin may be treated with erythromycin in total dosages of 20 to 30 Gm. over a period of 10 to 15 days. Tetracycline (Aureomycin or Terramycin), up to a total of 30 to 40 Gm., may be given orally over a period of 10 to 15 days.

Allergic and anaphylactic reactions to penicillin necessitate precautions such as questioning of all patients about previous allergic reactions, keeping all patients under observation for a minimum of 15 to 30 minutes following treatment, and at times simultaneous administration of either antihistamines or corticosteroids with penicillin. Anaphylactic reactions may be anticipated with prodromal symptoms of vertigo, nausea, flushing, itching, or even abdominal pain. The presence of any of these warrants the administration of two or three inhalations from an epinephrine Medihaler. If bronchial spasm or laryngeal edema is not immediately relieved, intravenous epinephrine is administered slowly with frequent checking of the blood pressure. An emergency tracheotomy set should always be available for emergency treatment.

Syphilis during pregnancy

During the antepartal period a serologic Wassermann test is done on the first visit and a few weeks prior to term to rule out syphilis. Prenatal syphilis is transmitted to the fetus in utero from the mother. The incidence of fetal infection varies according to the stage of the disease in the mother at the time of pregnancy. Eight percent of children born to untreated syphilitic mothers (in an early stage of the disease) will be affected in utero. Of these, 25% die prior to delivery as a result of the infection, and a high percentage of infants born alive die of the infection or of prematurity. Of all the infected untreated children who survive infancy, 40% will develop symptoms of syphilis sometime during their lives.

Transfer of organisms. Organisms may pass from the maternal to the fetal circulation without lesions in the placenta, or lesions may be found on the maternal side of the placenta, extend to the fetal side, and invade the fetal circulation, infecting the fetus. Whatever the mode of infection, the fetus is seldom involved prior to the fourth month of pregnancy. It is thought that the well-developed Langhans layer of the chorion serves as a protective barrier against the spirochete. This layer, however, atrophies and disappears after the sixteenth week, and then infection begins. The infected placenta may be of normal size and weight or enlarged, weighing 25% to 30% of the infant's weight, rather than the normal weight (25% of that of the fetus). If the infant dies before birth, the placenta appears pale, greasy, and bulky.

Clinical manifestations. Primary lesions or chancres of acquired syphilis are not seen in prenatal syphilis.

Early manifestations. Most infants appear well at birth and develop early lesions between 2 and 6 weeks, and rarely in a year or two, postpartum. When symptoms appear early the prognosis is not as good as when they appear later. The infant is usually well formed but underweight. Cutaneous lesions of the chin, circumoral region, palms, soles, and anogenital area similar to those of secondary acquired syphilis are common. There are also lesions of the mucous membranes with rhinitis (sniffles). The discharge is frequently profuse, bloody, or blood-tinged and is highly infectious. The nasal obstruction may cause difficulty in feeding.

On roentgenographic examination, epiphysitis is apparent, with irregularity and thickening of the epiphyseal line. Osteochondritis results, with pain on movement and local tenderness over one or more epiphyses. Also associated with early prenatal syphilis are generalized lymphoadenopathy, hepatosplenomegaly, meningitis, hemolytic anemia, saddle nose, nephritis, and iritis.

Late manifestations. Infants with prenatal syphilis who survive the early stage of the disease experience a stage of latency that may be brief or may last many years. The child may not have active lesions but yet be left with characteristics, scars, and malformations known as stigmata. Some of these are permanent—Hutchinson's teeth, destruction of nasal bones and cartilage (saddle nose), saber shin, perforated palate, and nasal septum.

With syphilis, as early as the second month of life or as late as 30 to 40 years, gumma type lesions attacking bone, skin, and viscera may be found. These involve the central nervous system in the form of meningitis, juvenile paresis or tabes dorsalis, eighth nerve deafness, and bilateral hydroarthritis (Clutton's joints).

A negative serologic test for syphilis (S.T.S.) at birth does not rule out prenatal syphilis, since the untreated fetus infected late in pregnancy may not show a positive test until after delivery. If the infection occurred in utero, the serology would be positive with a progressive rise for the first 6 months of life. A positive serology in the newborn may be a result of fetal infection (antibodies produced by the fetus), or it may be due to passively transferred maternal antibodies.

Treatment. Treatment of the mother prior to the fourth month will prevent infection of the fetus. Treatment after 16 weeks will effect cure of the fetus in utero but does not assure prevention of permanent osseous or dental stigmata. The longer the treatment of fetal infection is delayed, the more damage will be seen in the infant.

Treatment of choice in prenatal syphilis is penicillin G. One dose of 2,400,000 units of penicillin G given to the mother will prevent or cure infection of the fetus provided the mother is not reinfected during the same pregnancy. Following delivery, the infant is given 50,000 units of intramuscular penicillin G per kilogram of body weight in ten equally divided doses. When penicillin sensitivity exists, broad-spectrum antibiotics are given. Erythromycin does not completely cross the placenta, and tetracycline has an effect on dental enamel. Therefore, they are avoided.

Treated newborns are followed by qualitative S.T.S. tests every month for 6 months and then every 3 months for a year. Spinal fluid evaluation is performed 12 months following treatment. A report to the health department for epidemiologic investigation is essential to eradicate the disease.

INFECTIONS OF THE VULVA

Pruritus vulvae. Although pruritus of the vulva is a symptom of *pruritus vulvae,* it has many causes, some obvious, some obscure. Itching is often caused by bacterial invasion (as by *Candida albicans* or *Trichomonas vaginalis*); eczematous dermatitis; leakage of urine with stress incontinence; or use of detergents, powder, perfume, deodorants, nail polish, or douche preparations; irritation by vulvar pads; diabetes; intertrigo; condylomas; herpes genitalis; leukoplakia; kraurosis of the vulva; ringworm; pediculosis; scabies; vitamin deficiency; uremia; and leukemia. When no lesion is present, pruritis vulvae is known as neurodermatitis.

The itching may be so severe as to disturb sleep and interfere with activities of daily living. Pruritus is often severe with no skin lesions, and less severe with extensive skin lesions. There may be redness, edema, dryness, and scaling of the vulva area.

Determining the cause is often difficult, and treatment is geared toward providing comfort by relieving itching. Soap and water are avoided. The area is sponged with cool water with the legs as far apart as possible. Urging the patient to refrain from scratching reduces the incidence of secondary infection. A vaginal tampon keeps the area dry. Mild sedation, such as phenobarbital or a tranquilizing drug, is helpful.

Local therapy includes baths, wet dressings, lotions, and ointments. Baths and wet dressings are used in acute and moist lesions. Prolonged use, however, may produce skin maceration.

Oatmeal, starch, and bicarbonate of soda baths, boric acid and magnesium sulfate soaks, calamine lotion, zinc oxide ointment, olive oil, liquid paraffin solutions, and boric acid and bacteriostatic ointments are helpful.

For a discussion of Bartholin cyst, condylomas, and syphilitic lesions, see Chapters 25 and 27.

Folliculitis. Inflammation of the hair follicles is common in the vulvar region due to moisture and organisms from the vaginal secretions. Often following perineal shaving skin trauma may produce folliculitis. In many obstetric units vulvar shaving for delivery is not being done. Diagnosis is made when a small pustule appears encircling a hair follicle.

Treatment consists of keeping the area clean and dry and application of bacteriostatic ointments. The nurse may prevent folliculitis by great care in following the line of hair growth and in keeping the razor close to the skin to prevent skin breakdown.

Furuncles and carbuncles. Furuncles and carbuncles are deeper infections of the hair follicles of the vulva, caused by a staphylococcus organism. They are multiple and cause pain, swelling, and difficulty when sitting. The area is usually reddened and tender and has a central yellow region or core.

Local application of heat and antibiotic therapy prevent the spread of the infection. Incision and drainage is done only after the infection has become localized.

Pediculosis pubis. Pediculosis pubis is transmitted by direct contact with an infected person, contact with clothing belonging to an infected person, or through use of a toilet seat used previously by an infected person. The eggs of the crab louse, found at the hair shaft, are difficult to detect. Diagnosis is made by microscopic examination of the hair shaft.

Most effective in treatment are local application of Freon (DDT and pyrethrum) and gamma benzene hexachloride (Kwell).

Scabies. Scabies is a parasite that produces severe pruritus, especially at night. When it is present on the vulva there are burrows, vesicles, pustules, excoriation, and dermatitis. A 25% benzyl benzoate emulsion applied twice a day proves effective for 24-hour intervals.

NURSING CARE

Infections of the reproductive organs are directly related to feelings associated with womanliness, reproduction, and sexual competency. It is not uncommon to find reluctance in seeking health care when infections occur. Particularly during pregnancy women may anticipate danger to the baby and their own health status.

The anxiety that usually accompanies diseases of the reproductive system has a great deal of implication for teaching and health care. Reiterating the importance of follow-through on treatment is imperative for therapeutic effects.

Hand washing before and after treatments such as insertion of suppositories, douches, etc. needs to be emphasized. In monilial and trichomonal infections changing undergarments often is essential to prevent reinfection. The gonococcus has an affinity for the eyes and may cause blindness with conjunctival infection. Utensils and linens soiled with vaginal secretions should be handled carefully to prevent transmission.

A known fact that gonorrhea is a disease transmitted through sexual contact may produce varied reactions in patients. It is difficult to trace all contacts since sexual contacts may be members other than marital partners. However, the nurse, in promoting health, needs to be aware that treatment is essential for all contacts. Case finding and reporting contacts are just as important as treating known patients.

Syphilis in the acute chancre or latent gumma stage is infectious, and the active spirochete is found in the blood system and in the lesion. Therefore, open skin lesions in contact with the blood or the lesion of an active syphilitic patient could transmit the disease. Strict asepsis in caring for the active syphilitic patient is essential. As a public health service, all contacts should be traced and treated to prevent spread of the disease. Since syphilis is a known social disease, expertness in interviewing is essential in tracing contacts. Referral to public health agencies and the social caseworker is essential for community control of venereal diseases.

SELECTED REFERENCES

Behrman, S. J.: Fundamentals of gynecology, New York, 1963, Oxford University Press.

Burnette, S.: An odyssey toward veneral disease education, J. Sch. Health **34:**378, 1964.

Hallock, J., and Tunnessen, W. W.: Congenital syphilis in an infant of a Seronegative mother, Obstet. Gynec., vol. 32, no. 3, September, 1968.

Hodge, C. H., and Murdoch, D.: Treatment of vaginal discharge by sulfonamide pessaries, Amer. J. Obstet. Gynec. **86:**742, 1963.

Kozinn, P. J., and Taschdjian, C. L.: Candidiasis, Amer. J. Nurs. **61:**52, January, 1961.

Moore, M. B., Jr., Price, E. V., Knox, J. M., et al.: Epidemiologic treatment of contacts to infectious syphilis, Public Health Rep. **78:**966, 1963.

Novak, E. R., and Seegar Jones, G.: Novak's textbook of gynecology, ed. 7, Baltimore, 1965, The Williams & Wilkins Co.

Shapiro, L. H., and Lentz, J. W.: Kanamycin as treatment of acute gonorrhea in female, Obstet. Gynec., vol. 35, no. 5, 1970.

Willson, J. R., Beecham, C. T., and Carrington, E. R.: Obstetrics and gynecology, ed. 3, St. Louis, 1966, The C. V. Mosby Co.

World forum on syphilis, Public Health Rep. **78:**295, 1963.

Zacharias, L. F., Salzer, R. B., Gunn, J. C., and Dierksheide, E. B.: Trichomoniasis and metronidazole, Amer. J. Obstet. Gynec. **86:**748, 1963.

Questions for study

1. Name the organisms responsible for invading the reproductive organs.
2. Relate the effect of the invading bacterium to the physiology of the reproductive organs.
3. What are the nursing responsibilities in caring for women with infections of the reproductive tract?
4. Make a survey in your local community of services available for control of venereal disease.
5. What is the nurse's responsibility in your community related to communicable disease?

CHAPTER 26

CHILDBIRTH INJURIES

During delivery there is often trauma to the soft tissues of the birth canal. The primigravida with a firm perineum and resistant muscles may have a considerable amount of tissue damage, affecting the bladder anteriorly and the rectum posteriorly. Multigravidas, on the other hand, may deliver with little or no noticeable damage since there is much elasticity of tissue.

INJURIES TO BIRTH CANAL AND PERINEUM

Injuries and lacerations to the birth canal and the perineum, when evident following delivery, need immediate repair for adequate healing and prevention of infection.

Hematomas

Hematomas of the reproductive tract are rare during pregnancy. They may occur with spontaneous rupture of the tubo-ovarian veins, in the broad ligament and vagina during labor, as a result of operative pelvic delivery, or following delivery because of faulty hematostasis with an episiotomy repair.

The most serious is the broad ligament hematoma, since its origin is uncertain. Broad ligament hematomas may occur from spontaneous rupture of a broad ligament vein or with rupture of the lower uterine segment. In either origin, life is threatened and immediate supracervical hysterectomy is indicated. Symptoms include pain lateral to the uterus a few hours following delivery, marked tenderness on palpation, and abdominal distention. Rectal examination reveals tenderness and a high lateral fullness in the cul-de-sac. Hematoma of the broad ligament differs from uterine rupture since there is absence of vaginal bleeding.

The possibility of uterine rupture is always explored in the operating room with necessary preparation for unpredictable blood loss. If laparotomy and exploration are indicated, ligation of the internal iliac and ovarian vessels is often necessary to control bleeding and is followed by hysterectomy and bilateral oophorectomy.

Occasionally extrusion of blood into the loose tissue of the labia or an oozing blood vessel following episiotomy repair may develop into a large hematoma. Observation of the perineum following delivery cannot be overstressed. Often following spinal or saddle block anesthesia, the usual complaints of pain and pressure in the perineal area are marked. On examination the area is edematous, ecchymotic, and painful to touch. Cold applications will give temporary relief. Small ice chips in a sterile glove provide comfort against a painful perineum. Under sterile precautions the hematoma is evacuated, the blood vessel is ligated, and the episiotomy is resutured.

Episiotomy

Episiotomy is an incision into the perineum prior to delivery. It facilitates delivery and prevents laceration and overstretching of the pelvic floor. Since it is a clean, smooth incision, healing occurs rapidly. Episiotomy causes less pressure of the occiput against the anterior vaginal wall and preserves the surrounding perineal tissues and supporting structures of the bladder.

Indications for episiotomy are the following: (1) protection of the head from pressure and trauma during premature delivery; (2) abnormal flexion or position of the presenting part as in face presentation or posterior position of the occiput; and (3) forceps application, breech delivery, or when rapid delivery is indicated for fetal distress.

Episiotomies are of two types (Fig. 12-5), median or midline and right or left mediolateral, each having advantages and disadvantages. A midline episiotomy heals rapidly and causes less discomfort since there is natural direct skin line proximity. With a short perineal body, however, extension into the rectal sphincter may occur. Dyspareunia is a complaint of some women following a midline episiotomy. The mediolateral type involves the bulbocavernosus and transverse perineal muscles and is the method of choice when delivery is difficult. Episiotomies of this type cause discomfort as the thigh is in close proximity to the incision.

Lacerations

Lacerations of the birth canal occur more often during difficult or precipitate delivery. If bleeding persists following delivery and if the uterus is firm, inspection of the cervix, vagina, and perineum is indicated.

Lacerations of the cervix are commonly found on the sides where the descending branches of the uterine arteries are located. If the cervix is lacerated at the apex, exploration of the lower uterine segment is done to rule out extension.

Lacerations of the vaginal fornices are repaired with ease, whereas those occurring behind the pubic arch are difficult to repair since they are not visible. Vaginal tissue is friable, and often continuous oozing following repair necessitates packing the area firmly to control bleeding.

Lacerations of the perineum and the introitus are more likely to occur when episiotomy is not performed. Lacerations are classified into four categories depending upon extent and depth of tissues involved:

First degree lacerations (Fig. 12-6, *A*) involve the vaginal mucous membrane and skin of the perineum at the posterior fourchette.

Second degree lacerations (Fig. 12-6, *B*) involve the skin, endopelvic fascia, levator ani muscles, and perineal body.

Third degree lacerations (Fig. 12-6, *C*) involve the entire perineum and the external sphincter of the rectum, either partially or completely.

Fourth degree lacerations are complete, involving the entire perineum, rectal sphincter, and some degree of the mucous membrane of the rectum.

Nursing care. Discomforts of the perineum are common as edema of the suture line occurs with the healing process. With episiotomies of the mediolateral type, walking, friction of the perineal pad, and sitting may be uncomfortable. Nursing measures include teaching perineal exercise to improve circulation to the area, thereby preventing edema. Applying a heat lamp following perineal care produces the same effect. Occasionally commercial sprays containing menthol and benzocaine are ordered, and they produce a soothing anesthetic effect. Instructing the mother to wear a girdle relieves discomfort as the buttocks are brought closer together.

Lacerations are treated as episiotomies; however, healing is slower since the skin edges are uneven. Third degree lacerations cause much discomfort during bowel evacuation. It is a common practice to order a low-residue diet for a few days to allow for primary healing. Cathartics that are lubricant in nature are helpful to relieve discomfort during bowel evacuation.

Perineal care in which the area is cleansed from the vagina toward the rectum will prevent introduction of organisms into the repaired episiotomy or laceration. Keeping the suture line clean and dry hastens healing.

RELAXATION OF THE VAGINAL OUTLET

A relaxed vaginal outlet is usually a result of overstretching of the perineal supporting tissues as a result of childbirth. Although trauma occurs during childbirth, the damage is not apparent until the fifth or sixth decade when generalized muscular atony and loss of tissue elasticity are common.

A cystocele is a herniation of the anterior vaginal wall. There is a resulting descent and protrusion of the bladder floor into the vaginal canal (Fig. 26-1).

Rectocele is a similar condition in which the pararectal fascia protrudes at the vaginal orifice.

Signs and symptoms. Relaxations of the vaginal outlet may be entirely symptomless or, on the other hand, they may produce a feeling of looseness or heaviness in the vaginal region, especially after prolonged standing. Some women describe a feeling of "everything dropping out." Backache and a "bearing-down" feeling in the lower abdomen are common complaints. With marked relaxations, urinary incontinence and constipation are experienced. Another common complaint is difficulty in emptying the bladder. Often the bladder needs to be pushed back with the finger to facilitate emptying. In severe cases, in which the bladder retains

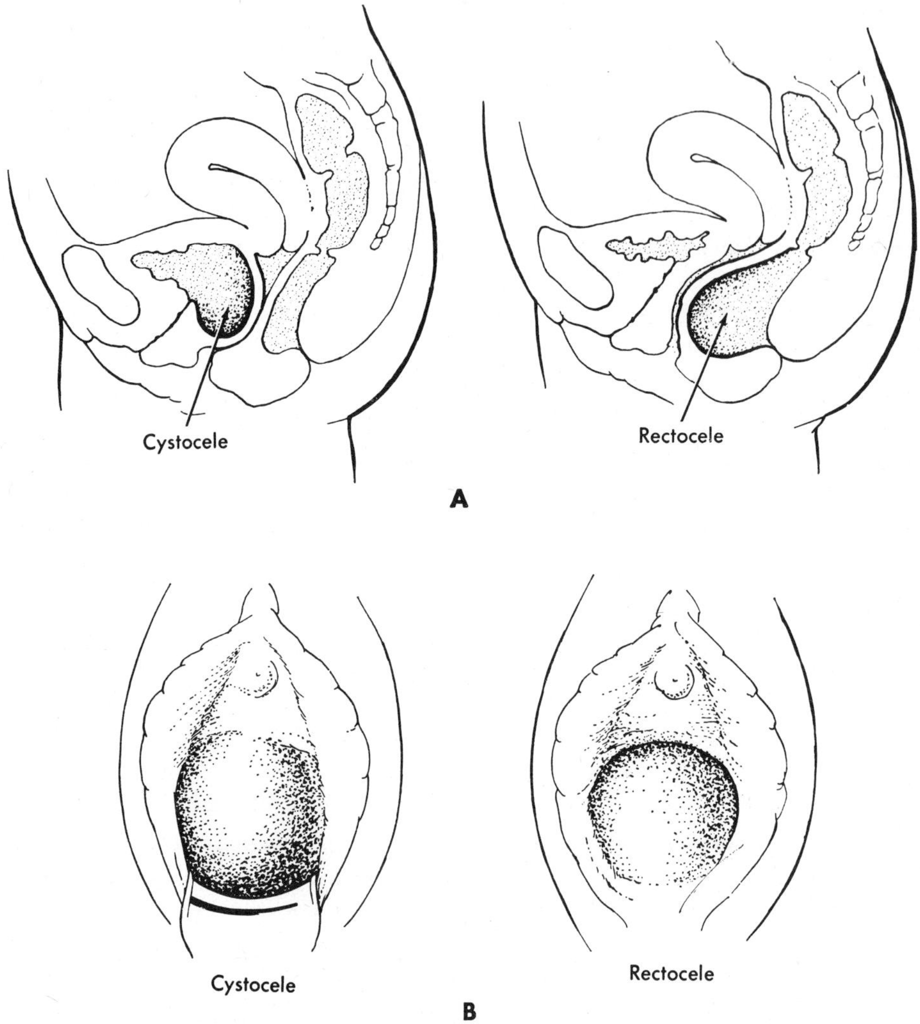

Fig. 26-1. A, Cystocele and rectocele (internal genitalia). **B,** Cystocele and rectocele (external genitalia).

residual urine, cystitis is common. With cystitis there is increased frequency of urination with tenesmus, the symptoms being troublesome during the day and improved at night with the patient in a recumbent position. With urethrocele, stress incontinence occurs with escape of urine on coughing, sneezing, laughing, or any muscular effort.

Often some women complain of stress incontinence at the 6-week postpartum visit, but this complaint disappears as involution progresses. It is essential for the nurse to understand the physiology of micturition so that she can instruct the mother who complains of stress incontinence following delivery. There are two urethral sphincters, the external and the internal. The external sphincter is striated voluntary muscle. The internal sphincter is an involuntary smooth muscle. When the bladder is distended, parasympathetic nerve impulses are stimulated, with a resulting urge to micturate. The cut sphincter muscle relaxes, permitting urine to enter the upper urethra. Distention of the upper urethra produces the urge to void. Since the voluntary external sphincter muscles are relaxed, urination occurs. With stress incontinence there is no control of the external or internal urethral sphincter.

Direct air urethrocystoscopy is done by using an optic instrument that allows for inspection of the female bladder and urethra as an office procedure. For the patient with stress incontinence, a closed air system allows for the female bladder to be deflated so that the trigone and retropubic areas may be inspected.

Perineal exercises introduced by Kegal are commonly used to correct symptoms of stress incontinence. Teaching exercising of the perineal muscles has eliminated the necessity for surgical repair in many women. Kegal devised a perineometer that, when introduced into the vagina, measures the force with which the perineal and vaginal muscles are contracted. Women are instructed to practice contraction of the perineal and vaginal muscles 75 to 100 times daily over a period of 3 months—it has been found that this relieves symptoms of stress incontinence. The physician often teaches the patient to contract these muscles against his examining fingers. The patient then follows through and learns to do this on her own.

Prolonged protrusion at the introitus results in chafing of the mucosa with ulceration and bleeding. Often with postmenopausal atrophy and relaxation, dyspareunia is experienced.

Treatment. Correction for cystocele and rectocele may be deferred until the childbearing period is complete, unless severe symptoms warrant immediate repair.

When possible, pessaries are inserted until the family has been completed, and then surgery is performed. Hysterectomy with repair of cystocele or rectocele by the vaginal route may be indicated in older women. If removal of the uterus is not indicated, tubal ligation is often done to preserve a functionless uterus, but this has the disadvantage of possible predisposition to myoma or carcinoma.

VAGINOPLASTY

Nursing care. Preoperatively the vaginal and rectal areas are shaved to remove surface bacteria. A soap solution enema is often ordered to cleanse the lower bowel of remaining stool. At times an indwelling three-way Foley catheter (Fig. 26-2) is inserted to empty the bladder before, during, and after surgery.

A new method for management of urinary drainage after vaginal plastic surgery is the insertion in the operating room of a suprapubic catheter (Figs. 26-3 to 26-5). The catheter remains open for drainage until 6:00 A.M. on the first postoperative day. It is then clamped off for 4 hours, opened for drainage for 5 minutes throughout the first postoperative day; it is left opened all night until 6:00 A.M. On the second postoperative day the catheter is clamped continually as

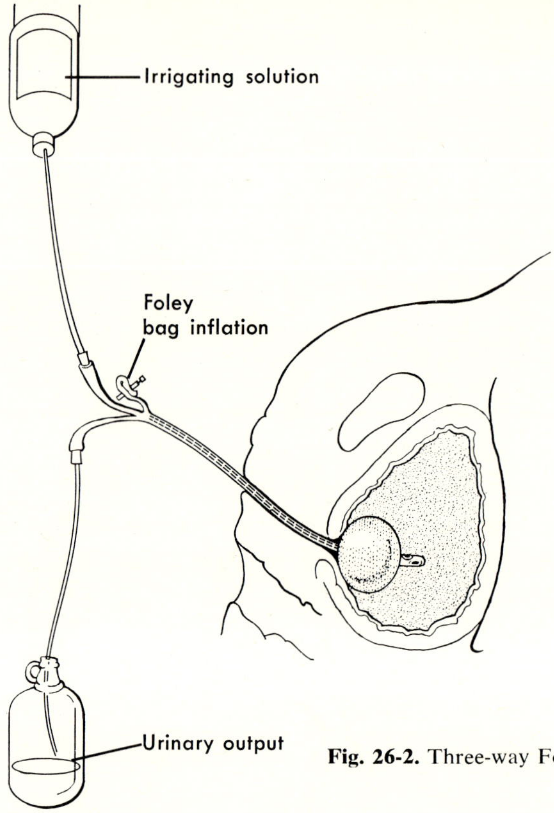

Fig. 26-2. Three-way Foley catheter.

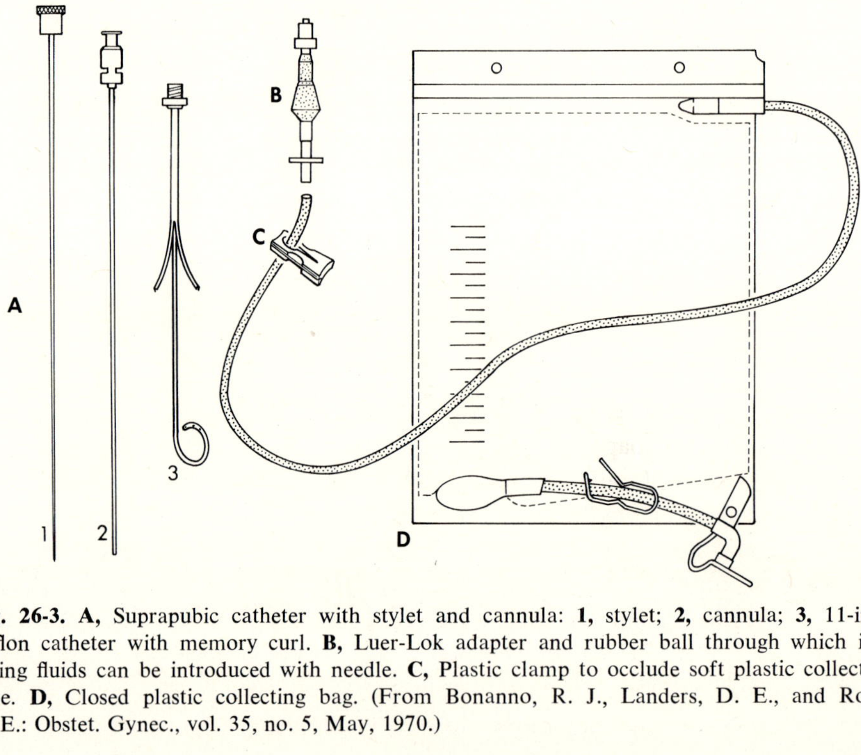

Fig. 26-3. A, Suprapubic catheter with stylet and cannula: **1,** stylet; **2,** cannula; **3,** 11-inch Teflon catheter with memory curl. **B,** Luer-Lok adapter and rubber ball through which irrigating fluids can be introduced with needle. **C,** Plastic clamp to occlude soft plastic collecting tube. **D,** Closed plastic collecting bag. (From Bonanno, R. J., Landers, D. E., and Rock, D. E.: Obstet. Gynec., vol. 35, no. 5, May, 1970.)

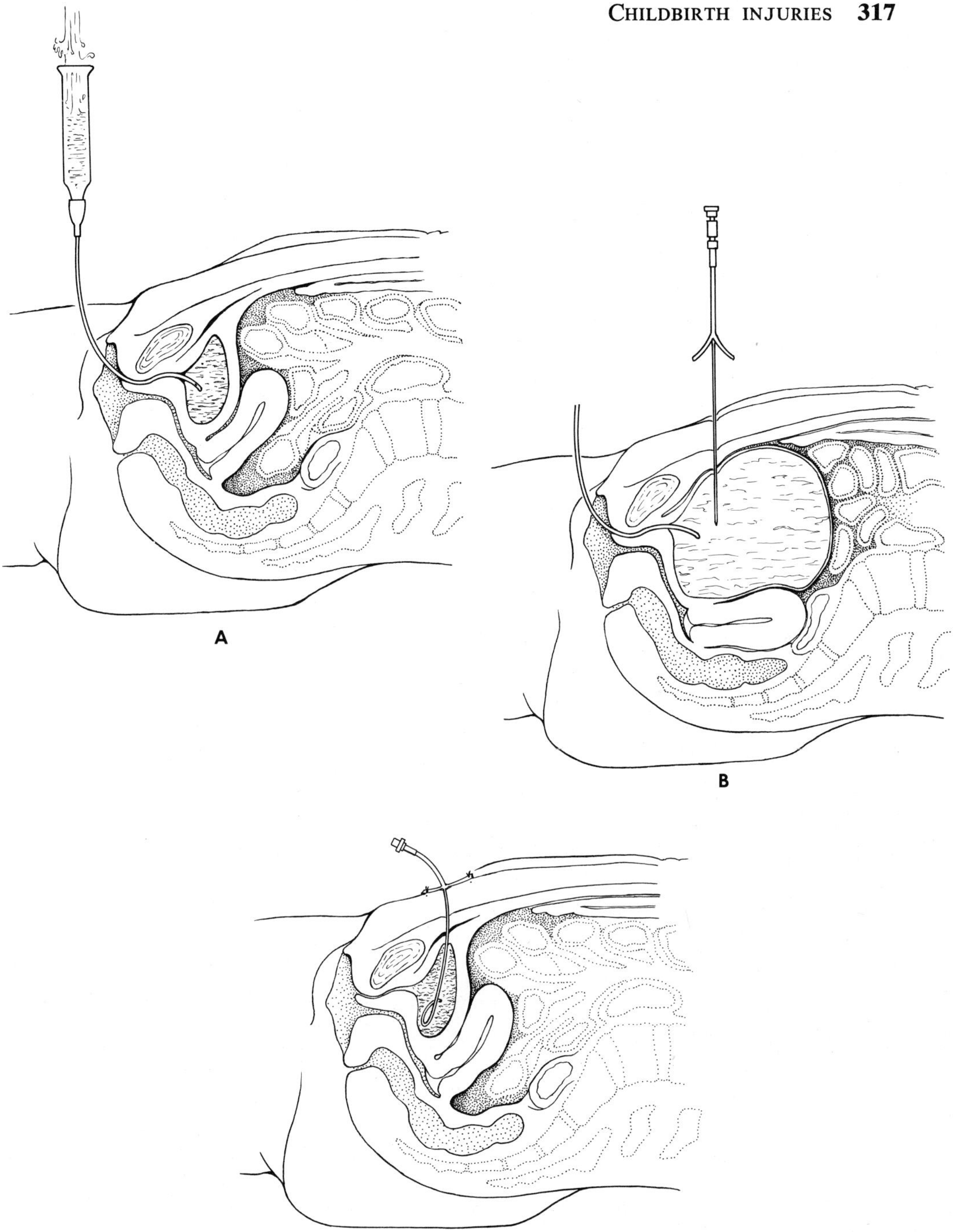

Fig. 26-4. Insertion of suprapubic catheter. **A,** Bladder is distended by 500 ml. of saline introduced through large-bore plastic urethral catheter. **B,** Stylet, with cannula and catheter, is introduced through abdominal wall into bladder. **C,** After withdrawal of stylet and cannula, catheter wings are fixed to skin with two fine silk sutures. (From Bonanno, R. J., Landers, D. E., and Rock, D. E.: Obstet. Gynec., vol. 35, no. 5, May, 1970.)

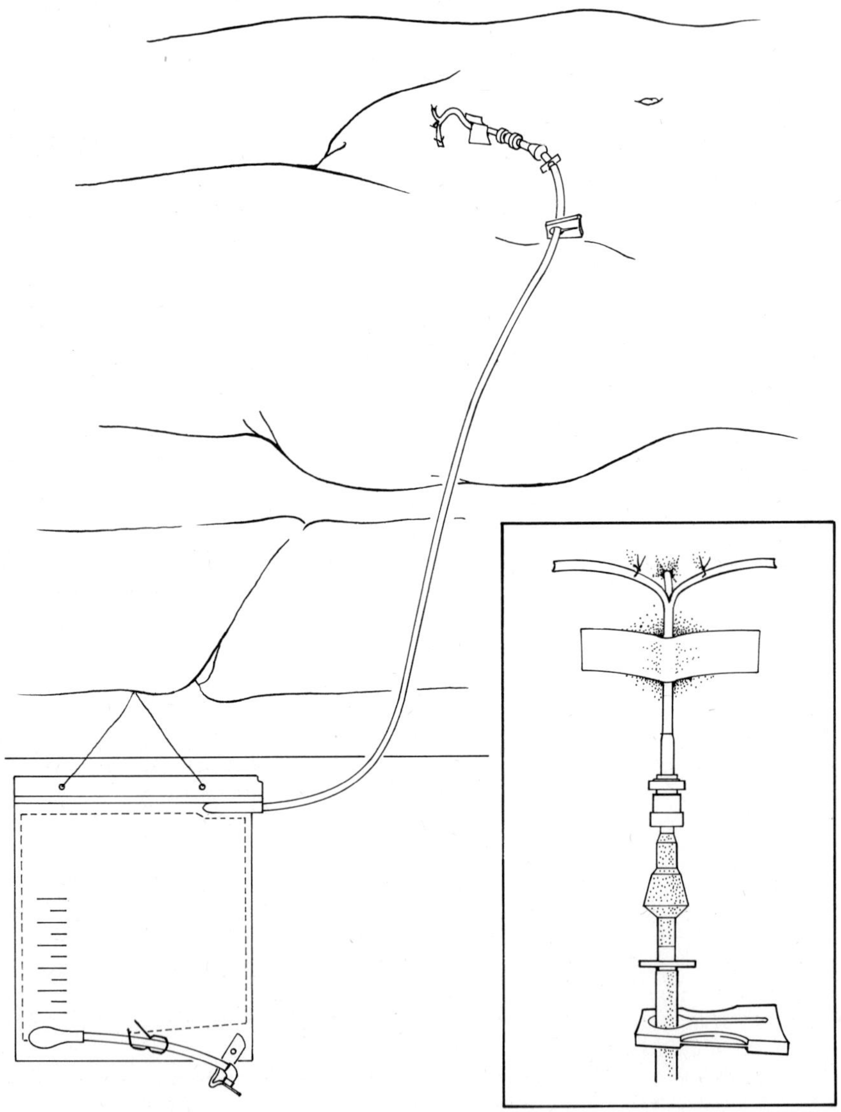

Fig. 26-5. Suprapubic catheter with collecting tube and bag in place. Inset shows detail of catheter wings sutured to skin near catheter and paper tape for additional fixation. (From Bonanno, R. J., Landers, D. E., and Rock, D. E.: Obstet. Gynec., vol. 35, no. 5, May, 1970.)

tolerated. If the patient becomes uncomfortable and cannot void, the catheter clamp is reopened for 5 minutes and left open during the night. When the patient begins to void, residual urine specimens are collected following three voidings by opening the catheter for 5 minutes after the patient voids and measuring the amount. (It has been proved that a catheter can drain up to 100 ml. per minute.)

When the patient is voiding well, the catheter may be clamped continually; it is removed when residual urine specimens are less than 120 ml. on two consecutive occasions. Through the Luer-Lok opening, 5 ml. of a genitourinary irrigating solution (Neosporin) is instilled twice daily and allowed to remain in the bladder for 20 minutes. The catheter is then drained for 5 minutes.

Hot sitz baths are given three or more times a day as soon as the vaginal drain and packing are removed. Mineral oil (Kondremul) or other stool softener is often given twice daily. For pain, dextropropoxyphene hydrochloride (Darvon), 65 mg., with hydroxyzine pamoate (Vistaril), 50 mg., is given orally every 4 hours. Antibiotics most often used are azo-sulfisoxazole (azo-Gantrisin) and methenamine mandelate (Mandelamine). Sterile urine specimens are obtained from the catheter for urinalysis, culture, and sensitivity.

Explaining the purpose for this preparation will alleviate much anxiety. Allowing the patient to ventilate her fears is therapeutic prior to surgery. Reassurance that medication will be available for discomfort is an adjunct to adequate preparation. Teaching the patient to contract and relax the pubococcygeus muscles will help when the patient is experiencing stress incontinence.

Spiritual attendance should be offered all patients prior to surgery regardless of religious faith.

Postoperatively, astute observation of vital signs and checking urinary output via the catheter are essential. Intake and output are recorded to rule out dehydration and urine retention. Keeping the perineal area clean and dry provides comfort and promotes healing. A diet high in protein assures rapid tissue repair with return to optimum health. Deep breathing and leg motion are encouraged to prevent circulatory stasis. Often ambulation is delayed to promote healing and relieve pressure on the perineal sutures. Instructing the patient against straining with bowel evacuation prevents discomfort and damage to sutures. Lubricating cathartics are helpful in promoting bowel evacuation.

UTERINE PROLAPSE

A condition in which the uterus is found in a lower position than is normal or is found entirely protruding the vaginal canal is known as uterine prolapse. The extent of the prolapse is expressed in degrees. First degree prolapse indicates that the cervix is at some level between its normal position and the introitus. When the uterus projects beyond the hymenal ring and can be seen at the introitus, this is a second degree prolapse. Third degree prolapse indicates that the entire uterus is outside the vulva. This is also called complete prolapse or procidentia. Another term used is descensus.

Causes. Although stretching and tearing of the tissues during childbirth is the cause of uterine prolapse, it is also believed that there is possibly some congenital tissue insufficiency. This often occurs upon severe exertion in nulliparous women who are acrobats, dancers, etc.

Symptoms. The condition is usually insidious in onset or may occur quite abruptly. Symptoms include a bearing down sensation and a feeling of a dropping of pelvic organs. With marked procidentia frequency with retention of urine and difficulty in walking or sitting are common. Leukorrhea with marked congestion of the cervix or an ulceration of the exposed vaginal walls may occur. Cystitis is common with prolonged frequency and residual urine. Often the woman needs to replace the uterus with her hand in order to void.

Treatment. Treatment depends upon the woman's age, her desire for more children, the severity of symptoms, and the degree of prolapse. With women who desire more children or those whose symptoms are not of a marked degree, wearing a vaginal pessary that is removed, cleansed, and replaced each month is all that is necessary. The Gellhorn pessary (Fig. 26-7, *D*) of lightweight Lucite is commonly used.

In women past childbearing age with distressing symptoms, surgical intervention offers complete relief. Usually vaginal hysterectomy is the method of choice. However, if the woman is young and desires more children, or is elderly and a poor surgical risk, a Manchester-Fothergill operation is done. This operation is done vaginally; the uterus is preserved by elevation and support with fixation of the parametrial tissue. In young women who have had a Manchester-Fothergill operation, subsequent deliveries are by cesarean section.

Colpocleisis (Le Fort operation), obliteration of the vagina, is done in elderly widowed women who will no longer have sexual relations.

DISPLACEMENTS OF THE UTERUS

Anterior (Fig. 26-7, *A*), upright or horizontal (Fig. 26-7, *B*), and retrodisplaced (Fig. 26-7, *C*) are the three fundamental positions of the uterus.

Retrodisplacements are results of lesions of the pelvic organs or stretching and relaxations of the ligaments that support the uterus. These displacements may be congenital or acquired, resulting from the trauma of childbirth. Occasionally pelvic infection, endometriosis, and uterine and ovarian tumors may cause retrodisplacements.

Signs and symptoms. The most common complaint is backache providing backache is not postural or genitourinary in origin. Excessive bleeding during menstruation may be due to retrodisplacement. To prove this as the cause, a pessary is inserted. If abnormal bleeding is relieved and recurs after removal of the pessary, retrodisplacement is definitely the cause.

A mild sense of pressure or fullness may be the result of pelvic venous congestion. Sterility is rarely caused by retrodisplacements. However, depending upon the degree of displacement conception may be delayed.

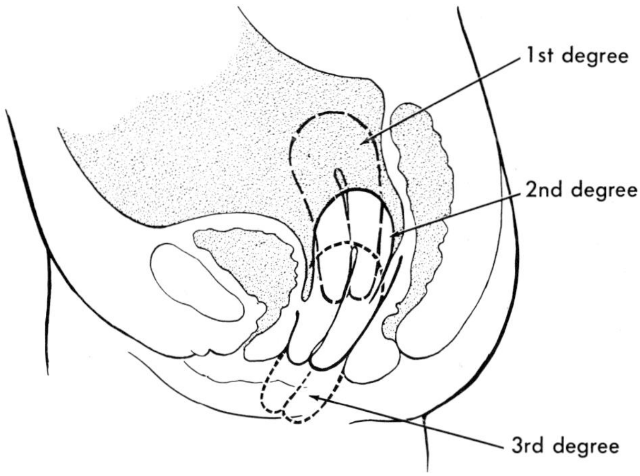

Fig. 26-6. Prolapse of the uterus.

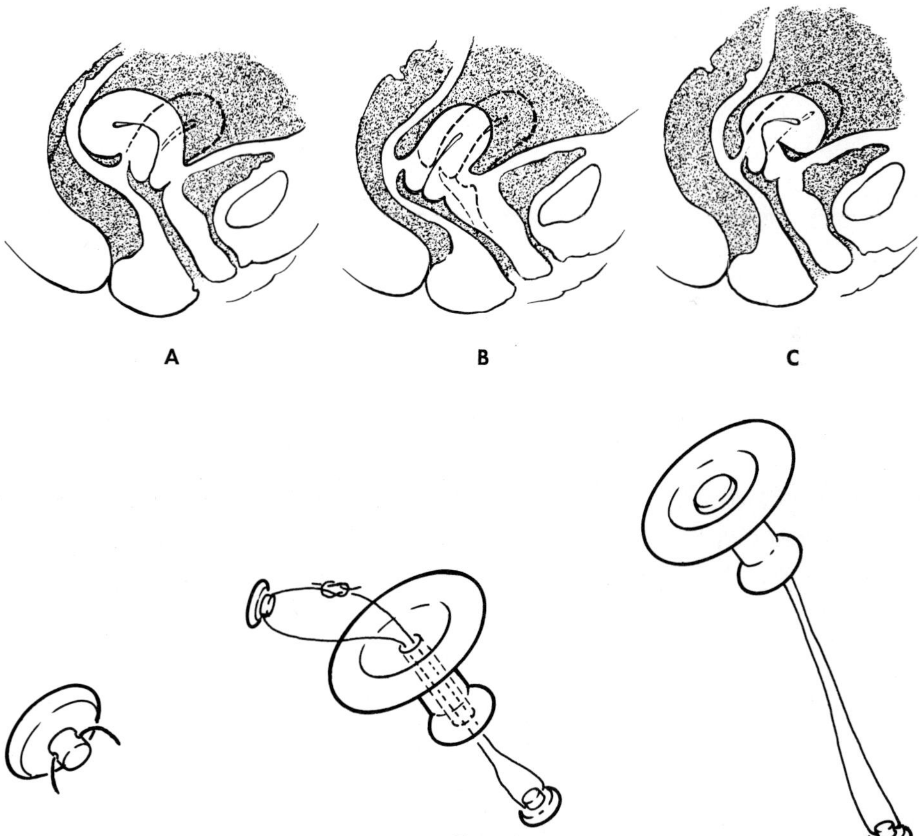

Fig. 26-7. Retrodisplacement of the uterus. **A,** Anterior. **B,** Upright. **C,** Retrodisplacement. **D,** Gellhorn pessary.

Diagnosis. The diagnosis of a retrodisplaced uterus is made by vaginal, rectal, or rectovaginal examination. If the uterus is softer and larger, a pregnancy may be suspected.

Treatment. Inserting a Smith-Hodge pessary for 1 month may be all that is needed to relieve symptoms. Only symptoms that are severe warrant surgical intervention. Often with severe symptoms, repeated abortion directly related to the retrodisplacement, or severe dysmenorrhea, a Baldy-Webster operation is done. This operation is done by plication of the uterosacral ligaments and advancement of the cervicovesical peritoneum.

RUPTURE OF THE UTERUS

Rupture of the uterus occurs after the period of viability of the fetus. Ruptures due to trauma, such as perforations in attempted abortion or rupture of interstitial pregnancies, are not included.

Causes. Rupture of the uterine wall is a serious injury of childbirth occurring more often during labor than during pregnancy. Ruptures may be etiologically classified into the following: (1) rupture of a previous uterine scar, (2) spontaneous rupture of an intact uterus, and (3) traumatic rupture of an intact uterus.

A previous cesarean section scar is the most common cause. Classical scars in the upper portion of the uterus are dangerous since rupture expels the baby and the placenta into the peritoneal cavity. Scars of the lower uterine segment are less dangerous since the bladder lies anterior to the uterus, preventing the expulsion of the baby into the abdomen and separation of the placenta.

Disproportion between the presenting part and the pelvis with ongoing contractions and retractions of the uterus is a common cause of spontaneous rupture. During induction, uterine sensitivity to oxytocics followed by tetanic contractions is dangerous with uterine overdistention or abnormal positions. Spontaneous rupture of the uterus is likely to occur in women of great parity; therefore oxytocics are given judiciously with this in mind.

Traumatic rupture of an intact uterus is quite uncommon but may occur in the latter part of pregnancy. A blow or fall on the abdomen or an automobile accident can result in uterine rupture. An attempt at version with extraction and injudicious use of strong fundal pressure to hasten delivery are other causes.

Prevention. Preventive measures include (1) a practice of repeating cesarean section with cephalopelvic disproportion before labor commences, (2) determining the cause of prolonged labors, (3) adequate anesthesia for effective relaxation during operative deliveries, and (4) the cautious use of oxytocic preparations for labor induction.

With previous cesarean sections for purposes other than malpresentation or cephalopelvic disproportion, a trial of labor is indicated. Should no progress be made within a designated time with occurrence of effectual labor contractions, cesarean section is repeated.

Nursing care. Immediate shock is the sequela to rupture of the uterus. Nursing care is the same as with bleeding. Emergency surgery is performed to control bleeding and prevent further shock. Whether partial or complete removal of the uterus or repair is done depends upon the degree of rupture.

SELECTED REFERENCES

Bonanno, R. J., Landers, D. E., and Rock, D. E.: Bladder drainage with suprapubic catheter needle, Obstet. Gynec., vol. 35, no. 5, May, 1970.

Bourne, A. W.: Recent advances in obstetrics and gynecology, New York, 1963, McGraw-Hill Book Co.

Brewer, J. I., and De Costa, E. J.: Textbook of gynecology, Baltimore, 1967, The Williams & Wilkins Co.

Eastman, N. J., and Hellman, L. M.: Williams obstetrics, ed. 13, New York, 1966, Appleton-Century & Appleton-Century-Crofts.

Kariher, D. H., et al.: Use of suction with suprapubic bladder drainage, Obstet. Gynec., vol. 35, no. 3, March, 1970.

Novak, E. R., and Seegar Jones, G.: Novak's textbook of gynecology, ed. 7, Baltimore, 1965, The Williams & Wilkins Co.

Robertson, J. R.: Air cystoscopy, Obstet. Gynec., vol. 32, no. 3, September, 1968.

Williams, G. A.: Gellhorn pessary modified to facilitate removal, Obstet. Gynec., vol. 33, no. 6, June, 1969.

Questions for study

1. Define episiotomy.
2. What nursing measures alleviate discomforts following episiotomy repair?
3. Define rectocele and cystocele.
4. What are the essential nursing needs following vaginoplasty?
5. Describe retrodisplacement of the uterus and its effect on the menstrual cycle and reproduction.

CHAPTER 27

ABNORMAL UTERINE AND VAGINAL BLEEDING

Bleeding before the menarche and after the menopause is especially significant since bleeding from the uterus does not normally occur during these phases of life. During the adolescent and mature ages, abnormal uterine bleeding is a frequent symptom. In the former, it is frequently dysfunctional (endocrine) in nature; in the latter, with advancing years it is often a result of pathologic lesions.

The bleeding may be excessive or prolonged menstrual flow *(menorrhagia, hypermenorrhea, or polymenorrhea),* bleeding between menstrual periods *(metrorrhagia),* or a combination of these two types *(menometrorrhagia).* Metrorrhagia may be profuse or solely spotting. *Gushing* bleeding is a term to indicate that blood spurts forth in a large quantity from the uterine cavity. It usually suggests an intrauterine lesion, as in complications of pregnancy, fibroids, cancer, and, on occasion, dysfunctional bleeding.

Abnormal uterine bleeding is a common symptom in women with palpable pelvic tumors. Although the two occur together, bleeding may not be the result of the tumor but a result of another pathologic lesion that may go unnoticed. For example, a small cervical polyp may appear to be the cause of bleeding, but endometrial biopsy may reveal carcinoma of the uterus. Therefore, any abnormal uterine bleeding is carefully and promptly investigated and demands immediate attention.

Since bleeding during the maternity cycle has been discussed in Chapter 19, it will not be considered here.

Abnormal uterine bleeding may be classified into two major etiologic types: *dysfunctional,* due to ovarian dysfunction and anovulation, and *anatomic,* a lesion in some part of the reproductive system.

DYSFUNCTIONAL UTERINE BLEEDING

Dysfunctional uterine bleeding is most often caused by abnormal function of the endocrine glands. It is more common in adolescent girls or in preeclamptic women, but it may occur throughout menstrual life.

The two principal causative factors are an endocrine dysfunction and the inability of the endometrium to respond in the usual manner. Often failure to ovulate, irregular shedding with prolonged menstrual flow or prolonged and irregular regression, and involution and sloughing of the endometrium are present. A so-called "mixed endometrium" exists in which the entire endometrium does not respond to ovarian hormonal stimulation, and a portion of the endometrium may be in the progestational phase while other portions are in the estrogenic phase. Bleeding, therefore, may occur from atrophic changes as well as from hyperplasia of the endometrium.

During adolescence

Excessive bleeding during adolescence is caused by abnormal endocrine activity. The ovarian cycle involves the seven basic structures: higher centers, endometrium, adrenal glands, thyroid gland, hypothalamus, hypophysis, and ovaries and at least seven different hormones: follicle-stimulating, luteinizing, luteotrophic, estrogen, progesterone, thyroid, and adrenal hormones. Often the actual quantitative change in hormones is minute, and yet dysfunctional bleeding occurs.

Dysfunctional bleeding is frequently associated with failure to ovulate. Not all adolescent bleeding is dysfunctional. Organic lesions such as pregnancy, estrogen-producing tumors, infections, or sarcoma and carcinoma are always ruled out. When necessary, examination under anesthesia or rectal palpation may suffice. When pelvic examination is done under anesthesia, curettage and cervical biopsies are performed at the same time.

Medical examination includes history, physical and pelvic examination, complete blood study, and evaluation of thyroid function (basal metabolic rate and protein-bound iodine uptake).

Treatment. The objectives of treatment are (1) to control bleeding, (2) to reestablish normal ovulatory menstrual cycles, (3) to maintain the cycle, (4) to preserve fertility, and (5) to correct abnormal conditions associated with or caused by the bleeding, such as anemia, vitamin deficiency, dysfunction of the thyroid, or emotional disturbances.

Often diagnosis of dysfunctional bleeding can be established only by curettage, which is sometimes curative as well as diagnostic. Curettage is believed to cure through the following mechanisms: scraping the uterus affects the hypothalamus—pituitary axis, correcting the abnormal cycle; growth of the endometrium following curettage alters estrogen-progesterone balance.

With endocrine therapy in which androgens are used, hirsutism or voice changes occur.

During childbearing years

Abnormal uterine bleeding is common in women 18 to 45 years of age. A thorough history is taken, and complete physical examination and cervical smears are done. It is often necessary to perform a cervical biopsy, and curettage is best done just prior to the expected onset of menstruation. Occasionally colpotomy or culdoscopy (page 362) is done for visualization of the ovaries.

Treatment. Treatment depends upon the severity of symptoms, the age of the woman, family size, and the desire for additional pregnancies. It is always necessary to exclude organic causes prior to treatment.

For women desiring more children, conservative treatment of a transfusion with severe bleeding is followed by curettage. Anemia and iron deficiency are treated by giving iron compounds along with estrogens, progestogens, and androgens, or various combinations of these that may effectively control the dysfunctional bleeding.

Should conservative efforts fail, hysterectomy is performed. Continued persistent dysfunctional bleeding is associated with a relatively high incidence of adenomatosis, hyperplasia, and cancer of the uterus.

At the climacteric

The climacteric begins around 45 years of age and ends 1 year after the last menstrual period. However, the actual menopause occurs around 50 years of age, but some women menstruate as late as their mid-fifties.

Benign organic lesions such as polyps, endometriosis, and myomas may cause or be associated with bleeding. Diagnostic curettage is essential and often curative. If bleeding recurs, hysterectomy is performed. Endocrine therapy to control bleeding is not recommended.

ANATOMIC ABNORMAL UTERINE BLEEDING

Anatomic factors associated with abnormal uterine bleeding are lesions and growths of the uterus, tubes, and ovaries.

Cervical erosions

Erosions of the cervix are characterized by replacement of the normal squamous epithelium with columnar epithelium (Fig. 27-1, *A*). They are common when the normal acidity of the vaginal canal becomes altered. With erosions, the tissue is quite vascular, and a common symptom is an increased mucous discharge and bleeding of the tissue to touch. With bleeding, a biopsy is indicated to rule out carcinoma.

When malignancy is not suspected or reported, the cervix is cauterized to promote healing. Cauterization destroys the eroded tissue, which results in sloughing and healing by granulation. Vinegar douches are then ordered to improve the vaginal pH, remove the sloughed tissue, and prevent infection.

Cervical polyps

Polyps are small growths of the cervical mucosa usually located at the external os (Fig. 27-1, *B*). At times polyps do not cause bleeding and are found accidentally.

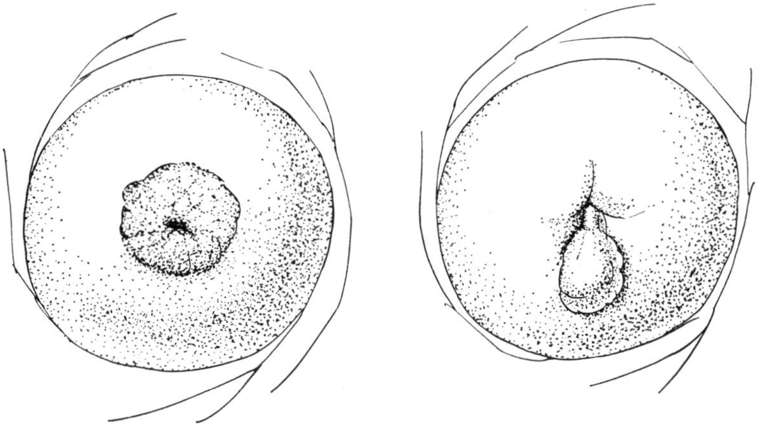

Fig. 27-1. A, Cervical erosion. **B,** Cervical polyp.

Usual symptoms are slight intermenstrual bleeding and bleeding provoked by muscular exertion such as with defecation and especially by coitus. These are the same symptoms suggestive of cervical carcinoma, and malignancy should always be ruled out.

The treatment for cervical polyps is hospitalization and surgical removal. At the same time a diagnostic dilatation and curettage of the uterus is done to rule out malignancy. Follow-up gynecologic examination is routine every 6 months during the premenopause and menopause.

Endometrial polyps

Endometrial polyps often are less likely to cause bleeding since they are hidden in the uterus. Many small polyps are found only accidentally at the time of curettage or when hysterectomy is performed for other reasons. Occasionally the larger polyps are attached to a pedicle, and these may be visible, protrude into the vaginal canal, and cause bleeding.

Condylomata acuminata

Condylomata acuminata are benign, wartlike growths that may involve the vulva, vagina, and cervix. Leukorrhea is the prominent symptom, and bleeding results from trauma and ulceration of the lesions. Treatment consists of cautery with an application of 25% podophyllum resin to the lesions or removal with an electrocautery. During pregnancy podophyllum resin is contraindicated. It is predominantly toxic and is highly laxative in nature. Its absorption into the maternal circulation may affect the vessels of the decidua basalis, with resulting vasospasm and embarrassment of fetal circulation and oxygenation. Abortion, premature labor, and intrauterine deaths have been reported. Studies also show that almost all patients with vulvar carcinoma following condyloma had had podophyllum resin therapy. The best treatment is electrodesiccation and curettage, which control lesions promptly with little pain or scarring.

Uterine myomas

A myoma is a neoplasm (growth) that originates in the muscle tissue of the uterus. Myomas are often referred to as "fibroid," "fibromyoma," and "fibroleiomyoma." They are usually multiple. Their sizes vary during the childbearing years, they seldom grow following the cessation of menstruation, and they do not occur after the menopause. It is assumed that estrogen stimulation is an important etiologic factor. Long-term therapy with progestogens stimulates the growth of myomas. During pregnancy myomas often enlarge since there is a markedly enhanced blood supply, increased cell growth, and an increase in estrogen levels. Growth in myomas is relatively slow in a nonpregnant woman. It is increased in a pregnant woman and decreases after the menopause. In the absence of pregnancy or following the menopause, enlargement of the tumor suggests degenerative change or sarcoma (malignancy).

The location of the myoma within the uterine wall designates the type of myoma. A *submucous* myoma is one found immediately beneath the endometrium, and it may protrude into the abdominal cavity. When the tumor is located within the muscular wall of the uterus, it is *intramural.* A tumor on the outer peritoneal covering and protruding into the abdominal cavity is known as a *subserous* myoma. A *pedunculated* myoma is one projecting into the abdominal cavity, connected to the uterus by a pedicle, or attached by a pedicle within the uterine cavity. This is designated as a *fibroid polyp* (Fig. 27-2). Occasionally a myoma develops in the wall of the cervix and is called a *cervical myoma.* A tumor projecting laterally from the uterus between the sheaths of the broad ligaments is of the *intraligamentous* type. The intraligamentous and the pedunculated myomas may twist and become completely detached, adhering to adjacent abdominal tissue and becoming *parasitic myomas.*

Signs and symptoms. Most myomas are asymptomatic and are detected only on routine pelvic examination. Some myomas produce symptoms, usually during the fifth decade of life and less often in the 30-year-old to 40-year-old woman.

Bleeding, either menorrhagia (increase in both amount and duration of menstrual flow) or metrorrhagia (frequent periods of bleeding) may occur. Spotting, continuous flow, or hemorrhage is common with the submucous or polypoid type of tumor. The occurrence and amount of bleeding are not related to the size and number of tumors.

Abnormal bleeding is usually a result of one of the following: (1) necrosis and sloughing of the endometrium overlying the surface of a submucous or polypoid myoma; (2) disturbed endocrine function such as failure to ovulate with excessive or prolonged estrogen stimulation of the endometrium or irregular regression of the corpus luteum with irregular shedding of the endometrium; (3) marked in-

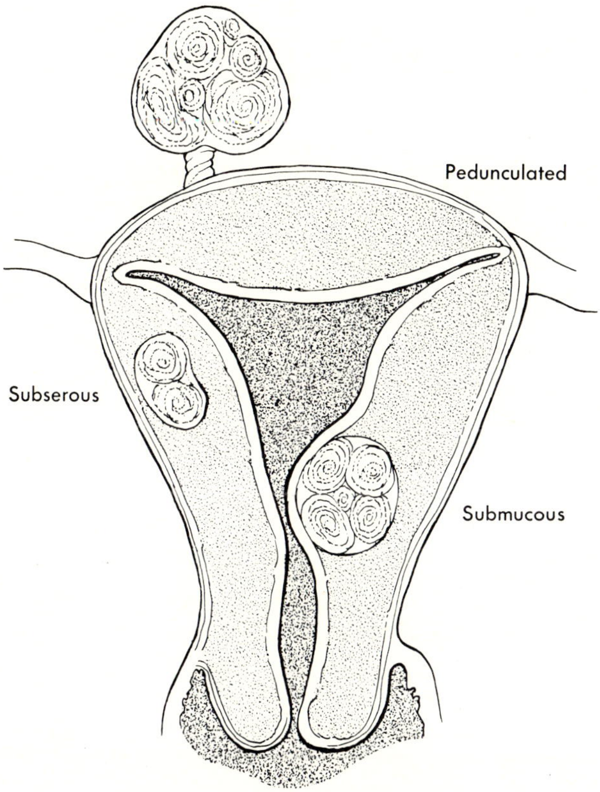

Fig. 27-2. Fibroid polyps of the uterus.

crease in the endometrium surface as it becomes stretched and thin with growth of the myoma; (4) mechanical interference with blood supply to the muscles of the uterus; or (5) inability of the endometrium to respond to ovarian stimulation. Bleeding during the menopause rarely occurs with myomas; therefore, malignancies should always be suspected and ruled out.

Although tumors are large, the woman experiences only mild *pressure* symptoms. Urinary symptoms (frequency and dysuria) are more common if the myoma is causing pressure on the bladder or ureter, such as occurs with the intraligamentous type of myoma. Rectal pain is rarely caused by myoma. More often it is a result of pelvic inflammatory disease or endometriosis.

Pain is rarely a symptom of uncomplicated myoma. When pain occurs it is usually a result of (1) torsion of the pedicle of the pedunculated type, (2) an attempt on the part of the uterus to deliver a fibroid polyp through the cervix, (3) degenerative changes in the tumor or adhesions resulting from these changes, and (4) complications such as appendicitis, endometriosis, urinary tract infections, or pregnancy.

Disturbances related to childbearing are more often those of mechanical interference with delivery of the baby rather than the ability of women to become pregnant. Tumors located in the lower portion of the uterus, close to the cervix, are prone to interfere with delivery. Myomas within the uterine musculature may interfere with efficiency of contractions, cause faulty separation and expulsion of the placenta, and prevent effective uterine contractions postpartally, thus causing hemorrhage.

Tumors may distort the uterus, causing malpositions of the fetus and interfering with implantation of a fertilized ovum. However, although some tumors are multiple and large, they often do not interfere with the maintenance and completion of a pregnancy.

Treatment. Treatment for uterine myomas depends upon the presence and severity of symptoms, the future risk to the woman, and the development of coexisting lesions that require treatment.

Conservative treatment requires a pelvic examination every 6 months for women who are asymptomatic and every 3 months for women who have mild symptoms. A cervical smear for cancer is done yearly or more often when indicated. When bleeding occurs, blood counts are done to detect anemia. When there is mild anemia, iron therapy is indicated. Blood transfusions are given if severe anemia occurs. Cervical biopsy or conization and curettage may be required. At times curettage is done not as a treatment but rather as a means to control bleeding. In very young women large doses of estrogen are administered to control bleeding. In women 50 years of age or older, surgical intervention is indicated only when symptoms are severe or when degenerative changes occur in the myoma.

When conservative treatment cannot be used, operative procedures include myomectomy or hysterectomy. Myomectomy, in which only the growths are removed, is indicated in young women who still desire to have children. Growths such as myomas that are of the fibroid polyp type and myomas associated with endometriosis are removed in this way. Hysterectomy is the procedure of choice when salvaging the uterus is not essential for reproductive function and when there is no surgical risk. In premenopausal women, the ovaries are conserved when lesions are found. In older women, complete hysterectomy is done. Vaginal route hysterectomies are done only if coexisting extensive endometriosis, pelvic inflammatory diseases or malignancies are present.

Radiation therapy is reserved only for the relatively few women in whom there may be surgical risk.

When myomas are diagnosed during pregnancy, treatment is extremely conservative, and operative procedures are avoided if possible. The pregnancy receives primary consideration; the myoma is secondary. If the tumor impedes delivery, cesarean section is performed. With cesarean section, the myoma is not removed unless the growth is pedunculated or in the line of incision. Myomas may so distort the uterine cavity that malposition interferes with implantation or early abortion follows. Further study should be done since infertility may be related to a functional cause. Studies indicate that an increase in the number of pregnancies occurs following myomectomy. Infertility is not due solely to myomas; however, there may be a relationship.

In the second trimester an asymptomatic myoma may cause pain, tenderness, fever, and leukocytosis and may reveal a surgically acute abdomen. This usually occurs since there is impaired or inadequate circulation in the myoma. If conservative treatment fails, surgical exploration and myomectomy are done.

In the last trimester of pregnancy and at delivery, myomas can cause premature bleeding, uterine inertia, or mechanical blocking of the birth canal. Postpartum hemorrhage and infection are common following atony of the uterus. With multiple myomas, cesarean section with hysterectomy is often indicated. Myomas of the lower uterine segment and cervix that impede the birth canal warrant cesarean section.

Malignant growths

The frequent sites of cancer in the female reproductive tract in order of occurrence are the breast, cervix, uterus, ovary, and vulva. The professional nurse is responsible for inclusion of preventive measures as an integral part of health teaching of all women. The early childbearing years bring women in close contact with the members of the health team, and self-examination of the breasts and a yearly health examination, including a cervical smear, are essential for women over 30 years of age.

In the United States, the rate of cancer in women is 245 per 100,000 population yearly.

Cancer of the cervix

Next to cancer of the breast, cancer of the cervix is the most common malignancy found in women. The incidence is highest in women 45 to 55 years of age, but the disease may occur in the early twenties as well as after the menopause.

Etiology. Although the etiology is unknown, there are several factors associated with cancer of the cervix. There are also factors that predispose to cancer of the cervix, and they must be identified and treated as a preventive measure.

There is a correlation between parity and cancer of the cervix, and the incidence is higher among those who have early and frequent sexual activity. However, statistics reveal that nulliparous women and virgins are also subject to cancer of the cervix. Jewish and Moslem women are relatively free of the disease, and the incidence is higher in Negroes and Puerto Ricans. It is speculated that circumcision in men and modes of hygiene are factors to be considered.

Untreated cervical infections and postpartum lacerations are precursors to carcinoma. Therefore, the prompt treatment of any cervical lesion is a preventive measure. There is some evidence that heredity may be a predisposing factor.

Invasive cancer of the cervix does not develop suddenly. However, the symptoms do not occur until the lesion is in an advanced stage and its curability is uncertain. Invasive cervical cancer is preventable if the growth is stopped at the in situ stage.

Pathology. The cell structure of the cervix has primarily two types of tissue cells. That portion of the cervix that extends into the vaginal canal, known as the external os, is covered with stratified squamous epithelium continuous with that of the vagina, while the internal os is lined with columnar epithelium. The point at which these tissues meet, known as the squamocolumnar junction, is the most common site of cancer cell growth. The majority of cancer cells originate in the squamous epithelium, while a few originate in the columnar epithelium.

In its earliest form the cancer may not be grossly apparent but rather may be a bleeding area of cervical erosion. With growth and progression, the lesion becomes *exophytic* (a cauliflower-like growth), *endophytic* (ulcerative lesion), diffuse (infiltrative type), or *polypoid* (growth from the endocervix).

The most common direct cause of death as the malignancy spreads is urinary tract invasion and obstruction. Urinary stasis, infection, and obstruction eventually lead to uremia and death. In other cases pulmonary metastases with pulmonary edema, pneumonia, or embolism may occur. Occasionally gastrointestinal tract invasion, obstruction, perforation, and peritonitis are sequelae.

Classification. The following classification proposed in New York City in 1951 by the International Federation of Gynecology and Obstetrics is being widely used:

Stage O	Carcinoma in situ, also known as preinvasive carcinoma, intraepithelial carcinoma, and similar conditions.
Stage I	The carcinoma is strictly confined to the cervix.
Stage Ia	Cases of early stromal invasion.
Stage Ib	All other cases of Stage I.
Stage II	The carcinoma extends beyond the cervix, but has not reached the pelvic wall; the carcinoma involves the vagina, but not the lower third.
Stage IIa	No parametrial involvement.
Stage IIb	Parametrial involvement.
Stage III	The carcinoma has reached the pelvic wall (on rectal examination no "cancer-free" space is found between the pelvic wall); the carcinoma involves the lower third of the vagina.
Stage IV	The carcinoma involves the bladder or the rectum or both, or has extended beyond the limits previously described.

This classification clinically estimates the extent of involvement and does not change once therapy is initiated.

Signs and symptoms. There are usually no signs and symptoms in early cancer of the cervix. As the disease progresses, the most common symptom is *bleeding.* This may occur intermenstrually or postcoitally, and occasionally there may be excessive bleeding at the time of the menstrual period.

At times a serosanguineous malodorous discharge is noted, suggesting a cancerous growth. Pain is a rather late symptom and suggests infiltration as the nerves and bones become involved. Later symptoms are similar to those of most malignancies. These include loss of appetite and loss of weight, resulting in cachexia.

Prevention. Cancer of the cervix could be eliminated by mass screening, which potentiates early diagnosis. Health teaching by the nurse of all women in the child-bearing years as to the importance of the Papanicolaou smear is imperative. Routine postpartum examination, Papanicolaou smear during pregnancy, and prompt treatment of any cervical lesion assure early detection.

The wide use of "the pill" in our society by young people has brought Papanicolaou smears into wider use. It is often during this routine examination that early lesions are detected. Much of the health teaching by the nurse in family planning clinics can be focused on preventive gynecology.

Fewer women between 30 and 40 years of age attend an obstetric or gynecologic clinic than in other age groups. It is during this time that premalignant lesions are advancing toward the invasive stage. Therefore, premalignant lesions are usually found among the obstetric population since these women are checked frequently during pregnancy.

Diagnosis. Any history of vaginal discharge or bleeding warrants pelvic examination and visualization of the cervix. All lesions of the cervix should be categorized as "suspicious."

The methods for early detection of cervical cancer are cytologic study by Papanicolaou smear, the Schiller test, biopsy, and conization.

For *cytologic study by Papanicolaou smear,* Papanicolaou's classification of vaginal smears is followed:

Class 1 Smear containing only normal cells.
Class 2 Smear containing cells having some atypical features, such as vacuolization, cytoplasmic granules, double nuclei, and nuclear enlargement, but none suggestive of a malignant cell.
Class 3 Smear containing cells having features suggestive but not diagnostic of malignant cells.
Class 4 Smear containing malignant cells.
Class 5 Smear containing malignant cells more bizarre than Class 4.

The *Schiller test* is a simple test done by applying iodine solution (Lugol's solution) to the cervix. Since cancerous epithelium does not contain glycogen, the area remains unstained. Normal epithelium, rich in glycogen, reveals a deep brown mahogany color reaction. At times inflammatory processes may produce a positive Schiller test, necessitating follow-up with biopsy and smear.

Cervical *biopsy* may be done as an office procedure when a suspicious lesion exists. Since the Schiller test outlines suspicious areas, it is usually done prior to biopsy so that these areas may be studied. The newest technique makes use of a cervical punch biopsy with forceps that provide tissue from the entire cervical circumference.

Conization is best done in the operating room using a knife rather than an electrocautery. Cone-shaped specimens of the cervix are excised to remove the entire lesion therapeutically or to determine the amount of cervical involvement. Often Gelfoam or Oxycel is placed against the coned area, and a vaginal packing is inserted for 24 hours to control bleeding. If bleeding persists beyond 7 days, ligation may be needed.

Treatment for carcinoma in situ. The treatment for carcinoma in situ depends upon the age of the woman and her desire to bear more children. In the very young woman anticipating more children, conization of the cervix may be the only treatment, realizing that the remaining cervix is a potential hazard. Conservative treatment warrants cervical smears and biopsies every 6 months.

Treatment for invasive carcinoma. The treatment for invasive carcinoma of the cervix is total removal of the diseased area, including its lymphatic system, and the immediate adjacent uninvolved tissue. This may be accomplished by a combination of external and internal irradiation or by radical surgery. The choice of treatment depends upon the extent of the disease, the facilities available, and the abilities of the surgeon.

For Stages I and II carcinoma of the cervix, hysterectomy and lymphadenectomy are done. Often irradiation of the lymph nodes is the method of choice postoperatively. In the more advanced Stages II and III, radical surgery necessitates removal of all pelvic structures, including the rectum and the bladder. This is known as pelvic exenteration. A wet colostomy in which the ureters empty into the bowel completes the surgery. This radical operation is done only with careful explanation to the patient regarding the risk and the 5-year survival rate.

Radiation therapy is a method of treatment at any stage of the disease. It is commonly used for the very obese, the elderly, or those of poor medical risk. Although irradiation complications can occur, there is a lower morbidity and mortality rate than that associated with radical surgery.

Management of terminal carcinoma. With women in this advanced stage, palliative treatment includes irradiation for pain relief or hemostasis, the use of sedatives and narcotics for pain, and the blocking of sensory pathways by anterolateral cordotomy or intrathecal injections of alcohol.

Radiation therapy for cancer of the cervix is done by first giving external irradiation. Total dosage depends upon the woman's size and the extent of the neoplasm and whether or not a radium applicator can be inserted into the cervix. If internal treatment cannot be given, external treatment is intensified. Internal treatment necessitates the insertion of a tandem into the uterine cavity for a period of 100 hours. At this time the vagina is measured for the second internal application. This consists of inserting two rubber Manchester ovoids containing radium for approximately another 100 hours.

Some of the factors that may limit radiotherapy are (1) previous radiotherapy with persistent or recurring lesions, (2) pelvic sepsis, (3) vaginal stenosis or severe uterine prolapse, and (4) a very young or pregnant woman.

Pregnancy complicated by cancer of the cervix. Approximately 1% of carcinomas of the cervix (or 1 in each 2,000 or 3,000 pregnancies) occur in pregnant women. Since most women seek medical supervision during pregnancy, cancer of the cervix may be detected and treated early because cytology study is a part of the prenatal visit.

Cancer of the cervix is difficult to diagnose during pregnancy. Delay in diagnosis is a result of attributing atypical bleeding to obstetric complications such as placenta previa, abruptio placentae, or a friable cervical erosion. Physicians are reluctant to perform vaginal examinations in first and second trimester bleeding, yet the cervix could be exposed carefully for cytology study or biopsy without endangering the pregnancy. If the malignancy remains untreated, successful treatment is diminished by 15% with each month's delay. Whether the woman is pregnant or not, the longer the cancer is present without being diagnosed, the poorer the prognosis.

Treatment of cancer of the cervix that is diagnosed during pregnancy depends upon the stage of the lesions and the weeks of gestation. During the first and second trimesters, radiation therapy is begun and the pregnancy is ignored. Abortion usually follows. If the uterus does not empty itself, the fetus is removed by total hysterectomy 2 to 4 weeks following irradiation. If cervical carcinoma is found in the last trimester, elective cesarean section is done to deliver a viable fetus. A classical incision is preferred to avoid the risk of cutting into the malignant cervical tissues. Following elective cesarean section, radiation therapy is instituted.

The religious doctrines of parents may stipulate that the life of the fetus must not be interrupted or endangered. However, no church (including the Roman Catholic Church) considers it sinful to treat cancer by irradiation or surgery even though treatment results in the death of the baby—the *primary* purpose of treatment is to cure the cancer and not to kill the fetus.

Cancer of the uterus

Cancer of the uterus occurs more often in postmenopausal women. There is a higher incidence of cancer of the uterus in obese, diabetic, hypertensive, and nulliparous women. Histories of women indicate that menstrual disturbances are common with this disease.

Etiology. The etiology of carcinoma of the endometrium is obscure, but there are speculations. Women who have received estrogen therapy have been known to develop a hyperplasia of the endometrium. Estrogen stimulation of the endometrium is favored as being a predisposing etiologic element in cancer of the uterus. Women who are obese, diabetic, hypertensive, nulliparous and have postmenopausal bleeding should always be screened carefully.

Classification. The following classification is recommended by the International Federation of Gynecology and Obstetrics:

Stage O	Histologic finding suspicious of malignancy but not proved.
Stage I	The carcinoma is confined to the corpus.
Stage II	The carcinoma has involved the corpus and the cervix.
Stage III	The carcinoma has extended outside the uterus but not outside the pelvis.
Stage IV	The carcinoma has extended outside the true pelvis or has obviously involved the mucosa of the bladder or rectum.

Signs and symptoms. Abnormal uterine bleeding is the complaint of 95% of women who have cancer of the uterus. Most of these women are postmenopausal and may experience intermenstrual bleeding, hypermenorrhea, and polymenorrhea. With postmenopausal bleeding or any recurrent bleeding 1 year following the last definite menstrual period, immediate investigation is warranted. Leukorrhea that is blood-stained on pelvic examination or bleeding with pain connotes invasion of the uterine wall and metastasis.

Diagnosis. Any vaginal bleeding following the menopause should arouse suspicions of cancer of the endometrium. Complete history and physical examination, including pelvic examination, are mandatory. The tests discussed in the following paragraphs are done as a diagnostic measure.

The Clark test is done as an office procedure. Under aseptic precautions, the endometrial cavity is probed with a uterine sound or narrow probe. A substantial amount of bright red bleeding suggests endometrial carcinoma and a positive Clark test.

A Papanicolaou smear of the posterior fornix and external os is done for cytologic study. A negative Papanicolaou smear does not, however, rule out cancer of the endometrium. Papanicolaou smears are more accurate for cancer of the cervix.

Suction biopsy may be done as an office procedure. Endometrial tissue is obtained from various areas within the uterus for cytologic examination.

Dilatation and curettage is done under aseptic technique in the operating room. Tissue from various areas of the uterus is obtained for microscopic examination.

Pelvic lymphography permits direct radiographic visualization of the lymphatic channels and lymph nodes of the parailiac and caudal para-aortic areas. It is a technique used as a preliminary to operation for lymphatic metastasis in women with invasive carcinoma of the cervix, uterine fundus, vagina, and vulva. It evaluates the extent of the spread. Prior to lymphography, 0.5 ml. of an equal part mixture of sky blue dye and 1% procaine hydrochloride is injected intradermally between the first and second toes. Three hours later, pentobarbital hydrochloride, 100 mg., is given orally, and a skin preparation with hexachlorophene is used. Following a nerve block with 1% procaine hydrochloride over the visible blue-streaked lymphatics, an incision is made, and the stained lymphatics are dissected. The lymphatic vessel is cannulated with a 27-gauge or 29-gauge needle, and a No. 10 or No. 20 polyethylene catheter is attached by two chromic catgut sutures. A 5 ml. syringe is used to inject into both legs a solution of 1% procaine hydrochloride with a test dose of Hypaque. The patient may experience temporary pain migrating from the site of the injection to the groin. X-ray films are taken of the thighs, pelvis, abdomen, and chest.

Treatment. The method of choice in treatment is individually evaluated, and consideration is given to the health of the woman. For early lesions total hysterectomy and bilateral salpingo-oophorectomy with a generous excision of the vaginal cuff are the treatment of choice. Some surgeons close the cervix and ligate the fallopian tubes prior to removal of the uterus to prevent possible spillage of the tumor cells.

If the lesion is not confined to the uterus, radiation therapy may be followed by surgery, or in advanced stages external irradiation and intrauterine radium insertion are done. Preoperative external irradiation has been found advantageous because the cells are devitalized, preventing spillage and spread, and irradiation decreases the size of the tumor, facilitating surgery. Since some women are surgical risks because of age, radiation therapy alone would be the chosen treatment.

Chemotherapy for advanced neoplasms is now being used as a palliative measure. Synthetic progestins such as Delalutin, 2,500 mg., are given weekly for 3 months and have been found to arrest secondary infections, control bleeding, and inhibit metastases. The major benefit is palliative, resulting in relief of pain and discomfort, elimination of ascites and edema fluid, an increased feeling of well-being, and a limited prolongation of life. Occasionally there is a dramatic response exhibited in the regression and disappearance of the tumor.

Tumors of the ovary

There are numerous types of tumors of the ovary because the ovary is an organ in which potentiality for growth of neoplastic tissue is particularly great. Ovarian tumors are usually classified according to their source of origin or tissue types; however, there is no uniform classification. Only the most commonly found will be discussed in this text.

Symptoms. Most ovarian tumors are asymptomatic, whether benign or malignant. Malignant growths may enlarge and produce signs and symptoms. Tumors of a benign nature may undergo malignant change without warning.

Abnormal uterine bleeding may occur with ovarian tumors but is not caused by the tumor itself. It is usually a result of an endocrine dysfunction and may be unrelated to the tumor.

Amenorrhea may be associated with certain types such as follicular cysts, masculinizing tumors, and, on occasion, malignant tumors. Sterility is a symptom found when ovulation fails to occur.

Pain is not a common symptom, but when it occurs it is caused by extension of the growth and is a serious symptom. Pain may be caused by rupture of an ovarian cyst, hemorrhage into a cyst with peritonitis and infection, or twisting of a pedicle growth, causing compression of blood vessels.

Pressure on the urinary bladder may cause frequency and urgency. Compression of the ureter commonly results in a hydronephrosis. If the growth is large, compression on the lower extremities and vulva causes edema.

Diagnosis. Bimanual vaginal and rectal examination reveals the presence of a tumor. The location, size, shape, consistency, mobility, and tenderness on palpation may also be determined. After the diagnosis is made, differentiation of a benign tumor from a malignant tumor may be difficult. Usually malignant growths are solid, bilateral, fixed, rapidly growing, irregular, and nodular, with a resulting ascites. If there is suspicion of a malignancy, determining whether the growth is primary or secondary is indicated. The breast, gastrointestinal tract, and endometrium are examined because metastasis to the ovary is common from these sites. Tumors arising prior to puberty or after the climacteric are considered malignant until proved otherwise.

Follicular cysts. Follicular cysts are enlarged graafian follicles, frequently multiple and bilateral. They are located in the ovarian cortex, and the fluid is thin and clear. There are no characteristic symptoms, some women have normal menstrual cycles, some have abnormal bleeding, while others have amenorrhea. Anovulation and sterility may result.

Follicular cysts are treated by monthly bimanual examination since often the enlargement disappears. With excessive bleeding, large doses of estrogens and progestogens are given. If found during surgery for other reasons, they are enucleated when large or left undisturbed when there are no symptoms.

Corpus luteum cysts. A corpus luteum cyst is one in which there is a persistence of the cyclic corpus luteum, and withdrawal of the ovarian hormones is retarded, slow, or irregular. Symptoms include prolonged periods of amenorrhea or abnormal uterine bleeding. Serious hemorrhage into or from the cyst may cause pain and necessitate surgery. The pain may need to be distinguished from that caused by ectopic pregnancy. With surgical intervention the cyst is removed, and the ovary is left intact.

Bilateral polycystic ovaries. Polycystic ovaries result from an endocrine disturbance in which there are small multiple follicular cysts, absence of a corpus luteum, anovulation, and ovarian enlargement. Treatment is curative with surgical wedge resection of the ovary. At times, human gonadotropins or clomiphene citrate (Clomid) is the method of choice in treatment.

Endometrial cysts. Endometrial cysts of the ovaries are unilateral or bilateral and are insidious growths characterized by dense adhesions. Although many women have no symptoms, excessive or frequent uterine bleeding, pelvic pain, sterility, dyspareunia, and dysmenorrhea may occur. The cyst contains old blood and is often called a "chocolate cyst."

In women with no history of pelvic infection, endometriosis should be suspected. The severity of symptoms, size of the cyst, and suspicion of malignancy are indications for surgery.

Dermoid cysts. Dermoid cysts of the ovary arise from "rests" of embryonic cells that later become active and produce a tumor containing various kinds of tissue. Since the predominant tissue is skin, the tumor is designated as "dermoid." Dermoid cysts are partly solid and partly cystic. The tissue parts of a dermoid cyst often contain hair, teeth, or bone.

If a dermoid cyst is completely solid with the tissues in a more embryonic stage, the growth is called a "teratoma." If thyroid tissue is found, the cyst is called a strumous teratoma or ovarian struma. Treatment consists of surgical intervention.

Granulosa cell tumors. Granulosa cell tumors of the ovary are nonmalignant solid ovarian tumors. They arise from the embryologic rest of undifferentiated female sex cells. The cells retain their power of development, and their endocrine function causes premature sexual development. The child may grow pubic hair, show breast development, and menstruate very early. If this type of tumor develops in an aged person, menstruation may return. Surgical removal of the tumor is indicated.

Arrhenoblastomas. Arrhenoblastomas are also nonmalignant solid ovarian tumors. They develop from undifferentiated male sex cells in the ovary. Ordinarily the cortex of the ovary in the female contains ova, and the male elements in the medullary portion atrophy and disappear. At times remnants of the male sex cells remain without causing trouble, or they may secrete male hormones. If this happens menstruation ceases, male distribution of body hair appears, the breasts flatten, the voice deepens, and the clitoris enlarges, resembling the male glans. Removal of the tumor inhibits abnormal endocrine influence, and feminine characteristics return.

Fibromas. Ovarian fibromas, another type of solid ovarian tumor, are rare, varying in size from a few grams to 40 kg. They are usually unilateral and always benign. Mechanical irritation of the fibroma causes ascites and an unexplainable hydrothorax commonly known as Meig's syndrome. Treatment consists of unilateral salpingo-oophorectomy and hysterectomy. In older women, bilateral salpingo-oophorectomy and hysterectomy are done.

Brenner tumors are smaller in size, less nodular on palpation, and are often mistaken for fibromas. They are treated conservatively.

Malignant ovarian tumors. Most of the carcinomas of the ovary arise from papillary cystadenomas. They are usually cystic but with rapid growth become solid. Primary cancer of the ovary is insidious and symptomatic. Symptoms such as gastrointestinal disabilities, anemia, loss of weight, and pain develop late in the disease. Visible growth and ascites occur when the disease is well advanced.

Cancer of the ovary is classified as primary if it originated from normal tissue within the gonad or from a preexisting benign tumor of the gland. It is considered secondary if metastasis occurs from a primary site elsewhere. An example is Krukenberg tumor, which results from metastasis from the gastrointestinal tract. Bilateral involvement occurs in 50% of women with cancer of the ovary, with the second ovary becoming affected years later.

Cancer of the ovary is more common in women over 50 years of age. Cystic neoplasms that are hosts to carcinoma are serous and pseudomucinous cystadenomas, papillary cystadenomas, and dermoid and endometrial cysts.

Treatment. The treatment for unilateral or bilateral cancer of the ovary is removal of both ovaries, uterus, fallopian tubes, and omentum. If peritoneal metastasis and extensive lesions are present, external irradiation is begun 2 to 4 weeks following surgery. Radioactive gold suspended in a salt solution and placed within the peritoneal cavity, followed by rotating the patient, has been found to reduce the rate at which ascites redevelops.

Chemotherapeutic agents such as nitrogen mustard, triethylenemelamine (TEM), and triethylenethiophosphoramide (Thio-TEPA) have been used to relieve the ascites and are used in advanced stages. TEM and Thio-TEPA are used as palliative treatment and are worthwhile if toxic effects are not too severe.

Lesions of the vulva

Fibroma, myoma, and lipoma are all benign tumors of the vulva involving various tissues; a fibroma involves connective tissue, a myoma involves muscle or fibrous tissue, and a lipoma involves fatty tissue.

They do not produce symptoms but may interfere with walking, sitting, or intercourse. Excision is the method of treatment.

Carcinoma of the vulva is rare, comprising 3% to 4% of all gynecologic cancers. Of all vulvar cancers, 80% to 90% are of the squamous type. Occasionally they are adenocarcinomas and rarely melanocarcinomas. The malignancy may originate in the skin or mucous membrane of the vulva, in preexisting leukoplakia or kraurosis, or in a pigmented nevus. This is a disease of old age, occurs rarely in women under 40, and the maximum incidence is at the age of 60.

There are no symptoms in early vulvar cancer except a persistent pruritus. Pain is not experienced until the lesion is extensive. There is seldom discharge or bleeding, although there may be an ulcerative lesion.

In squamous carcinoma, which comprises 80% of the cases, 60% involve the labia majora, 20% the labia minora and vestibule, and 12% the area around the clitoris. The growth is usually superficial. Once extension into the vagina occurs, the prognosis is grave because the lymph nodes are involved.

The superficial lesion may appear to be an ordinary wart that is brownish and flat but bleeds with minimal trauma, or the lesion may be hard or a nodular elevation of smooth, shiny skin. As the lesions become extensive, they may be cauliflower-like or excavated and ulcerlike in appearance.

In all suspected cases of vulvar carcinoma a biopsy is done to determine the type and existence of malignancy. The inguinal regions are palpated to detect lymph node involvement. Palpation of a solid, fixed mass indicates extensive involvement, and surgery is not attempted.

Radical vulvectomy, a bilateral resection of the deep and superficial inguinal, femoral, iliac, and obturator nodes, is the surgical procedure recommended. Since most women having the disease are elderly, the surgery is done in stages. For advanced stages, irradiation with radium or roentgentherapy may be done; however, the results are not entirely satisfactory.

Lesions of the vagina

Inflammation and vaginal infections are discussed in Chapter 25.

Inclusion cysts are small cysts located in the posterior and lateral walls of the vagina close to the introitus. They are produced when the normal integrity of the vaginal epithelium is interfered with, such as in obstetric tears, episiotomies, and other gynecologic surgical procedures. No symptoms are produced. Inclusion cysts are rarely removed unless discovered during delivery.

Squamous cell carcinoma of the vagina is rare and may be located at any site. It is more common on the posterior wall. Fistulas are common sequelae due to the thin tissue between the vaginal mucosa, rectum, and bladder. Lesions in the lower portion of the vagina invade the lymph nodes rather early and those in the upper portion of the vagina spread to the paracervical, hypogastric, iliac, and inguinal nodes.

Bleeding, the chief symptom, may be spotting, a continuous flow, or hemorrhage. Early lesions are localized, red, and nonelevated. Later they become papillary, soft, and friable. Diagnosis of early lesions is made by cytosmear examination. In any suspicious lesion, biopsy and rectal, rectovaginal, proctoscopic, and complete urologic examination are performed.

Treatment for carcinoma of the vagina is radical. Malignancy involving the lower portion of the vagina extending to the vulva is treated by radical vulvectomy, removal of superficial and deep lymph nodes, femoral, iliac, and obturator nodes, and removal of the vagina and uterus. Lesions of the upper vagina necessitate radical abdominal hysterectomy, bilateral node dissection, and vaginectomy.

Radiation therapy includes both roentgen and radium therapy either individually or in combination. The method used depends upon the location and extent of the lesion. Exteral irradiation may be used alone or in conjunction with radium application vaginally. Radium is applied by plaques, by a tandem in a vaginal applicator, or by a suitable colpostat. The common complication with radium therapy is bladder and rectal fistulas.

NURSING CARE

The psychologic trauma of the removal of any part of the reproductive system is as great and at times greater than the physiologic changes. Each women has feelings about her femininity and the ways in which there will be alterations in appearance, her biologic makeup, and her performance as a woman. The removal of a breast involves disfigurement, a hysterectomy is followed by many hormonal changes and incapability of reproduction, and a radical vulvectomy signifies termination of sexual activity. With their fears of malignancy and of a shortened lifespan, women admitted to a gynecologic unit are in need of a highly skilled professional nurse.

The professional nurse in turn is also a woman, and her own feelings come into play. The nurse needs to be able to talk with the physician, the radiologist, the gynecologist, the clergyman, and the dietitian, in order to be able to meet the woman's needs. The nurse works closely with family members so that they too understand the feelings of the woman who has had surgery of the reproductive organs.

Prior to surgery, letting the woman talk through her feelings, discussing the possible postsurgery course, will alleviate fear and anxiety. Women find the nurse easier to talk with and may discuss the most delicate subjects with her. Often the nurse shows understanding simply by listening, by encouraging verbalization of fears and feelings, or by referral to another member of the health team.

In some units patients who have had the same kind of surgery may be supporting to another woman prior to surgery. Group discussions are valuable for ventilating feelings and clearing up misconceptions when women are ready to verbalize.

Preoperative preparation

Prior to surgery skin preparation is done only for major surgery so that pruritus and inflammation associated with shaving and regrowth of hair are eliminated. For extensive vaginal or abdominal surgery, however, the abdominal, vaginal, and rectal areas are shaved. Small-quantity enemas (such as Travad) or suppositories are ordered when necessary, since there is less bowel distention following surgery. In selected women, vaginal douches are ordered and given to cleanse the vaginal canal before surgery. Whenever possible a midstream urine is used instead of unnecessary catheterization.

For extensive surgery (lymphadenectomy), an indwelling three-way Foley catheter is inserted to keep the bladder empty during and following surgery. A continuous solution of 1,000 ml. of normal saline with 40 mg. of neomycin and 20 mg. of polymyxin keeps the bladder irrigated, reducing chances of bacterial invasion. Since the urinary system is so closely related to the reproductive system, supsceptibility to infection is common; therefore strict aseptic technique is imperative. When vaginoplasty is anticipated, the patient is instructed to refrain from smoking because excessive coughing may prove painful following surgery and may cause strain of the suture line. Preoperative medication the night and morning prior to surgery alleviates much anxiety and tension. Spiritual attendance is offered to all patients before surgical intervention.

Postoperative care

Nursing care following surgery of the reproductive system promotes repair and restoration of body tissue, return of natural body functions such as circulation, digestion, and excretion, and comfort measures. Following surgery, observation of vital signs and frequent checking of the operative site for bleeding are essential. The abdominal dressing is checked carefully on either side since bleeding may not penetrate the top of the dressing. Observing for bleeding, redness, irritation, and foul odor is essential when vaginal surgery has been done. Parenteral fluids to prevent dehydration until nausea and vomiting cease may be necessary. When liquids are started, they produce less nausea and vomiting when given at room temperature. Ice chips have a tendency to damage the mucous membrane, and small portions of food help initiate peristalsis.

Checking and irrigation of the indwelling catheter for effective urinary drainage will facilitate healing at the operative site and will cause less discomfort. For the first 48 hours, sedatives for the relief of pain are given freely when necessary. Frequent changes in position and deep breathing improve circulation and increase lung expansion. Early ambulation prevents blood stagnation that could result in thrombosis or embolism. In the operating room the legs are removed from the stirrups slowly and simultaneously so as not to change the blood pressure suddenly. When varicosities are present, Ace bandages are applied immediately following surgery to prevent blood stasis. Leg dangling is discouraged, and while the patient is sitting up in a chair pressure is kept off the popliteal space. Keeping the bed flat eliminates much discomfort following lithotomy position and extensive vaginal repair. When early ambulation is not feasible, frequent changes of position will improve circulation and prevent skin breakdown.

Following vaginal repair, tub baths are ordered on the second or third day to improve circulation, relieve discomfort, provide comfort and cleanliness, and promote healing. The water should be lukewarm because hot water may weaken the patient. To promote adequate bladder drainage, toilet facilities are far better and more comfortable with the patient in an upright position.

A diet high in proteins and carbohydrates is essential for adequate tissue repair. Antibiotics are frequently ordered to prevent infection.

Care following vulvectomy

Radical surgery of the vulva and vagina requires special care of the operative site. Often Hemovac suction may be used with inguinal node dissection. The tubes are attached by a Y tube to the Hemovac apparatus and are held in place by sutures. Minimal dressings are placed over the groin areas so that they may be observed frequently to assure adherence of the skin flaps. It is important to make sure these tubes remain patent for adequate drainage following surgery. It is common practice to culture the drainage and to do sensitivity tests if microorganisms are found. Tetracycline and chloramphenicol (Chloromycetin) are given prophylactically to prevent infection. The woman should be kept immobile in bed to minimize lymph flow and drainage from the groin. Suction is maintained for a period of 4 to 5 days until the drainage becomes scant.

A Foley catheter or suprapubic polyethylene tube into the bladder prevents wound contamination and maceration by urine. The catheter and tube are removed only when vulvar healing is certain. The bowels are emptied by enema or cathartic on the third day and every other day thereafter.

The most common complication is necrosis of the skin flaps. It is important to keep the wound dry. Keeping the woman flat and elevating the legs prevent tension on the sutures. Edema of the mons veneris, thighs, and entire legs is another complication. Cellulitis caused by streptococcal invasion is treated promply with antibiotics. Elastic bandages or stockings are often applied following surgery to aid in return of blood flow.

Nursing care following radiation therapy

Irradiation of cancer cells destroys aberrations in cell growth. This results in tissue fibrosis and control of growth of new cells. Irradiation is given by roentgen ray or by implantation of radium.

Radium therapy. Radium, a white crystalline substance, throws off alpha, beta, and gamma rays. Alpha rays are not used because they are the least effective. Beta rays can produce caustic effects in which tissue destruction is necessary. For deep penetrating effect the gamma ray is used. Radium may be used in its natural state, a salt, or in a gaseous state (radon produced by immersion of salt in acidulated water). Radium is used more often in its gaseous form because this preserves the salt element.

For irradiation of the reproductive tract, radium is commonly enclosed in silver, platinum, or brass containers inside of which is a glass tube containing the element. These containers are usually inserted into the uterus or cervical canal. Radium needles made of steel alloy produce a gamma ray and are used when destruction of tissue by sloughing is desired. Radon seeds are small glass, gold, or platinum tubes embedded in the tumor, causing eventual necrosis or sloughing of the tissue. Radon seeds lose their radioactivity in a month.

The effectiveness of irradiation depends upon the amount used, the time of tissue exposure, and the distance between the radium and involved tissue. In order to have effective results and preserve healthy tissue, materials such as rubber, brass, and platinum are used to screen the element from the tissue involved.

Since irradiation destroys tissue, the handling of radium becomes of primary concern to personnel working with patients receiving therapy. Radium is handled with long forceps and placed in lead containers to prevent irradiation of healthy tissue. Careful inspection of bed linens and bedpans for radon seeds or needles is important. Charting the exact time and type of radium implant is important for safe care of the patient. Any elevation in basal temperature should be reported at once and may necessitate removal of radium.

X-ray therapy. Gamma rays are also produced by x-ray equipment and are used singly or combined with radium therapy. Since the gamma rays penetrate the skin areas with this form of therapy, skin changes, such as reddening, blistering, and exfoliation of superficial epithelium, occur. Skin erythema may result, with an eventual deep purple discoloration. Pruritus due to drying is a common complaint. Skin care consists of keeping the area clean and dry. Excessive water is unnecessary, and soap should be avoided. Bland powders may be soothing following a moist sponge cleansing. Creams, ointments, alcohols, tub baths, and showers are contraindicated. Exposing the skin area daily will allow for drying. Clothing should be soft, light, and nonconstricting.

Digestive disturbances such as anorexia, nausea and vomiting, and diarrhea are common with therapy. Frequent small meals and drugs to control diarrhea are necessary for comfort. Frequency due to bladder irritability may also occur.

With radium insertion, a liquid low-residue diet is given until the radium is

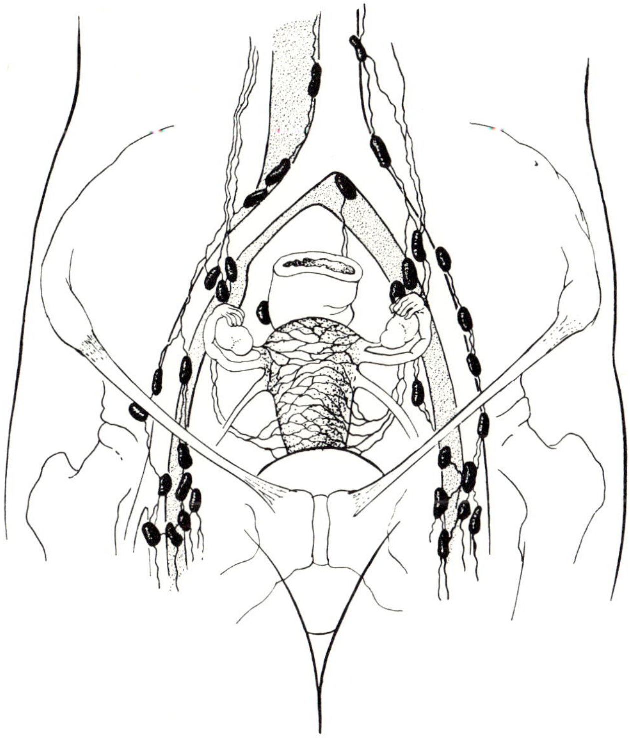

Fig. 27-3. Lymphatics of the utcrus.

removed. This eliminates bowel evacuation, which may displace the radium implant. In selected patients, if bowel evacuation is desired suppositories are used. Enemas are contraindicated because they produce some degree of lower bowel inflammation. A Foley catheter keeps the bladder empty, decreasing the damage of radiation. Often a packing is inserted vaginally to increase the distance between the radium and the rectum or the bladder. The patient should be kept flat so as not to displace the radium. Preferably women are put in a single room, or at a sufficient distance in a double room with postmenopausal women.

Professional nurses in the childbearing years should remain at a safe distance and should limit their time in giving bedside care. This may prove most trying to the patient and should be explained adequately. Nurses who are pregnant (especially in the first trimester) should be barred from these clinical areas to protect their unborn infants.

SELECTED REFERENCES

Alpenfels, E.: Cultural clues to reactions—cancer in situ of the cervix, Amer. J. Nurs. **64:**83, April, 1964.

Baird, Sir D.: Combined textbook of obstetrics and gynecology, London, 1962, E. & S. Livingstone, Ltd.

Behrman, S. J., and Gosling, J. R. G.: Fundamentals of gynecology, ed. 2, London, 1966, Oxford University Press.

Bourne, A. W., and Williams, L. H.: Recent advances in obstetrics and gynecology, New York, 1963, McGraw-Hill Book Co.

Brewer, J. I., and De Costa, E. J.: Textbook of gynecology, ed. 4, Baltimore, 1967, The Williams & Wilkins Co.

Corscaden, J. A.: Gynecologic cancer, Baltimore, 1962, The Williams & Wilkins Co.

Ellison, R. R.: Treating cancer with antimetabolites, Amer. J. Nurs. **62:**79, November, 1962.

Craytor, J. K., and Fass, M. L.: The nurse and the cancer patient, Philadelphia, 1970, J. B. Lippincott Co.

Gusberg, S.: Treatment as preventative medicine, Amer. J. Nurs. **64:**76, April, 1964.

Hodari, A. A., and Hodgkinson, P. C.: Lymphography as a diagnostic aid in female genital malignancy, Obstet. Gynec., vol. 29, no. 1, January, 1967.

Kroeger, W. and Fried, C. S.: Psychosomatic gynecology, Philadelphia, 1951, W. B. Saunders Co.

Lewis, G. C., et al.: New concepts in gynecological oncology, Philadelphia, 1966, F. A. Davis Co.

Lewis, G.: Screening and diagnosis, Amer. J. Nurs. **64:**72, April, 1964.

Lewison, E. F.: Breast cancer, Amer. J. Nurs. **62:**107, October, 1962.

Lucci, A. F., Jr.: Carcinoma of the cervix and pregnancy: an analysis of 111 cases in carcinoma of uterine cancer, endometrium and ovary, Chicago, 1962, Year Book Medical Publishers, Inc.

MacGillis, A.: To tell or not to tell, Nurs. Sci. **2:**444, 1964.

McGowan, L.: Nursing care of the patient with vaginal surgery, Amer. J. Nurs. **64:** 73, February, 1964.

Novak, E. R., and Seegar Jones, G.: Novak's textbook of gynecology, ed. 7, Baltimore, 1965, The Williams & Wilkins Co.

Papanicolaou, G. N.: A general survey of vaginal smear and its use in research and diagnosis, Amer. J. Obstet. Gynec. **51:** 316, 1946.

Pettit, M. D.: Gynecologic diagnosis and treatment, New York, 1962, McGraw-Hill Book Co.

Robbins, L., and Walker, E.: Problems of control, Amer. J. Nurs. **64:**80, April, 1964.

Rodman, M.: New drugs in the fight against cancer, RN **27:**79, November, 1964.

Sturgis, S. H.: The gynecologic patient, New York, 1962, Grune & Stratton, Inc.

Taylor, S. E.: Essentials of gynecology, Philadelphia, 1962, Lea & Febiger.

Winterton, W. R.: Aids to gynecology, Baltimore, 1960, The Williams & Wilkins Co.

Wolf, E. S.: Where hope comes first. Nurs. Outlook **12:**52, April, 1964.

Wright, R. C.: Hysterectomy: past, present and future, Obstet. Gynec., vol. 33, no. 4, April, 1969.

Questions for study

1. What are the causes of abnormal bleeding?
2. What is a myoma? What are the symptoms and treatment of myomas?
3. How do fibroids affect pregnancy?
4. What are the most common sites for malignant growths of the reproductive system?
5. What are the diagnostic measures used for prevention and detection of malignant growths?
6. What are the psychologic implications for women with surgery of the reproductive organs?
7. What are the nursing care needs of women prior to and following surgery of the reproductive organs?
8. What community agencies are concerned with detection and prevention of malignancies? What kinds of services do they give?

CHAPTER 28

CANCER OF THE BREAST

About one fourth of the female population has a lifetime probability of cancer developing in any site. Approximately one-fourth of this portion of the female population will develop cancer of the breast. Seventy-five women die of cancer of the breast daily, and 1,300 new cases are found each week. Early diagnosis of a localized tumor without spread to the adjacent lymph nodes assures women the greatest likelihood of survival.

Breast cancer is significantly less frequent in married women who have borne children than in single nulliparous women. Women who did not breast-feed infants for longer than 3 months have a higher risk of breast cancer. The highest incidence of breast cancer is seen in women between 45 and 55 years of age. The statistic likelihood of women having breast cancer increases with each decade even when women are safely past the menopause. Although oral contraceptives have an impact on breast anatomy and physiology, the relationship of oral contraceptives to cancer of the breast has not been ascertained. If a woman has had cancer of the breast and has been treated, oral contraceptives are forbidden since estrogens and progestogens stimulate growth of dormant cells. If pregnancy is to be avoided, a mechanical or intrauterine device should be used.

SELF-EXAMINATION

Women need to be motivated to perform self-examination of their breasts so that lesions are identified while they are still small. Using models and a testing score improves the technique in screening the disease.

In teaching self-examination of the breasts, the nurse may use various methods. A film on self-examination may be obtained from the American Cancer Society and from local health departments. The film, followed by group discussions, is most valuable in early detection of breast cancer.

The breasts are examined regularly each month a few days after the menstrual period. Some women have engorgement, soreness, and often small lumps prior to ovulation. Women past the menopause should examine the breasts on the same day each month, as outlined by the American Cancer Society:

1. Sit before a mirror; with the arms relaxed at the sides, note the contour of the breasts.
2. Raise both arms high above the head and observe the breasts through the mirror for any change in size, shape, or abnormal puckering or dimpling of the skin.
3. Lie flat on the bed with a small folded towel under the shoulder and raise the right arm above the head on the side to be examined. With the left hand, feel the inner half of the breast gently with the flat of the fingers.
4. Bring the right arm down to the side and feel gently the outer half of the breast, giving special attention to the upper outer section.
5. Examine the other breast the same way.

Any suspicious outer skin changes or lumps in the breasts warrant immediate examination by the physician. Mass screening of all women during routine gynecologic examinations is the only method of reducing the incidence of breast cancer.

CLINICAL DIAGNOSIS

Diagnostic measures, besides physical examination, include mammography, thermography, xerography, and biopsy. Other measures are under investigation.

Mammography, x-ray examination of the breasts, helps locate the specific area in which biopsy is needed. This is done for both breasts, since the most frequent precancerous lesion of the breast is cancer of the opposite breast.

The skin temperature of the breast in which a palpable mammary cancer is present is usually higher than that of the other breast of the same woman. To test skin temperature of the breast, a new technique, known as thermography, is now being used along with mammography. As a diagnostic measure, it is not as effective when there is considerable fatty tissue in the breast.

Xerography of the breast is considered to be superior to conventional film mammography. It requires less radiation, provides good visualization of the breast structures, permits more efficient and economical operation, and is easier to interpret.

Biopsy of the breast, followed by histologic study, determines the mode of treatment. In women who refuse biopsy, angiography may be performed. Angiography is done preoperatively to determine the source and nature of blood supply to the tumor and to distinguish highly vascularized areas from poorly vascularized areas. It may also serve as a guide for chemotherapeutic perfusion techniques. Angiography is done following radiographic examination of the breast. The patient is sedated. Under local anesthesia the brachial artery on the side of the lesion is punctured. A dye is injected, and filming is done.

A blood determination test is under much experimentation. Findings demonstrate that particles of monocytes are significantly different in the individual with breast cancer. Also plasma protein-bound fructose levels are found to be significantly elevated. Along with blood determinations, ultrasonics, transillumination, tracer isotope uptakes, and the laser beam may prove to be helpful in diagnosing mammary cancer.

SYMPTOMS

Most breast cancers are discovered by the individual. The earlier the lesion is found and cared for, the better the prognosis. It is a universal fact that most patients delay reporting the lesion because they fear cancer will be found.

In some women recurrent lumpy breasts resulting from chronic cystic mastitis make diagnosis of breast cancer most difficult.

The classification of breast cancer by Haagensen follows:

Class A Limited local tumor.
Class B Minimal nodal palpable metastases.
Class C Locally advanced tumor invasive in the breast or excessively metastatic to lymph nodes despite absence of remote metastases.
Class D Tumors with established blood-borne metastases.

TREATMENT

Surgery and irradiation

In Class A and Class B types of breast cancer, mastectomy and axillary dissection are performed. In Class A, with histologic negative axillary lymph nodes, there is an 80% to 90% survival rate. If axillary lymph nodes are involved, postoperative irradiation is necessary for the axillary, supraclavicular, and internal mammary areas but not for the operative site. If the patient is still menstruating and is within 5 years of spontaneous menopause, oophorectomy is done along with postoperative irradiation. The cyclic estrogenic stimulation of the first half of the normal menstrual cycle is associated with stimulation of the growth of breast cancer. Oophorectomy (also called postoperative castration) is done to remove this cyclic stimulation of the tumor. In postmenopausal women, estrogens are frequently used to arrest cell growth.

In Class C patients, local irradiation is done. Simple mastectomy may precede irradiation only when the breasts are pendulous, making irradiation difficult. Mastectomy is contraindicated because cutting through the lymph system only spreads malignant cells.

Chemotherapy is the method of choice in Class D patients or in patients in whom cancer cells are found in the blood during surgery.

Chemotherapy

Fluorinated pyrimidines were synthesized in 1957 and have an inhibitory effect against the growth of bacteria, transplanted solid tumors, and human tumor cells in vitro. Commercially available 5-fluorouracil is being used for a variety of neoplasms, particularly for adenocarcinoma of the breast, large bowel, and ovary.

Considerable variations have been reported in rate of response, drug toxicity, and drug mortality. The course of treatment is rapid injection with 15 mg. per kilogram every 2 or 3 days until mild toxicity occurs. Courses of palliative treatment are given at monthly intervals because they often produce severe morbidity and some mortality.

Prerequisites for therapy with fluorouracil are the following: (1) a diagnosis of incurable malignancy for which no other standard treatment is available; (2) one or more tumors that are palpable or visible roentgenographically, or hepatomegaly directly due to metastasis; (3) no other chemotherapy or radiotherapy for 3 weeks prior to 5-fluorouracil treatment; (4) white blood count above 4,500 and platelet count above 150,000; and (5) no concurrent therapy. The only contraindication to treatment is bleeding and infection.

Newer methods include giving 5-fluorouracil on an outpatient basis. The dose is 15 mg./kg. of body weight weekly for 4 weeks, then 20 mg./kg. from 5 to 8 weeks, and then additional monthly increments of 5 mg./kg. of body weight. The drug is stopped when mild toxicity occurs and then is resumed at lower dosages when the toxicity subsides.

Follow-up treatment

The most frequent precancerous lesion of the breast is cancer of the opposite breast. The opposite breast should always be considered a "high-risk" premalignant organ and should be observed carefully and routinely. Following surgery of one breast, examination is done every 3 months for the first year, every 4 months for the second year, every 5 months for the third year, and every 6 months thereafter. Routine chest roentgenograms are done every 6 months for the first 3 years and then annually thereafter, since the most common site for metastases in breast cancer is the lungs. Mammography of the contralateral breast is recommended periodically, depending upon physical findings.

NURSING CARE AFTER MASTECTOMY

The postoperative nursing care following mastectomy centers upon meeting the psychologic needs of the woman who has undergone breast removal, facilitating healing of the wound, and maintaining function of the arm on the affected side. With radical mastectomy the entire breast, the lymph channels, the lymph nodes, and the pectoral muscles are removed. Since this is a highly vascular area, fluid exudates and wound drainage necessitate copious dressings of the chest and upper arm. The wound may be allowed to drain into an applied pressure dressing, or a drainage tube may be attached to a Hemovac or to a gentle suction machine. With the Hemovac, the pressure gradually equalizes as the wound exudate is suctioned. To maintain suction, the Hemovac is emptied periodically, and negative pressure is reestablished. Care should be taken to maintain sterility while emptying contents and not to dislodge chest tubes. Maintaining the tubes in alignment by using adhesive tape and periodic checking to avoid pressure and kinking of tubes are essential for adequate drainage. The catheter may be left in place for a few days and is then removed. Hemovacs are discarded after use.

Elevation of the head of the bed increases comfort and encourages drainage from the chest wound. Position of the arm depends upon the surgery performed. Some physicians order the arm to be abducted at the shoulder, the forearm flexed at the elbow, and the hand elevated above the head. When there is extensive surgery (as with skin grafting to close the wound), the arm may be bandaged across the chest to prevent tension and permit adequate wound healing. In either position, the woman will feel more comfortable with a pillow supporting the arm and a pillow elevating the shoulder on the affected side. In order to allow for adequate drainage of the wound, the hand should be higher than the elbow and the elbow higher than the shoulder. Improper positioning causes discomfort and edema of the arm. If a pressure bandage has been applied, it is necessary to examine the hand for swelling since this is an indication of interference with circulation. The dressing is periodically checked by examining the undersurface that is toward the patient's back. If this is not done, hemorrhage may go unnoticed.

Analgesics that are ordered may also be given for comfort following surgery. It is imperative to move the patient postoperatively to promote drainage and prevent pneumonia. Encouraging deep breathing, coughing, and leg motion restores circulation and prevents respiratory complications. To prevent undue tension on the suture line, the patient may wear a sling to support the arm, or support with a pillow is comforting while sitting.

Arm movement is essential following mastectomy to prevent and limit arm edema and restore arm motion as healing occurs. The type of exercises and when they are started are determined by the physician. The nurse plans carefully with the physician so that there is optimum restoration of arm function. Most women have a great deal of fear and discomfort in beginning to restore arm movement. The patient should be urged to start with such simple exercises as feeding herself, washing her own hands and face, and combing her own hair, in order to restore arm function and improve morale. Encouraging the patient by telling her that the pain will subside and explaining the necessity for exercise are important and reassuring. Later, exercises such as wall climbing, pendulum swinging, rope turning, and broom raising may be started.

Wall climbing. While standing close to the wall, with feet spread apart slightly, the patient places both hands against the wall at shoulder level. Then using the fingers, the hands gradually climb the wall until both arms are fully extended. This is done each day, with a gradual increase in the number of times it is done. Full arm extension may be achieved in a few days depending upon the patient's motivation, amount of pain, and extent of wound tension.

Pendulum swinging. In a standing position, the patient bends forward with feet slightly apart and swings both arms back and forth, allowing the arms to hang downward. With practice the arms may be swung in circles.

Rope turning. This consists of turning a rope attached to a door knob without turning elbows or wrists. The patient is encouraged to form larger circles through continued practice. To maintain balance, the arm on the unaffected side is placed on the hip when doing this exercise.

Broom raising. Using a broomstick or a stick of similar weight, the patient grasps it with her hands two feet apart; she raises it progressively to extend above her head.

Psychologic aspects. Removal of the breast poses many psychologic threats to women. Since the breast is a part of the reproductive process and is associated with womanliness, its removal is coupled with feelings of disfigurement and being less a woman. Allowing the woman to express her feelings is paramount in relieving anxieties.

Appearance is a factor most women worry about, and arranging for a comfortable prosthesis as soon as wound healing permits is helpful. Most department stores carry appropriate prostheses that are fitted to resemble the contours of the opposite breast. The newer prostheses are filled with a fluid that resembles a breast, and the fluid shifts with changes in body position. Until the wound heals, a soft temporary prosthesis may be inserted into the brassiere cup to lessen embarrassment.

Family support should be encouraged. For the woman who anticipates radiation therapy following surgery, there may be added anxiety. Allowing the patient to ask questions and supporting the other family members are functions of the health team. Collaboration with the physician is essential so that the nurse knows what information the patient has been given and can plan her care accordingly.

For the patient who needs help financially for treatment, medications, dressings, etc., community agencies such as the American Cancer Society, American Red Cross, and oncology clinics may be helpful.

Questions for study

1. What preventive health measures would you implement in the care of young women in relation to breast cancer?
2. What kinds of diagnostic measures are used in cancer of the breast?
3. What psychologic preparations would you plan preoperatively and postoperatively?
4. Visit a department store where prostheses are sold so that you are better able to help women in need of one.
5. What are the essential components in the care of a woman postoperatively following a radical mastectomy?

UNIT V MISCELLANEOUS

Marriage has a biological basis and would be far more often a success if its biology were generally understood and the knowledge acted upon.

J. B. S. Haldane

CHAPTER 29

INFERTILITY AND STERILITY

Infertility and sterility problems have concerned people from primitive days to our present society. Ten percent of all newly married couples are incapable of reproducing.

Sterility is the term applied to a person who has some absolute factor preventing procreation. Infertility is the inability on the part of a couple to initiate the reproductive process after a desired or attempted 1-year period. Infertility is primary and absolute when pregnancy never occurs, when the causative factor cannot be corrected, or when there is absence of genital organs; it is secondary and relative if at least one pregnancy has occurred and the causative factor can be corrected.

Infertility is not an individual problem—rather it involves two people. Physician, nurse, and both individuals need to be cognizant of the social, economic, psychologic, personal, and marital relationships involved in the problem of infertility. Each couple is unique, and their reactions, desires, attitudes, and apprehensions must be considered.

The couple consulting the physician for infertility have varied motivations. Often the physician, although most skilled, may never find the couple's reason for investigating their infertility problem.

The drive to reproduce, although instinctive, is often associated with social and family problems. An unstable marriage with a motive that a child will save the marriage is not uncommon. In other families the wife may be looked on as barren by in-laws who had hoped for grandchildren.

Studies by a psychiatrist at the Sloane Hospital for Women Infertility Clinic revealed some interesting facts. Of the patients admitted for infertility study, 25% expressed desires for a cure but had no desire for children. Others desired assurance of knowing they were definitely infertile so that they could abandon the use of contraceptives. With some women it was not their desire for children but rather pressure from within the family that prompted them to investigate their barrenness. The latter women were really not ready in maturity for motherhood, and bearing a child would complicate matters.

The couple who are investigating their infertility with a sincere desire to beget children are concerned with why they are infertile and what the chances are for future pregnancies. The answer to why they are infertile can be solved by frank discussions and education relating to the anatomy and physiology of the reproductive organs. Only when this is done will the couple understand the reasons for the varied diagnostic tests and examinations proposed by the physician. What the chances are for future pregnancies can be determined by the cause of infertility and whether or not it is amenable to treatment.

The major causes of infertility are the following: cervical factors, 20%; tubal factors, 30% to 35%; male factors, 30% to 35%; and hormonal factors, 15%. One of the most common deterrents to adequate diagnostic evaluation of infertility is lack of cooperation of the male partner. Unless both marital partners are involved in the investigation, the subsequent treatment is futile. An expensive, time-consuming study of the woman is useless if the male is azoospermic. It is therefore essential and necessary that the male partner be evaluated first.

PREVENTION OF INFERTILITY

The following measures would reduce infertility:

1. Education for sex, marriage, and parenthood.
2. Adequate resources for effective contraception, as best preventive measure for illegal abortions and their complications. (The new liberalized abortion law in New York City is an example.)
3. Avoidance of pelvic surgery unless absolutely necessary.
4. Conservative surgery of the female reproductive tract.
5. Prevention of venereal disease.
6. Early and adequate treatment of cryptorchidism.
7. Varicocelectomy to improve impaired fertility of sperm.

MALE GENITAL FACTORS

A complete and thorough history includes the following: (1) questioning as to previous illnesses such as mumps, orchitis, and childhood diabetes; (2) occupational hazards such as exposure to roentgen rays or to other radioactive substances; (3) sexual habits such as infrequent coitus; (4) social habits such as excessive smoking and alcoholism; and (5) the use of precoital lubricants. The physician frankly discusses with the husband coital positioning, premature ejaculation, and his knowledge of the sexual act. At times lack of knowledge of the sexual act may be a causative or related factor to infertility. Occupations in which metals such as lead, iron, zinc, and copper are used as in painting, plumbing, and printing may be a causative factor. The fact that heat affects spermatogenesis needs to be considered because men who work at sitting jobs most of the day often have excessive heat at the scrotal area.

The male genital factors are composed of the following: (1) a disturbance in spermatogenesis; (2) an obstruction in the seminiferous tubules, ducts, or vesicles;

(3) changes in the amount and quality of seminal fluid; and (4) anomalies concerned with the ejaculatory process.

Physiology of spermatogenesis

At the time of puberty, the germinal cells lining the seminiferous tubules are stimulated by the pituitary gonadotropic hormones to produce spermatozoa. At the same time the pituitary gonadotropic hormone also stimulates the interstitial cells of the testis to secrete androgens. In the male, changes occur in the epithelium of the germinal layers after 55 or 60 years of age, reducing fertility.

Disturbances of spermatogenesis

Physical systemic diseases are known to have an effect on spermatogenesis. A high basal temperature elevation associated with infection will temporarily reduce sperm formation. Infections, such as mumps, gonorrhea, syphilis, or tuberculosis with resulting orchitis (inflammation of the testes), often cause occlusion of the epididymis and the ductus deferens, inhibiting passage of the sperm.

Endocrine imbalances of the pituitary and the thyroid glands affect the development of the genitalia and inhibit spermatogenesis. Excessive coitus is known to reduce the number of mature and motile sperm greatly. To improve the number of sperm ejaculated, the male is counseled to engage in coitus less frequently, thus improving chances of fertility.

Previous surgical intervention for herniorrhaphy may cause impairment of circulation, resulting in degenerative changes in the tubules affecting sperm production. Absolute sterility is not uncommon with massive and continuous exposure to radiation.

Obstruction of sperm ducts

Infections such as gonorrhea result in occlusion of the lumen of the duct. Occasionally there may be a congenital stricture or absence of the ducts.

Changes in seminal fluid

Infectious processes decrease the concentration of spermatozoa and change the viscosity of the seminal fluid. Often there is hyperviscosity, pyospermia, hypospermia, or hyperspermia. Any disturbance or infection of the prostate gland is directly related to sperm transport. The prostatic fluid, alkaline in nature, neutralizes the acidity of vaginal secretions, thereby protecting the sperm.

Anomalies of ejaculation

Improper ejaculation occurs with congenital hypospadias. With hypospadias the male ejaculates prior to intromission. The reason for this may be psychologic. In hypogonadism, surgery of the prostate, diabetes, drug addiction, or latent syphilis, there may be absence of ejaculation. Often with urethral obstruction, the sperm is ejaculated into the bladder and later voided with urine.

FEMALE GENITAL FACTORS

A complete and thorough history of the female includes menstrual history (age of onset, duration and frequency of flow, amount of bleeding, presence or absence of pain, periods of amenorrhea or irregularities). The physician is also concerned about premarital and postmarital coitus, especially with relation to frequency and the time practiced during the female's ovarian cycle. Added information related to previous occupations, use of cigarettes and alcohol, surgical history, accidents or illnesses, and the use of contraceptive measures such as mechanical devices, intravaginal medications, or douches is essential for diagnostic purposes.

The physical examination includes observation of body contour, hair distribution, fat deposits, and breast development. A complete pelvic examination is done. An enlarged clitoris with male distribution of hair may be related to adrenal or ovarian tumors. Beginning vaginal infections causing dyspareunia may be a causative factor in infertility.

Causative factors

Congenital anomalies of the vagina and the vulva, such as lesions or malformations, interfere with coitus. Bacterial invasion of the vagina so alters the acidity that the spermatozoa become inactive due to toxic effects. Often violent orgasm in highly erotic women causes spasm of the levator ani muscles with expulsion of semen during coitus.

In the female, developmental anomalies of the reproductive organs, such as retroversion of the uterus, an imperforate hymen, or dyspareunia (painful intercourse), may prevent the sperm from meeting the ovum. Any blockage of the cervical os or the fallopian tube and endocrine dysfunction, such as amenorrhea, anovulatory cycles, decreased progesterone activity, or dysfunctional uterine bleeding, must also be considered. The incidence of infertility increases with functional organic diseases, nutritional deficiencies, and in women past 40 years of age. Emotional factors related to marriage compatibility and the sincere desire for children are important.

Cervical factors involving the position of the cervix, the patency of the external os, and the quality and quantity of cervical secretions are studied thoroughly.

DIAGNOSTIC MEASURES IN INFERTILITY

Often the gynecologist may refer the male partner to a urologist interested in infertility. This referral is often made when the male partner does not want to be examined by a gynecologist. It is only recently that board-qualified gynecologists are permitted to treat the infertile couple.

Semen examination of the male is done by collecting a semen specimen after 5 days of abstinence from coitus. The semen is collected in a wide-mouthed glass jar either by masturbation or by coitus interruptus (withdrawal of the penis prior to ejaculation at the time of coitus). Instruction to collect the entire specimen is important, since the first semen contains the greatest concentration of sperm. The specimen should be kept at room temperature and taken for examination within a 3-hour period. The semen is examined 1 hour following ejaculation when complete liquefaction has occurred. The quality of sperm motility, the number of sperm, and the morphology are evaluated. Normally 20 million to 60 million are considered normal sperm counts. Motility and progression of sperm are intimately correlated with density. A high sperm count has great motility and progression, whereas a low sperm count has poor motility and progression. At least two semen analyses are performed for proper evaluation of the male factor.

The laboratory procedures for diagnosis in the female include: (1) serology for syphilis, (2) complete blood count and sedimentation rate, (3) urinalysis, (4) serum protein-bound iodine, (5) chest roentgenogram, and (6) basal metabolic rate. The serum protein-bound iodine is always done prior to the Schiller test or a false positive reaction results. With a history of menstrual irregularities, the following tests are done to rule out endocrine abnormalities: (1) urinary 17-ketosteroids and 17-hydrocorticoids, (2) urinary follicle-stimulating hormone, and (3) a roentgenogram of the sella turcica.

Diagnostic procedures commonly done in the physician's office are postcoital examination of cervical mucus (Sims-Huhner test), endometrial biopsy, and tubal insufflation.

Basal body temperature

Basal body temperature (B.B.T.) is taken by the woman before she arises each morning. She also notes whether she had a good night's sleep and is free of infection.

Each patient is given the following instructions:

1. In the left-hand margin of your temperature record, note whether the temperature is oral or rectal, and the time it is usually taken.
2. If, on any morning, your waking time varies by an hour or more, be sure to record the time on that date line.
3. Take your temperature on awakening in the morning before you get out of bed and before talking or any other activity. Temperatures may be taken either orally or rectally, but consistently one way or the other. Take the temperature for a full 5 minutes by the clock.
4. Read the temperature to within one-tenth of a degree, at your convenience. The mercury remains stationary until shaken down provided the thermometer is kept at room temperature. However, be sure to chart the temperature as soon as it is read; do not trust your memory.
5. Any known cause for temperature variation should be noted on the chart: for example, if sleep has been interrupted or shortened, if you have a cold, flu, indigestion, a severe emotional disturbance, or if you have indulged in alcohol.
6. After you have read the thermometer, it should be shaken down and replaced at your bedside, ready for use the next morning. Do not wash the thermometer in hot water.
7. If you notice an increased, slippery vaginal discharge, slight staining, or discomfort (pain or gaseous bloating) in the lower abdomen, note these on the chart as well.
8. Your menstrual period ends one cycle and begins a new one. Mark the onset of your period (M) at the end of the old cycle. The same date is charted over day 1 of the new cycle. Write in the dates for the entire new cycle.*

*Kleegman, S. J.: Infertility in women, Philadelphia, 1966, F. A. Davis Co.

Ovulation takes place within a 24-hour to 72-hour period of the temperature change. In some women the span may be 3 days. A woman who ovulates has a biphasic curve, because estrogen depresses the basal temperature, whereas progesterone elevates it. Therefore the temperature is lower prior to ovulation, is elevated with the production of progesterone, and drops when the corpus luteum regresses; therefore before menstruation there is a drop in temperature. A woman who menstruates without ovulating does not have a biphasic curve.

The basal body temperature is accurate only when taken as instructed. Advantages of this method are that it is simple, there is no expense, it evaluates estrogen and progesterone phases, it evaluates results of endocrine therapy given to stimulate ovulation, and it is an early diagnostic test for pregnancy.

Vaginal smears

Since the mucosa of the vagina undergoes cyclic changes in response to the biphasic ovarian hormones, the character and degree of change can be determined by taking daily vaginal smears. The daily smears are done in conjunction with the basal body temperature.

Before arising the woman introduces a pipette into the vault of the vagina and aspirates secretions. The secretions are aspirated onto a slide, spread into a thin layer, and *immediately* placed into a fixing solution. The jar is kept tightly covered to avoid evaporation of the fixing solution. The slides are taken each day from the first day of the menstrual period to the end of the cycle. A study is then made of the daily changes occurring during the entire cycle.

Sims-Huhner test

This test is usually performed at the time of ovulation. Prior to examination the woman is instructed to refrain from douching or using intravaginal medication for at least 48 hours.

Following coitus, a minimum of at least 6 hours is desirable prior to the study of sperm survival. The physician then collects a sample of mucus high in the endocervical canal where sperm motility and survival are at a maximum. On gross examination the cervical mucus at the time of ovulation forms a thin continuous thread as it is pulled apart. This is known as *spinnbarkeit.* When allowed to dry on a slide, the mucus forms a fernlike pattern known as *arborization.* Both these characteristics are indicative of increasing levels of estrogen and disappear with the progesterone phase that follows ovulation. Microscopic examination of the slide reveals motility, number, and morphology of spermatozoa. It is evident then that the Sims-Huhner test gives a picture of the cervical environment of spermatozoa and also the ovarian function controlling it. Often this test is substituted for semen analysis.

Endometrial biopsy

Endometrial biopsy is a test for ovulation. Secretory changes in the endometrium are presumptive evidence that ovulation has occurred. The biopsy is done on the first day of the menstrual period to determine whether the menstruation is of the anovulatory type. On the first day chances of disturbing a pregnancy are minimal. If biopsy is not feasible at this time, the estimated menstrual history is discussed, and biopsy is performed on or before the sixth postovulatory day. This is also a safe period because the ovum is in the oviduct, and if fertilization has occurred implantation has not yet taken place.

A pelvic examination precedes the biopsy, and the physician ascertains the position and size of the uterus. Tissue is then obtained with a tenaculum, starting high in the fundus and moving down toward the cervix. The tissue is immediately fixed in Bouin's solution and then examined microscopically. When biopsy reveals abnormal tissue, diagnostic curettage follows to rule out malignancy.

Tubal insufflation

The Rubin test for tubal patency is performed following thorough pelvic examination. Any acute or subacute pelvic infection is a contraindication for tubal insufflation. The test is performed with the woman in lithotomy position. The cervix, uterus, and tubes are insulated with carbon dioxide under pressure. Pressure readings with a gradual rise and fall indicate tubal patency. A sharp increasing rise with no decline indicates tubal obstruction. With tubal patency, the woman experiences shoulder pain due to pressure of carbon dioxide on the diaphragm. Auscultation of the abdomen with a stethoscope indicates patency when bowel sounds are heard.

Hysterosalpingography

Occlusion found by a Rubin test is followed by a hysterosalpingogram. A water-soluble solution of Skiodan acacia or Salpix, 12 ml., is introduced through the cervix with a sterile syringe. This is followed by fluoroscopy and roentgenologic examination to determine tubal patency.

Culdoscopy

Culdoscopy is a procedure performed under sterile precautions in the operating room (Fig. 29-1). It permits direct visualization of the organs of reproduction through a culdoscope inserted into the posterior fornix of the vaginal canal. With the culdoscope in place, a solution of methylene blue is injected into the cervix, and visualization of the fallopian tubes is possible. A newer instrument, the panculdoscope, permits photographing the internal reproductive organs for further evaluation.

TREATMENT IN THE MALE

Therapy in the male for oligospermia or azoospermia is controversial. Testosterone, desiccated thyroid, vitamin compounds, and radiation therapy have proved useless. Positive therapy consists of the following: (1) regulating hours of sleep, exercise, and work; (2) adequate nutritional diet; (3) avoiding excesses in alcohol, smoking, and coitus; (4) adequate social engagements; (5) avoiding

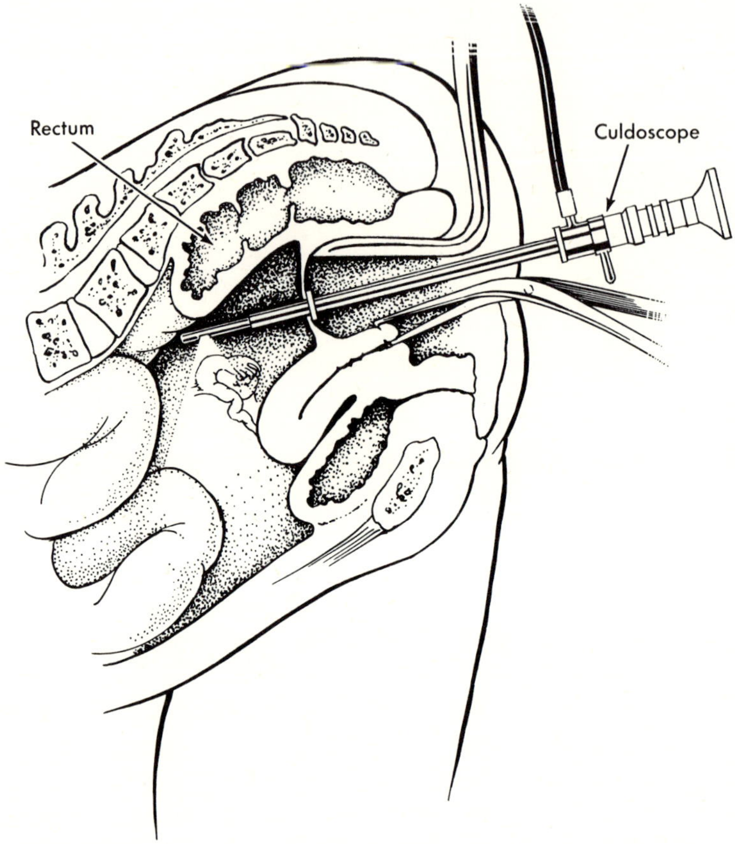

Fig. 29-1. Culdoscopic examination of internal reproductive organs.

prolonged heat interfering with the thermoregulatory mechanism of the scrotum; (6) correcting hypothyroidism with medication; (7) controlling and eliminating infectious diseases; and (8) prolonged continence to improve sperm count and motility.

Surgical intervention is indicated for obstructions in passage of sperm, correction of hypospadias, and correction of cryptorchidism (undescended testicles) before puberty.

TREATMENT IN THE FEMALE

Cervical factor

Hormonal, anatomic, and infectious factors are considered in treatment. With estrogen deficiency, small doses of estrogens are administered for several months. Anatomic defects such as malpositions of the uterus are corrected with pessaries. Often a closed cervix may be dilated to permit entrance of the sperm. It also may be traumatic to dilate the cervix with large instruments, subjecting the woman to subsequent cervical incompetence. Some physicians have instructed couples to practice knee-chest coitus following cervical dilatation, and successful subsequent pregnancy has followed. Cervical polyps or growths obstructing the vaginal canal and cervix are treated by cauterization or surgical excision. Inflammation and infections of the cervix are treated with antibiotics and sulfonamides.

Tubal factor

Blocked fallopian tubes are made patent by time, sexual rest, antispasmodics, and repeated tubal insufflations. Acute pelvic inflammatory disease is treated cautiously with large doses of broad-spectrum antibiotics to prevent scarring and narrowing of the fallopian tubes. A closed oviduct warrants surgical intervention when all other methods have failed. Tuboplasties with polyethylene are being done to reconstruct severely damaged oviducts. Hazards of tuboplasty are pelvic inflammatory disease and subsequent ectopic pregnancies.

Uterine factor

With endometrial biopsy progesterone activity is determined. Oral progestogens such as norethynodrel with mestranol (Enovid) or norethindrone (Norlutin) may be ordered in 5-mg. daily doses from the eighteenth day through the twenty-first day of a 28-day cycle. In some infertile women endometrial hypoplasia is treated with 10 mg. of norethynodrel with mestranol (Enovid) daily for 20 days (day 5 through day 25) for three consecutive cycles. Large submucous fibroids interfering with pregnancy warrant surgical intervention. Displacements of the uterus are corrected with insertion of a pessary (Smith-Hodge), which is left in place for 12 weeks if pregnancy occurs. Congenital anomalies such as bicornuate or septate uteri are treated surgically following diagnosis.

Ovarian factor

The endometrial biopsy or fern test has been described to determine whether ovulation occurs. If ovulation does occur, determining the time by the basal temperature method and practicing coitus at that time improve chances of fertility. With anovulatory cycles, further study needs to be made of pituitary, thyroid, and adrenal gland function.

IMMUNOLOGIC RESPONSE

ABO incompatibility may be a possible cause of infertility in some couples. Studies by Behrman show that spermatozoa may be blocked or immobilized by antibodies in cervical secretions in incompatible ABO matings. Normal postcoital findings do not rule out the immunologic factor. Another speculation is that the wife has a "naturally occurring" ABO antibody that is not specific to her own blood type but is specific to the antigen carried by the husband's sperm. Pregnancy has occurred in some couples because of a decrease in antibody titer. Whether the husband and the wife are heterozygous or homozygous is also important. Segal and his co-workers found sperm-agglutinating antibodies more frequently in subfertile couples.

Masters and Johnson postulated the existence of a vaginal spermicidal "lethal factor" in some couples who had no ABO or Rh incompatibilities. Scheinfeld's studies attribute infertility to a genetic factor that is carried. Genetics undoubtedly holds the clues to some of the unknown factors in sterility and infertility.

The treatment for infertility consists of advising the couple to abstain or use a condom during sexual relations for several months.

Further study in the field of immunology is necessary before clinical application is possible. In selected women with anatomic and physiologic insufficiency of the cervix, artificial insemination with the husband's semen is done. A polyethylene cervical cup attached to a plastic tube is inserted vaginally. This procedure affords close contact of the sperm with the cervix and eliminates the hostile environment of the vagina. Artificial insemination is done only when other methods fail and only when religious beliefs are given consideration.

Therapeutic husband and donor insemination will not be discussed in this text. It is discussed adequately by Kleegman.

PSYCHOLOGIC ASPECTS OF INFERTILITY

Clinical studies show that there are as many psychologic implications in infertility as there are in other diseases. The early successes, with pregnancy occurring in some women before therapy is begun, strongly support that psychologic factors were involved. Fertility and reproduction are so intimately associated with sexuality that often emotional feelings are greatly repressed. Often when there is evidence of psychologic factors, the gynecologist refers the couple for psychiatric consultation. The gynecologist who has psychiatric preparation is better able to work with problems of infertility. Psychotherapy may prove fruitful if there is no other apparent organic cause.

ROLE OF THE NURSE IN INFERTILITY

The nurse who works closely with the physician and with infertile couples needs a thorough understanding of human relations and psychology. The nurse is in a unique position since she is often the person to whom the female partner is comfortable is discussing womanly functions. She is an essential link between the doctor and the couple during infertility work-up. The woman who is to undergo study may have feelings of inadequacy in her role as a woman and mother, coupled with deeper feelings of guilt. The ability to reproduce is a maturing process leading to responsibilities of parenthood and is the strength of the family unit. Problems of sterility and infertility are stressful life crises, situations that often need therapeutic intervention for maintenance of optimum health. The nurse recognizes the need to listen, support, and give truthful answers, as couples crave information. Often the nurse finds herself reinterpreting what has been said time and time again to the anxious couple.

Diagnostic procedures are accepted with greater ease when explanations are offered. The suspense of waiting for the outcome is often a source of greater anxiety. The woman who is admitted to the hospital for infertility study is often most anxious since other studies have proved futile.

Nursing care prior to and following culdoscopy necessitates adequate preparation since it is a surgical procedure. The mixed hopes of most women produce anxiety because the procedure will reveal the answer to the problem. Explaining preoperatively the reasons for vaginal douching and shaving, the knee-chest position to be assumed, and the dark room for adequate visualization of the reproductive organs will alleviate anxiety of the unknown. The postoperative practice of sulfa cream vaginal insufflations to prevent infection is distressing to the woman who is not prepared for the treatment. The few days spent at the hospital may provide the opportunity for the woman to ventilate her feelings to the nurse who is prepared and ready to listen.

In many infertility clinics the nurse also works closely with the psychologist–marriage counselor. The major functions of the psychologist–marriage counselor are (1) screening and evaluating, (2) relationship improvement, (3) sexual compatibility guidance, and (4) supportive counseling. One or two of these functions may also be responsibilities of the physician and the nurse.

The couple who are receiving therapy on an outpatient basis would benefit from public health nursing service if the need exists. With problems of sterility, frank discussions on adoption are often conducted with members of the health team.

SELECTED REFERENCES

Behrman, S. J.: Immunological aspects of infertility, Int. J. Fertil. **6**:349, 1961.

Braz, J.: The infertile marriage, Haarlem, Netherlands, 1963, De Erven F. Bohn N. V.

Gilbert, H.: Love in marriage, New York, 1964, Hawthorn Books, Inc.

Hutton, I. G.: The sex technique in marriage, New York, 1961, Emerson Books, Inc.

Iorio, J.: Culdoscopy—nursing care, Nurs. Outlook **12**:35, September, 1964.

Kimbrough, R. A.: Gynecology, Philadelphia, 1965, J. B. Lippincott Co.

Kistner, R. W.: Gynecology—principles and practice, Chicago, 1965, Year Book Medical Publishers, Inc.

Kleegman, S.: Infertility in Women, Philadelphia, 1966, F. A. Davis Co.

Klemer, R. H., Rutherford, R. N., Banks, A. L., et al.: Marriage counseling with the infertile couple, Fertil. Steril. **17**:104, 1966.

Kroger, W.: Psychosomatic obstetrics, gynecology, and endocrinology, Springfield, Ill., 1962, Charles C Thomas, Publisher.

Masters, W. H., and Johnson, V. E.: Intravaginal environment: a lethal factor, Fertil. Steril. **12**:560, 1961.

Masters, W. H., and Johnson, V. E.: Human sexual response, Boston, 1967, Little, Brown and Co.

Masters, W. H., and Johnson, V. E.: Human sexual inadequacy, Boston, 1970, Little, Brown and Co.

Mayes, J. B.: Cervical incompetence, Amer. J. Obstet. Gynec. **84**:299, 1962.

Novak, E., and Seegar Jones, G.: Novak's textbook of gynecology, ed. 7, Baltimore, 1965, The Williams & Wilkins Co.

Penrose, L. S.: Genetical aspects of infertility, Proc. Roy. Soc. **159**:93, 1963.

Rothman, D., Kaplan, A. H., and Nettles, E.: Psychosomatic infertility, Amer. J. Obstet. Gynec. **83**:373, 1962.

Scheinfeld, A.: Your heredity and environment, Philadelphia, 1965, J. B. Lippincott Co.

Sturgis, S. H.: Treatment of ovarian insufficiency, Amer. J. Nurs. **64**:113, January, 1964.

Questions for study

1. Define infertility and sterility.
2. List the male and female causative factors in infertility.
3. What diagnostic measures are pursued in the male and female?
4. Following diagnostic outcome, what method of treatment is instituted to improve fertility?
5. What is the nurse's role as a member of the health team?
6. Visit an outpatient department in your community for infertility study. Discuss with members of the health team the diagnostic measures and treatment being used. How many members comprise the health team, and what is their function?

CHAPTER 30

THE MENOPAUSE

The menopause is that period in a woman's life in which there is a gradual cessation of ovarian function and cessation of menstruation. The average duration of menstrual life is approximately 33 years. Often some women menstruate at 48 and 50 years of age. Bleeding that continues after 55 years warrants a Papanicolaou smear at 6-month intervals.

The beginning of the menses is only one manifestation of a developmental process. So, too, the retrogressive changes occurring during the menopause are referred to as the climacteric or, in lay terms, "change of life."

PHYSIOLOGY OF THE MENOPAUSE

The origin of the changes occurring in the endocrine system during the menopause is unknown. Primary alterations are found probably in the ovary as it gradually loses its ability to respond to gonadotropic hormones. As ovulation gradually ceases, there is loss of progesterone. The failure of ovulation and the cessation of progesterone secretion, with the continued growth of follicles, account for the irregularity of the menses. Although all these changes occur, the quantity of estrogens excreted in the urine diminishes but never disappears. There is also an increase in gonadotropins in menopausal women, and it is not uncommon to find a falsely positive biologic test for pregnancy. The hyperactivity of the pituitary gland during the menopause is thought to be a result of gonadal inhibition, and gonadotropin is increased in the blood since it is not being utilized by the ovaries.

CESSATION OF MENSTRUATION

The average age at which menstruation ceases is under 50, yet there are wide variations. In some women the menstrual period ceases abruptly, while in others there is a gradual disappearance. Usually the phenomena occur with skipping one or two periods, a normal recurrence for a few months, and then another period of amenorrhea. This phenomenon occurs repeatedly until there is complete cessation.

The amount of flow and duration of the menstrual period may be normal until complete cessation or there may be diminution in both.

Normally there should be no excessive flow or intermenstrual bleeding at the menopause. Both of these symptoms are not normal and should be immediately investigated to rule out cancer.

CESSATION OF OVULATION

Although ovulation as well as menstruation ceases, the disappearance of the two functions is not always simultaneous. Often ovulation ceases prior to cessation of menstruation; the latter cycles are of the anovulatory type. The long periods of amenorrhea that often precede cessation of the menses make pregnancy difficult to diagnose at this time. Some women are more relaxed in trying to avoid pregnancy since they often associate amenorrhea with cessation of ovulation. Although ovulation rarely occurs following 6 months of consistent amenorrhea, it is safer to instruct women to use precautions for 1 year following the last menstrual period.

SYMPTOMS

Symptoms associated with the climacteric are somatic and psychic. The major physiologic change is failure of the ovary to produce a sufficient amount of estrogen. Some of the atrophic changes in the organs of reproduction are related to decreased hormonal action and the ageing process. Vasomotor symptoms include hot flashes involving chiefly the head, neck, and upper parts of the thorax, followed by profuse diaphoresis. In some women the skin texture loses its softness, there is a tendency to gain weight, there is noticeable facial hair growth, and the breasts become smaller and pendulous. All of these symptoms differ in frequency and severity and are variable in women.

Anatomic changes during the menopause are evident as the external genitalia become thinner and flattened, the amount of vaginal fluid decreases, and the endometrium becomes smooth and pale. These changes increase the susceptibility to infection and dyspareunia.

Often some women experience an increase in emotional irritability during the menopause. Complaints are those that affect visceral function, such as vertigo, headache, constipation, pruritus, faintness, and cardiac palpitation. These symptoms are usually more common in women of nervous temperament. Since the physiologic changes during the menopause are so complex, it is difficult to determine whether complaints are psychosomatic, due to endocrine imbalance, or due to dysfunction of the autonomic nervous system.

Although 75% of women stop menstruating with no ill effects, 25% have severe symptoms that warrant medical attention. It has been found that as estrogen levels decrease, pituitary gonadotropins rise in an effort to stimulate ovarian function.

Psychologically, the chief symptom of the menopausal syndrome is anxiety. Early symptoms of amenorrhea produce fears of possible pregnancy. Later symptoms of anxiety arise from feelings of loss of reproductive function, a decrease in sexual feelings and capacity, the loss of feeling womanly as alterations in the skin, abdominal muscles, and breasts occur, the decrease in the number of social contacts due to death of lifelong friends, and the economic insecurities felt with increase in age.

Not all women experience the menopausal syndrome to the same degree. In the well-integrated woman many of these symptoms are controlled and accepted as part of the physiologic changes that normally take place in the female reproductive system.

TREATMENT

The woman experiencing mild menopausal symptoms responds well to a mild sedative such as phenobarbital or a short-acting tranquilizer such as chlorpromazine. If the symptoms of the menopause are troublesome, estrogens are given as specific therapy.

Estrogen therapy minimizes the intensity and the frequency of flashes when given in adequate and intermittent doses. Small oral doses of estrogen given over a limited period of time are withdrawn gradually to produce the best results. Occasionally withdrawal bleeding may occur, obscuring symptoms of uterine carcinoma. If withdrawal bleeding occurs and does not cease after 10 days, diagnostic curettage of the cervix and uterus is essential. Estrogen therapy is contraindicated in women having irregular bleeding episodes during the menopause regardless of the severity of flashes.

In women who have been salvaged and have survived genital cancer, severe flashes are treated with androgen therapy. Unfortunately androgens are poor inhibitors of hypophyseal function, and large doses are needed to relieve flashes. Occasionally large doses of androgens produce virilization in women.

Atrophic vaginal changes are often followed by irritating vaginal discharge, introital discomfort, and dyspareunia. Vaginal creams containing estrogens are effective. Nightly vaginal applications for a 1-week period and then twice weekly have restored the vaginal epithelium to its former physiologic state. Often the physician may prescribe 0.1 mg. of stilbestrol orally as an alternative for the vaginal cream.

In women with postmenopausal frigidity, the use of combined estrogen and androgen produces a hyperemia of the vulva and clitoris. The hyperemia greatly increases the sensitivity of these organs and improves the female's response during coitus. This combined therapy is given intermittently under close supervision. Often frigidity in younger women is due to psychic factors rather than hormonal imbalance.

Studies by Wilson indicate that prophylactic doses of estrogen and progesterone to all menopausal women are advocated since vaginal smears reflect estrogen deprivation. Studies by Robinson and associates indicate that estrogens tend to lower elevated serum lipids, thereby preventing atherosclerosis. In fact, men with myocardial infarctions are being treated with estrogen therapy. These data have created two trends in therapy, the long-continued use of small doses of estrogens in postmenopausal women and preservation of ovaries during hysterectomy.

NURSING CARE

The woman approaching the menopause needs information concerning the many changes that will occur so that she is ready to accept these changes more readily. At times the husband needs to be a vital participator in the give-and-take of everyday married life. Changes that occur in women often occur earlier than in the sexual life of the male. A strong family unit in which there is free exchange of feelings between wife and husband is a great advantage.

The nurse is often the person women will confide in, and the person to whom feelings are directed. The nurse then needs to understand that the menopause is symbolic of reproductive cessation equivalent to castration. At a conscious level the menopause is indicative of beginning senescence with eventual social dependence. Along with this, the woman may not be needed by her children as a mother figure and loses much of the gratification she received from them. Perhaps these feelings are closely interwoven with friction between herself and daughters-in-law or sons-in-law. Women at this time may feel more masculine as changes occur, they may unconsciously have sexual fantasies, some may feel sexually less attractive, and some fear possibilities of cancer and insanity.

The nurse is a good listener who allows the woman to verbalize and works closely with the physician in planning for alleviation of symptoms. Perhaps referral and a visit to the home by the public health nurse will prove helpful in evaluating the home environment. Women need to verbalize about how they feel, and often the nurse is a good sounding board. The nurse may also help the woman who feels useless by directing her energies toward feelings of usefulness. Explaining the approach in therapy and why changes are occurring alleviates much fear and anxiety.

When vaginal creams are ordered, instruction as to insertion at bedtime will provide for effectual application. While lying prone, the woman introduces the vaginal applicator into the vaginal canal in a downward and backward motion. A perineal pad will collect any excess cream that escapes from the vagina.

Women on estrogen therapy should be made aware of the importance of medical supervision and the reporting of any withdrawal bleeding that occurs.

SELECTED REFERENCES

Kimbrough, R. A.: Gynecology, Philadelphia, 1965, J. B. Lippincott Co.

Kistner, R. W.: Gynecology—principles and practice, Chicago, 1964, Year Book Medical Publishers, Inc.

Kroger, W., and Freed, W. S.: Psychosomatic gynecology, Philadelphia, 1951, W. B. Saunders Co.

Lammert, A. C.: The menopause, a physiologic process, Amer. J. Nurs. **62:**56, February, 1962.

Marmorston, J., Magdison, O., Kuzma, O., and Moore, F. J.: Estrogen therapy in men with myocardial infarction; side effects with increasing dosage and time, J.A.M.A. **174:**241, 1960.

Novak, E., and Seegar Jones, G.: Novak's textbook of gynecology, ed. 7, Baltimore, 1965, The Williams & Wilkins Co.

Parker, E.: The seven ages of woman, Baltimore, 1960, The Johns Hopkins Press.

Robinson, R. W., Higans, N., and Cohen, W. D.: Effects of long-term administration of estrogens on serum lipids of postmenopausal women, New Eng. J. Med. **263:**828, 1960.

Sturgis, S. H.: Treatment of ovarian insufficiency, Amer. J. Nurs. **64:**113, January, 1964.

What every nurse should know about the menopause and postmenopause, 1968, Ayerst Laboratories.

Wilson, R. A.: The roles of estrogen and progesterone in breast and genital cancer, J.A.M.A. **182:**327, 1962.

Wilson, R. A.: Feminine forever, New York, 1967, M. Evans & Co., Inc.

Questions for study

1. What are the physiologic changes occurring during the menopause?
2. How do these changes affect women? What are the symptoms experienced during the menopause?
3. What methods in treatment are available to women with menopausal symptoms?
4. What is the nurse's responsibility in caring for women during the menopause?

CHAPTER 31

UNMARRIED PARENTS

INCIDENCE

The illegitimate birth rate increased steadily from 1940 to 1958, but then changed from 1958 to 1965. The rate for nonwhite women has declined slightly since 1960; for white women it has increased 25% from 1960 to 1965. Over 40% of the mothers are 15 to 19 years old. Rates are highest in the South Atlantic and South Central states (highest, Mississippi—64.3) and relatively low in New England and the Midwest. Recently the highest rate has been for first births—136 per 1,000 in 1964. White couples are more apt to marry soon after pregnancy is discovered; nonwhites may wait until after the birth of one or more children. This fact plus the lower incidence of induced abortions among Negroes raises the nonwhite illegitimacy rate somewhat.

CAUSES

The causes of pregnancy out of wedlock reflect the cultural patterns of a society. In the United States, adolescents are struggling to achieve a sense of self. The acceptance of the naturalness of sex as a basic human drive is prevalent in the mass media of communication and advertising. To young people the inconsistencies in attitudes toward sex are confusing as adolescents are in the process of setting down values. Unfortunately in our present-day society, pregnancy out of wedlock is censured only when the visible evidence appears, and it is often the woman who is exploited. Attitudes and reactions to the unwed mother range from those of punishment to those of forgiveness. It is often the unborn child who is punished when assistance and care are withheld.

PHILOSOPHY IN CARE OF UNMARRIED PARENTS

At the White House Conference on Children and Youth in 1960, Dr. Leontine Young stated:

> They [unmarried mothers] need something as simple and wonderful as human interest. They need someone strong enough to share the responsibility they cannot carry, to give the

direction they lack, and to provide the structure which can put controls on their destructive behavior and encourage what strengths they do have. In other words, they need protective authority that will keep them out of trouble instead of punishment after they are already in it.

Each unwed mother needs early and adequate prenatal care for her own health and that of the infant. Regardless of race or socioeconomic status, plans are made for a residence during pregnancy and for the baby following delivery. The social worker and the health team work together to meet the individuals needs of each mother.

The unmarried father, a partner in the premarital sexual relationship, often needs as much help as the mother. Services are now including the father as a responsible partner and offer help and guidance with his future responsibilities. The goals of prevention (of repetitive experiences) lie in the help available to young people who are faced with a pregnancy out of wedlock.

Social agencies are available to the unwed mother. The majority of agencies arrange for medical care of the mother, for living facilities when indicated (such as foster home or maternity shelter), for help in continuing the girl's education or in finding a job, and offer guidance and help in planning for the baby.

Approximately 130 maternity homes in 46 states care for 5,000 mothers. Of this total, 45 are nonsectarian, affiliated with the Florence Crittenton Association of America, 35 are supported through Salvation Army funds, and 50 are under Roman Catholic auspices. It has been estimated that 75% of all mothers in maternity homes place their infants for adoption; 90% of these are white infants.

NURSING CARE OF THE UNWED MOTHER

Prenatal care of the unwed mother needs special consideration for many reasons. Studies reveal a higher incidence of toxemia in girls less than 16 years of age since there is incomplete uterine development, late irregular prenatal care, and improper diet, with a resulting higher incidence of prematurity and fetal and perinatal deaths. Often these mothers receive little or no prenatal care as they try to conceal the pregnancy, fail or refuse to recognize that pregnancy has occurred, may have obligations to other children, or are financially unable to discontinue working. Clinic services are available to them, but the lack of privacy, long waiting periods, and the ever-changing medical and nursing staff do not provide the amount of support the unwed mother needs. In a number of clinics, the absence of qualified social workers and psychologists makes it difficult to meet total needs.

Maternity shelters are providing the kinds of service needed for complete rehabilitation of unmarried women. Often a doctor from the local hospital comes to the home and establishes a "constant" relationship and is often the doctor who is present at delivery. Nurses employed by the maternity home provide preparation for labor and delivery and conduct group discussions on reproduction and pregnancy. Informal group discussions are often therapeutic, for many of the girls have similar problems. A few maternity homes are beginning to experiment with having selected girls live in small groups in apartments close to the shelter to provide privacy and encourage likeness to family group living.

Education of the teen-age mother is recognized as an important and integral part of care. The young teen-ager has a need to experience achievement, and education has proved to be a fruitful outlet. Often the school administrator and the school nurse are the first to learn of the pregnancy. Both the administrator and the nurse may foster continuance of education through referral agencies providing medical supervision and social services.

Meeting the needs of the unwed mother during pregnancy is difficult since there is often great emotional turmoil. Although the unwed mother is superficially reconciled that she is pregnant, she has deep-seated feelings about herself, her baby, the father of her baby, her parents, and friends. The social stigma attached to an out-of-wedlock pregnancy is something only the girl experiences. Adolescents in dire need of self-assertion find themselves in rather precarious positions. Evaluation of the childbearing experience is made in light of the help and support received from the nurse, the physician, the social worker, and the welfare agency. Since childbearing is a maturing process, the experience greatly determines the outlook of future pregnancies.

Nutrition for these girls is a problem during pregnancy since they often overeat because of the anxiety and stress. Some of the girls do not follow a good diet because they feel guilty about the pregnancy and use starvation for self-punishment.

The prenatal period seems endless to the mother who has made definite plans to place her infant for adoption. Although she is cognizant that it is best for the infant, the motherly instinct is strengthened as she faces being separated from the infant, a part of self. The nurse needs to be a good listener because the unwed mother has a need to talk through her anxieties during this stressful period. While listening the nurse is given clues that she often shares with the doctor or social worker to provide effective continuity in care. Often it is difficult for the nurse to be understanding and nonjudgmental unless she is aware of her own feelings regarding out-of-wedlock pregnancy. The nurse may need to seek the help of persons in other disciplines and talk through some of her own feelings before she is better able to intervene therapeutically. It has often been found that, once a relationship has been established, the same persons at each clinic visit would ease embarrassment, provide for relaxed discussions, and add to supportive therapy.

The labor and delivery period should be one of added support. Support can be provided by sensitivity to needs, alleviation of discomfort, and constant attendance of a familiar person. The nurse needs to be aware that labor and delivery for the unwed mother is often a period of punishment for her wrongdoing and is not visualized as a reward and privilege of giving life. Therefore, sparing as much of the discomfort will ease the burden of that which is to follow delivery.

The postdelivery period is the most trying and stressful. Often the social worker has done extensive counseling, and the mother has planned not to see the infant and has made placement for adoption. Since the maternal instinct is so strong, the mother often asks questions such as, "Is my baby all right? What is it, a boy or girl? What does he weigh? May I see him?" The nurse is then in a dilemma. On the one hand she knows the mother has a right to see her infant, and yet she has specific orders from the maternity home not to show the infant to the mother. The mother who asks to see her infant after having decided against it really does not wish to see the infant. She is often expressing feelings of guilt and feels she should ask because all mothers do. The nurse might consult the social worker concerning the matter. This should be done immediately to relieve anxiety in the mother. One of the greatest comforts the nurse can convey to the mother is that giving up one's infant in its best interest is the greatest love a mother can have.

For the mother who chooses to keep her infant, the nurse gives assistance in planning for future care. The mother's age and maturity are of particular significance. For the adolescent unwed mother, perhaps planning that she care for the infant all day and return to school at night may be feasible. For the older working mother, placement of the infant in a foster home and weekends with the mother may be suitable. Each mother needs individual planning.

Referral to public health nursing service, baby keep-well clinic, social service, and social welfare is also made according to need.

THE UNWED FATHER

Consideration of both partners is essential in planning. Including the father often provides better planning for the child. It also improves the father's behavior and his future relationships. At a National Conference on Social Welfare, Arthur L. Johnson stated, "I trust we all agree the male contributes about 50% to the illegitimacy problem."

Vista Del Mar, an agency in Los Angeles, California, has done research and found that unwed fathers have as many problems as mothers. Male social workers (representing a father figure) hold discussions on attitudes toward sex and emphasize the responsibilities associated with the sexual act without condonement. Stress is placed on the differences between age, mature love, responsibilities of parenthood, and the need for security through family living. Research at Vista Del Mar indicates that the majority of boys have had disappointing and depressing sexual experiences and are concerned about future adjustments in marriage. It is a policy at Vista Del Mar that the boy is shown his baby to complete the reality of the experience. Parents of both partners are involved in sharing the responsibilities for medical care and living arrangements. Parent participation is therapeutic since it relieves guilt feelings.

ADOPTION

The child born out of wedlock is at a great disadvantage. The social stigma often deprives him of certain rights and responsibilities. Questions often asked are, "Can a minor unwed mother bring suit against the father for support of the child? Can a minor unwed mother freely place her child for adoption without the consent of her parents or guardians? If the mother is a minor, will this negate her rights to the child born out of wedlock?"

Nurses need to understand that these questions relate to specific state laws of the girl's residence. In some states, an out-of-wedlock birth is never indicated on the birth record in order to protect the child.

The sole consent of the mother is required for child placement. Frequently when the father has acknowledged the child as his own, his consent is mandatory. The Federal Children's Bureau requires that a minor's mother, parent, or guardian be notified at the termination of adoption proceedings unless another decision has been made at the court's discretion. The minor unwed mother may be given care only at the consent of her parents, since they have legal parental rights of their child.

A generally accepted court rule holds that a mother is the natural guardian of a child born out of wedlock and has the legal right to his care, custody, and control over that of the father or any other person. This right, however, is only absolute after the best interests of the child have been considered. A minor unwed mother, therefore, may be given the right to custody of her child by court action in the best interests of the child. This principle is twofold, however—the best interest of the minor unwed mother is also considered since she is also a child.

LONG-TERM GOALS

Community efforts are focusing on the broad social, moral, and psychologic problems associated with pregnancy out of wedlock. Adequate housing, education, job, and social opportunities are essential in strengthening the family unit. Provisions for adequate social services to unmarried parents are seen as a goal toward prevention of repetitive practices.

Educational systems that include sex education and moral and ethical values are spreading rapidly throughout the United States. There is a need for continued research on the effect of out-of-wedlock births on the future adjustment and happiness in marriage and childbearing of unmarried parents. Following placement of the baby, continuance of psychologic counseling is necessary for any unresolved conflicts. Unmarried mothers and infants born out of wedlock are high medical risks and are given high priority in maternal child health programs.

SELECTED REFERENCES

Adams, H. M., and Gallagher, U. M.: Some facts and observations about illegitimacy, Children **10**:43, March-April, 1963.

Beck, J.: The other face of the problem: the unmarried teenage father, Today's Health **43**:28, February, 1965.

Bernstein, R.: Gaps in services to unmarried mothers, Children **10**:49, March-April, 1963.

Brewer, T. H.: Good prenatal nutrition prevents toxemia of pregnancy, Postgrad. Med. **39**:119, February, 1966.

Claman, A. D., and Bell, H. M.: Pregnancy in the very young teen-ager, Amer. J. Obstet. Gynec. **90**:350, 1964.

Clark, A. L.: Maturational crisis and the unwed adolescent mother, Nurs. Sci. **2**:113, April, 1964.

Clark, A. L.: The crisis of adolescent unwed motherhood, Amer. J. Nurs. **67**:465, July, 1967.

Costello, M.: The unwed mother, Catholic Nurse **13**:52, December, 1964.

Davens, E.: A view of health services for mothers and children, Children **12**:47, March-April, 1965.

Day, G. A.: A program for teen-age unwed mothers, Nurs. Outlook **55**:978, 1965.

Fanshel, D.: An upsurge of interest in adoption, Children **11**:193, September-October, 1964.

Garland, P.: The community's part in preventing illegitimacy, Children **10**:71, March-April, 1963.

Garrett, B.: Meeting the crisis in foster family care, Children **13**:2, January-February, 1966.

Guttmacher, A. D.: Unwanted pregnancy, a challenge to mental health, Ment. Hyg. **51**:512, 1967.

Herzog, E.: Why so few Negro adoptions? Children **12**:14, January-February, 1965.

Herzog, E.: Who are the unmarried mothers, Children **9**:157, July-August, 1962.

Hornecker, A.: Adoption opportunities for the handicapped, Children **9**:149, July-August, 1962.

Isler, C.: When you asked about your adoption, RN **25**:44, December, 1962.

Katz, S. N.: Legal protection for the unmarried mother and her child, Children **10**:55, March-April, 1963.

Kelley, J. L.: The school and unmarried mothers, Children **10**:60, March-April, 1963.

Kelley, J. L.: The unmarried mother, Child and Family **2**:48, Summer, 1963.

Kimball, C. P.: Some observations regarding unwanted pregnancy and therapeutic abortion, Obstet. Gynec. vol. 35, no. 2, February, 1970.

Kotaska, J. G.: Prenatal classes for unmarried expectant mothers, Canad. Nurse **64**:35, January, 1968.

Laden, E.: Your approach to the teenage mother, RN **26**: 58, 98, September, 1963.

Lamers, W. M.: Understanding the teenager, Obstet. Gynec., vol. 33, no. 1, January, 1969.

Langer, T. E.: What nurses can do to prevent illegitimacy, Catholic Nurse **11**:18, June, 1963.

Larsen, V. L.: Stresses of childbearing years, Amer. J. Public Health **56**:32, January, 1966.

Mayo, R.: Social services for children and youth, Children **9**:66, March-April, 1962.

Montgomery, H. B.: Differential utilization of social work personnel, Children **11**:103, May-June, 1964.

Pannor, R.: Casework service for unmarried fathers, Children **10**:65, March-April, 1963.

Polk, L. D.: UNWED mother or unwed MOTHER, Nurs. Outlook **12**:38, February, 1964.

Rashbaum, W., Rehr, H., Paneth, J., and Greenberg, M.: Use of social services by unmarried mother, Children **10**:11, January-February, 1963.

Reed, E.: Unmarried mothers who kept their babies, Children **12**:118, May-June, 1965.

Services for unmarried parents: Florence Crittenton League, 307 East 12th St., New York, N. Y.; Salvation Army, 546 Avenue of Americas, New York, N. Y.

Shanahan, L.: Adoption—a work of careful love, Marriage **46**:10, February, 1964.

Stein, O. C., Rider, P. V., and Sweeney, E.: School leaving due to pregnancy in an urban adolescent population, Amer. J. Public Health **54**:1, January, 1964.

Steinmetz, M. A.: Role playing in a maternity home, Children **11**:61, March-April, 1964.

Questions for study

1. Visit a maternity shelter in your community. How is it supported? What services are offered?
2. As you care for unwed mothers, what do you see as common needs during pregnancy, labor, delivery, and postdelivery?
3. Visit a social service agency for unmarried parents in your community. What kinds of help are given? When is the service terminated?
4. What materials are available from government agencies for broadening your knowledge of unmarried parents and adoption?
5. What is the nurse's role in caring for the out-of-wedlock mother? How do her needs differ from those of the married pregnant mother?

CHAPTER 32

TRENDS IN MATERNAL CHILD HEALTH SERVICES

VITAL STATISTICS

Recording the birth of an infant entitles him to his rights of citizenship and rights of inheritance. Births are recorded on a local, state, and national level. The National Bureau of Vital Statistics in Washington, D. C., is concerned with a country's socioeconomic status based on its population rate.

Today there is less childlessness and a trend toward medium-sized families having two to four children, a decline from families having six or more children. In 1962, 97% of all deliveries were in hospitals, New England leading with 100%, the South lowest with 90%. The birth rate was highest in Alaska, New Mexico, and Utah and lowest in Oregon and Pennsylvania.

In 1963 there were 4,098,000 live births registered in the United States, a decline of 1.6% from that of 1962. By 1980 there will be 51,782 women of childbearing age, that is, between the ages of 15 and 44 years. A report from the Natality Statistics Analysis for the United States in 1962 by the United States Public Health Service indicates an expected 5.5 million births by 1970 and 6,000,000 by 1980.

In 1963 1,466 women died as a direct result of childbearing. There were 4,098,000 live births, making the maternal mortality rate 3.6%. Although the maternal mortality rate has dropped considerably, it is still higher in the nonwhite women. This is due chiefly to environmental factors rather than poor maternity care. Environmental factors include lack of medical attendant at delivery, lack of prenatal care, dietary deficiences, poor hygiene, and faulty health education. As unfavorable environmental factors improve, the maternal death rate in the nonwhite will be reduced.

The maternal mortality rate increases in women of advancing age because there is often hypertension, higher incidences of uterine neoplasm, and greater tendency to hemorrhage. The maternal mortality rate also increases in women of high parity.

The lowest maternal mortality occurs in mothers in the 20-year to 30-year age group because during this period the outlook for the mother and the baby is best. Decline in maternal mortality is due to widespread training and educational programs in obstetrics, well-qualified specialists approved by the American Board of Obstetrics and Gynecology (6,000 approximately), and expansion of prenatal facilities through financial aid or the Children's Bureau.

Maternal death rates differ in various parts of the country depending upon cultural and socioeconomic factors. Rates are higher in the South among the deprived nonwhites who deliver at home without prenatal care. The decided reduction in maternal mortality is a result of the increased number of deliveries in hospitals, the accessibility of blood, and the advent of chemotherapy to combat infection.

The leading causes of maternal deaths are the following: (1) hemorrhage, 33.4%; (2) infection, 28.3%; (3) other—anesthesia and embolism, 22%; and (4) toxemia, 16.3%. The leading causes of neonatal deaths (20 weeks to 1 month) are *prematurity, respiratory distress syndrome* (brain injury resulting from hypoxia in utero and trauma to the brain during delivery), and *birth defects.*

Perinatal mortality rates include all infant deaths before delivery or during the first month of life. Some institutions include total perinatal mortality on the basis of all deaths occurring after 28 weeks of pregnancy; therefore the perinatal mortality rate must be considered with this in mind. Fetal deaths are classified at the recommendation of the World Health Organization as follows:

Group I	Early fetal death, less than 20 weeks of completed pregnancy
Group II	Intermediate fetal death, 20 to 27 weeks of completed pregnancy
Group III	Late fetal death, 28 or more completed weeks of pregnancy
Group IV	Unclassified

Neonatal death rates include live-born infants who die in the first month of life. Most states require that all infant deaths occurring after 20 weeks gestation be reported; others require reporting deaths under 20 weeks gestation.

Improvement in Maternal Child Health Services includes the efforts of obstetricians, pediatricians, pathologists, social scientists, public health specialists, epidemiologists, researchers, biostatisticians, health educators, and medical economists. Closer relationships with professional nurses, nurse-midwives, social services, and rehabilitation are essential toward amalgamation of services for optimum health care of mother and infant.

THE EXPANDING ROLE OF THE NURSE IN MATERNAL CHILD HEALTH SERVICES

The area in which more work needs to be done in order to meet the mother's needs is in the antepartal outpatient units. Consideration needs to be given to broadening services so that mothers receive not only medical supervision but also help and anticipatory guidance in preparation for the parenthood role. Most prenatal clinics are overcrowded, and reallocation by setting up smaller clinics within a community has proved beneficial. In some areas night clinics are ideal for the woman who may be working during pregnancy or who may have small youngsters needing her care. Prenatal services need a team approach in which medical staff, nurses, nutritionists, social workers, homemaker services, and public health personnel plan for continuity in care toward optimum health for families.

Studies reveal there is a relationship between lack of prenatal care and the high incidence of prematurity and perinatal deaths. Obstacles to prenatal care are lack of transportation, clinics not being held in outlying neighborhoods close to the population groups needing care, problems of finding a baby sitter for the other children during the mother's absence, and a poor understanding by the mother of the need for prenatal care.

Recommendations for adequate prenatal services include the following:

1. Setting up neighborhood prenatal clinics to serve population groups that find it difficult to travel to a distant hospital clinic.
2. Waiving residency eligibility restrictions and admissions based on arbitrary stages of gestation.
3. Initiating a public health education program to motivate expectant mothers to seek early prenatal care, with the need and cultural differences of the economically and socially deprived being given special understanding.
4. Intensifying public health nursing programs of mothers and children in the low socioeconomic areas of the city.
5. Providing hospital care for high-risk maternity patients and their infants before emergency care is necessary.

In many outpatient departments the nurse has now assumed a role in which she is responsible for women who are having uneventful pregnancies. The woman is seen by the physician on her first visit and then only by the nurse on subsequent visits. The nurse weighs, does urinalysis, checks the height of the fundus, checks fetal heart rate after 20 weeks gestation, checks for danger signs of toxemia, and gives anticipatory guidance. She is prepared to teach the mother according to needs. Many mothers are finding this system one in which their needs are met, and the nurse becomes supportive in that she sees the same mothers at each visit.

WORLD HEALTH ORGANIZATION (WHO)

The World Health Organization, founded in 1948, is one of the specialized agencies of the United Nations. Through this organization the public health and medical professions of more than 100 countries exchange their knowledge and experience and collaborate in an effort to achieve the highest possible level of health throughout the world. WHO is not concerned with problems that individual countries can resolve themselves but rather with problems that can be solved through the cooperation of all countries. In many parts of the world improvement in maternal and child health is much needed. Many professional nurses work with WHO in giving aid to people of other countries.

CHILDREN'S BUREAU

Children's Bureau, under the Department of Health, Education, and Welfare in Washington, D. C., was founded in 1912. The Bureau was primarily set up to improve services for the maintenance of health in children of the nation through research, care, and teaching. In 1921 Congress appropriated another one million, two hundred thousand dollars to be used to improve the health services of infants and for mothers during childbearing. This act expired in 1929 but was again provided for in the Social Security Act in 1935. Children's Bureau to date has been delegated this responsibility of administering grants in promoting the improvement of Maternal Child Health Services.

Under the Social Security Act, federal aid was provided to develop suitable methods for locating crippled children and maintaining a registry. Crippled Children's Commission provides aid for orthopedic and muscular problems and rehabilitative services.

White House Conferences are a federal activity held every 10 years to identify health problems in maternal child health services. Through these conferences standards are developed to improve health services to mothers and children.

OTHER UNITED STATES GOVERNMENT AGENCIES

Bureau of Family Services

The Bureau of Family Services provides aid to dependent children by providing federal monies to the state for food, shelter, and medical services for mothers and infants. The objectives of the service are primarily to keep the mother at home so that she may care for her infant in those important early months.

Woman's Bureau

Under the Department of Labor the Woman's Bureau is concerned with the conditions existing in industrial plants in which pregnant women are employed.

National Institute of Health

Under the National Institute of Health monies are provided for research on child health and human development.

LA LECHE INTERNATIONAL

La Leche International is an organization interested in fostering, encouraging, and helping mothers who desire to breast-feed their infants. The organization started in 1956 as an interest of six mothers in Franklin Park, Illinois. The first meetings were held in private homes, and the topics of discussion were the following: (1) advantages of breast-feeding, (2) techniques in breast-feeding, (3) nutrition and breast-feeding, and (4) weaning the infant. Although the meetings were centered about breast-feeding, childbearing and child rearing practices were often discussed.

As interest progressed, groups in other areas in the United States spread rapidly. Although headquarters are still in Illinois, chartered chapters of La Leche include Africa. The organization has a membership of interested mothers, nurses, physicians, and members of the health team. Members receive a monthly newsletter covering new aspects of breast-feeding and an up-to-date bibliography. Publications such as *The Womanly Art of Breast-Feeding* are now available through the League.

Nurses and physicians have become interested in the services offered and are acting as consultants and liaison between the hospital and the home. In areas where La Leche groups are established, hospitals are referring mothers upon discharge. Many nurses and doctors attend the sessions to broaden their knowledge of breast-feeding and the needs of parents during the childbearing years. In some areas a member of La Leche telephones the mother on her first week at home to give added support. Public health agencies are also working closely with La Leche to foster continuity in care to families.

INTERNATIONAL CHILDBIRTH EDUCATION ASSOCIATION

International Childbirth Education Association is a federation of groups and individuals interested in family-centered maternity and infant care. Its purpose is to create interest in education for childbirth, emotional support during labor, delivery, and breast-feeding, and good physical maternity and infant care to meet the needs of each individual and to foster the closeness of father, mother, and baby during the important days that surround birth. The ICEA was started through the cooperative efforts of mothers and fathers who did not have special preparation such as medicine or nursing.

The organization upholds no one method. It strongly upholds and believes that cooperation and communication between lay and professional groups are essential. ICEA also has an advisory and consultant board of physicians, psychologists, and nurses.

NURSE-MIDWIFERY

The nurse-midwife in countries such as England, Italy, and Scandinavia delivers practically 70% of all pregnant women. In the United States, however, the nurse-midwife cares for women in the rural South or isolated mountain areas where medical personnel are not available.

In 1925, Mary Breckinridge established the Frontier Nursing Service in Kentucky by bringing English nurse-midwives to practice in the isolated rural areas. In 1939 she established and opened a school called the Frontier Graduate School of Midwifery, which provides public health services to families in the mountainous Kentucky area. The school is still in existence today and is affiliated with Hayden Hospital. There are at present five satellite clinics supervised by nurse-midwives.

The Maternity Center Association was founded in New York in 1918 and in 1932 started a school for nurse-midwifery for graduate nurses. In 1935 the Maternity Center and the Lobenstine Clinic consolidated under the name of the Maternity Center Association. The nurse-midwife is prepared to work within the

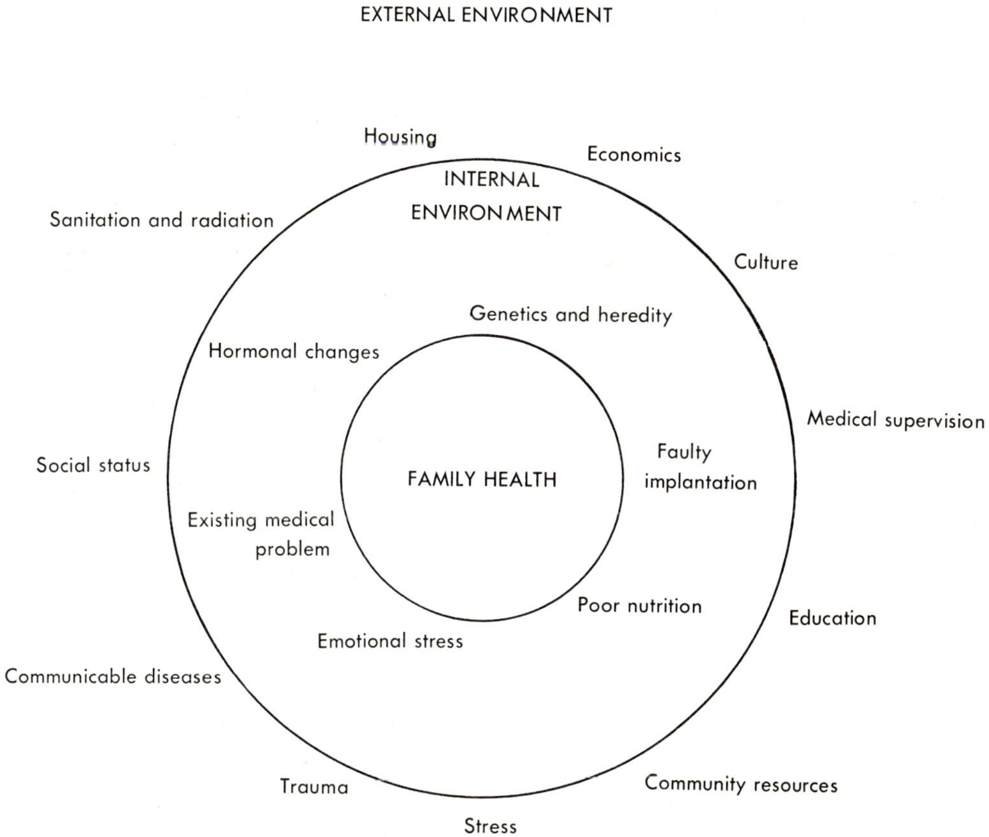

Fig. 32-1. Family health.

framework of an organized obstetric service and gives care to mothers prenatally, during labor and delivery, and in the home. She also teaches preparation for parent classes. The graduates of nurse-midwifery programs direct maternal child health services in government settings and teach undergraduate and graduate nurses. They are often professional nurses with bachelor's degrees, and many have master's degree preparation in public health.

Nurse-midwives at Maternity Center have been affiliated with Downstate Medical Center of the State University of New York and Kings County Hospital since 1958. Licensure of midwives is provided by the New York City Department of Health, and a few municipal hospitals now employ them.

In 1955 The American College of Nurse-Midwifery was established. Its purpose was to study and evaluate the role of the nurse-midwife and to plan programs for educational preparation. In 1957 the College became a member of the International Confederation of Midwives, which incorporates some thirty countries around the world.

In May, 1962, the College proposed the following definition of the nurse-midwife and nurse-midwifery:

The nurse-midwife is a registered nurse who by virtue of added knowledge and skill gained through an organized program of study and clinical experience recognized by the American College of Nurse-Midwifery, has extended the limits of her practice into the area of management and care of mothers and babies throughout the maternity cycle so long as progress meets criteria accepted as normal.

Nurse-midwifery is an extension of nursing practice into the area of management of care of mother and baby throughout the maternity cycle so long as progress meets criteria accepted as normal.

SELECTED REFERENCES

Preparation for marriage and a family

Brecher, R., and Brecher, E.: An analysis of human sexual response, ICEA, 208 Ditty Bldg., Bellevue, Wash., 1966.

Carroll, G. H.: First time parents, Child and Family, Spring, 1965.

Day, B., and Liley, M.: The secret world of the baby, ICEA, 208 Ditty Bldg., Bellevue, Wash., 1968.

Deutsch, R.: The key to feminine response in marriage, ICEA, 208 Ditty Bldg., Bellevue, Wash., 1968.

Eisenberg, L.: A developmental approach to adolescence, Child and Family, vol. 5, no. 4, Fall, 1966.

Geissler, E. S.: The meaning of marriage, Notre Dame, Ind., 1964, Fides Publishers, Inc.

Gruenberg, S.: The wonderful story of how you were born, ICEA, 208 Ditty Bldg., Bellevue, Wash., 1953.

Johnson, E. W.: Love and sex in plain language, ICEA, 208 Ditty Bldg., Bellevue, Wash., 1967.

Lowrie, S.: Early marriage—premarital pregnancy and associated factors, J. Marriage and Family, February, 1965.

Moss, J. J.: Teenage marriage cross national trends and sociological factors in the decision of when to marry, J. Marriage and Family, May, 1965.

Novak, M.: The experience of marriage, New York, 1964, The Macmillan Co.

Parker, E.: The seven ages of woman, Baltimore, 1960, The Johns Hopkins Press.

Pollack, O.: Family structures, Child and Family, vol. 5, no. 4, Fall, 1966.

Riker, A.: New parent blues, Child and Family, vol. 6, no. 2, Spring, 1967.

Shainess, N.: Motherhood: a tempering experience, Child and Family, Spring, 1965.

Simon, N. M.: Psychologic and social factors in family formation, Child and Family, Winter, 1964.

Treat, D. B.: Understanding the expectant father, Child and Family, Spring, 1964.

Vellay, P.: Childbirth and confidence, ICEA, 208 Ditty Bldg., Bellevue, Wash., 1969.

Pregnancy

Allen, S.: Nurse attendance during labor, Amer. J. Nurs. **64:**70, July, 1964.

Clark, A.: The adaptation problems and patterns of an expanding family, Nurs. Forum, vol. 2, no. 1, 1966.

Elliott, J. M.: Pica and pregnancy, Nurs. Clin. N. Amer. **3:**299, 1968.

Findlay, E., and Capes, M.: Figure control for your postpartum patient, R.N., January, 1969.

Hazlett, W.: The male factor in obstetrics, Child and Family, vol. 6, no. 4, Fall, 1967.

Heckerman, L. D., and Wolf, H. L.: Continuity of treatment as prevention of stress in high-risk maternity cases, ANA Clinical Sessions, New York, 1968, Appleton-Century-Crofts.

Hilliard, M. E.: The changing role of the maternity nurse, Nurs. Clin. N. Amer. **3:** 277, 1968.

Hogan, A.: The role of the nurse in meeting the needs of the new mother, Nurs. Clin. N. Amer. **3:**337, 1968.

Kelman, N.: The father, Child and Family, vol. 6, no. 4, Fall, 1967.

King, E.: The pregnant father, Bull. Amer. Coll. Nurse Midwifery **13:**19, February, 1968.

Matousek, I.: Fetal nursing during labor, Nurs. Clin. N. Amer. **3:**307, 1968.

Meek, L.: Maternal emotions and their implications in nursing, R.N., April, 1969.

Pappers, P. J.: Overventilation during labor, Bull. Amer. Coll. Nurse Midwifery **13:** 4, May, 1968.

Rodman, M.: The pituitary hormones, R.N. **31:**55, June, 1968.

Rubin, R.: Attainment of the maternal role, Nurs. Res. **16:**237, Summer, 1967.

Rubin, R.: Cognitive style in pregnancy, Amer. J. Nurs., vol. 70, no. 3, March, 1970.

Seyle, H.: The stress syndrome, Amer. J. Nurs. **65:** 97, March, 1965.

Simpson, J.: The medium for the message in maternal-child nursing, Amer. J. Nurs., vol. 67, no. 11, November, 1967.

Smith, E.: An oasis for pregnant teenagers, R.N., March, 1970.

Stephens, G.: Mind-body continuum, Amer. J. Nurs., vol. 70, no. 7, July, 1970.

Watkins, E. L.: Low-income Negro mothers—their decision to seek prenatal care, Amer. J. Public Health **58:**655, 1968.

Williams, B.: Sleep needs during the maternity cycle, Nurs. Outlook **15:**53, February, 1967.

Yeaworth, R.: Identification and maternity nursing, Nurs. Forum, vol. 7, no. 3, 1968.

Young, E. W.: Prepared childbirth: its impact on nursing, Canad. Nurse **64:**39, January, 1968.

Nutrition

Callahan, C. L.: The White House Conference on food, nutrition, and health, Nurs. Outlook **18:**58, January, 1970.

Cooper, L. F.: Nutrition in health and disease, Philadelphia, 1963, J. B. Lippincott Co.

Editorial: Human pregnancy nutrition: a clinical view, Obstet. Gynec. **30:**605, 1967.

Hubbard, E.: How we solve breastfeeding problems, R.N. **33:**46, March, 1970.

Moore, M. L.: The clay eaters, R.N., vol. 33, p. 44, August, 1970.

Moore, M. L.: When families must eat more or less, Nurs. Outlook **14:**66, April, 1966.

Peckos, P. S., and Heald, F. P.: Nutrition of adolescents, Children **11:**27, 1964.

Rubin, A.: Nutrition during pregnancy and lactation, Child and Family, vol. 5, no. 3, Summer, 1966.

Spindler, E. B.: Better diets for teenagers, Nurs. Outlook **13:**32, February, 1964.

Newborn

Arnold, H. W., et al.: The newborn—transition to extra-uterine life, Amer. J. Nurs. **65:**77, October, 1965.

Connolly, R. B.: Lactation, the lost art, Hosp. Top. **42:**99, September, 1964.

Davis, L.: Practical points in P.K.U. testing, Nurs. Outlook **14:**46, January, 1966.

Hervada, A. R.: Nursing evaluation of the newborn, Amer. J. Nurs. **67:**1669, August, 1967.

Breast-feeding

Applebaum, R.: Abreast of the times, ICEA, 208 Ditty Bldg., Bellevue, Wash., 1969.

Birchfield, M.: A mother's view on breast-feeding, Amer. J. Nurs. **63:**88, March, 1963.

Dyal, L., and Kahrl, J.: When mothers breast feed, Amer. J. Nurs. **67:**2555, December, 1967.

Evans, R.: Needs identified among breast-feeding mothers, ANA Clinical Sessions, New York, 1968, Appleton-Century-Crofts.

Evans, R.: Exploration of factors involved in maternal physiological adaptation to breast feeding, Nurs. Res. **18:**28, 1969.

Haire, D.: Instructions for nursing your baby (in English, French, and Spanish), ICEA, 208 Ditty Bldg., Seattle, Wash., 1969.

Heinstein, M. I.: Influence of breast feeding on children's behavior, Children **10:**93, May-June, 1963.

Iorio, J.: When your patient wonders about breastfeeding, R.N. **26:**44, November, 1963.

Iorio, J.: Breastfeeding mothers help each other, Amer. J. Nurs. **64:**119, October, 1964.

La Leche League International: The womanly art of breastfeeding, Franklin Park, Ill., 1963.

Newton, N., and Newton, M.: The management of lactation, Child and Family, January, 1964.

Newton, N., and Newton, M.: Psychologic aspects of lactation, Child and Family, Spring, 1968.

Nichols, M. G.: Breastfeeding: a nurse-mother discovers its joys, R.N. **31:**50, May, 1968.

Salbers, E. J. M. D.: Patterns of breast-feeding, Child and Family, October, 1963.

Stewart, B.: Breast-fed Babies, ICEA, 208 Ditty Bldg., Bellevue, Wash., 1961.

Parent-child relationships

Bunnell, P., and Henning, E.: Parent-child relationships. Implications for Nursing, New Brunswick, N. J., November, 1968, Rutgers University.

Crawford, M.: Physiological and behavioral cues to disturbances in childbirth, ANA Clinical Sessions, New York, 1968, Appleton-Century-Crofts.

Dutcher, I., and Hakerem, H.: Mother-child interaction in psychosomatic illness, Nurs. Forum **7:**173, 1968.

Kimball, C. D.: Mother-child relationships, Child and Family, July, 1963.

Rubin, R.: Maternal touch, Nurs. Outlook, November, 1963.

Rubin, R.: The family or child relationship and nursing care, Nurs. Outlook **12**:36, September, 1964.

Rubin, R.: Attainment of the maternal role —Part 1, Nurs. Res. **16**:237, Summer, 1967.

Family planning

Calderone, M. S.: Sexual health and family planning, Amer. J. Public Health **58**:223, February, 1968.

Corfman, P., and Segal, S.: Biologic effects of intrauterine devices, Amer. J. Obstet. Gynec. **100**:448, Feb. 1, 1968.

Fischman, S. H.: Choosing an appropriate contraceptive, Nurs. Outlook **15**:28, December, 1967.

Guttmacher, A.: Planning your family, New York, 1964, The Macmillan Co.

Hutchinson, H. A.: Patient education for low-income women in a family planning program, ANA Clinical Sessions, New York, 1968, Appleton-Century-Crofts.

Hutchinson, H. A.: Extending family planning services, Amer. J. Nurs., vol. 70, no. 7, July, 1970.

Jaffe, F.: A strategy for implementing family planning in the United States, Amer. J. Public Health, April, 1968.

Lumley, I. B., MacDonald, R. R.: Immediate postnatal family planning, Nurs. Mirror **127**:35, December, 1968.

Martin, R. M.: Teaching family planning, Nurs. Outlook, vol. 15, no. 12, December, 1967.

Milton, I.: Contraceptive practices, past and present, Canad. Nurse **63**:29, October, 1967.

Taylor, H., and Berelson, B.: Maternity care and family planning as a world program, Amer. J. Obstet. Gynec. **100**:882, 1968.

Wiedenbach, E.: The nurse's role in family planning—a conceptual base for practice, Nurs. Clin. N. Amer. **3**:355, June, 1968.

Cultural aspects

Bigham, G. D.: To communicate with Negro patients, Amer. J. Nurs. **64**:113, September, 1964.

Brown, A.: Understanding other cultures, Nurs. Sci. **2**:78, February, 1964.

Freiden, B.: The feminine mystique, Nurs. Sci. **2**:258, June, 1964.

Johnson, C. A.: Nursing and Mexican American folk medicine, Nurs. Forum **3**:102, 1964.

Lindner, E. M.: Childbirth practices in two primitive cultures, Nurs. Mirror **127**:29, July, 1968.

Loughlin, B. W.: Pregnancy in the Navajo culture, Nurs. Outlook **13**:55, March, 1965.

Paynick, M. L.: Cultural barriers to nurses' communications, Amer. J. Nurs. **64**:87, February, 1964.

Teaching

Beebe, J. E., et al.: Bench conferences in a large obstetric clinic, Amer. J. Nurs. **68**: 85, January, 1968.

Cochran, L., and Yeaworth, R.: Ward meetings for teen-age mother, Amer. J. Nurs. **67**:1044, May, 1967.

Golub, S.: How nurses reply to questions about sex, R.N. **30**:41, September, 1967.

Hillsman, G. M.: Genetics and the nurse, Nurs. Outlook **14**:34, January, 1966.

Juberg, R. C.: Heredity counseling, Nurs. Outlook **14**:28, January, 1966.

Kirkendall, L. A., and Cox, H. M.: Starting a sex education program, Children **14**:136, July-August, 1967.

Koldjeski, H. D.: Concerns antepartal mothers express in group teachings, experiences and implications for nursing practice, ANA Clinical Sessions, New York, 1966, Appleton-Century-Crofts.

Kotaska, J.: Prenatal classes for unmarried expectant mother, Canad. Nurse **64**:35, January, 1968.

Madore, E., and Deutsch, Y. B.: Talking with parents, Amer. J. Nurs. **62**:108, November, 1962.

McCaffery, M. S.: An approach to parent education, Nurs. Forum **6**:77, 1967.

Moore, L., and White, G.: Comparisons of teaching methods in maternal and infant care, Nurs. Outlook **13**:74, May, 1966.

Trends in maternal child health nursing

Anderson, E., and Lesser, A.: Maternity care in the United States, gains and gaps, Amer. J. Nurs. **66**:1539, July, 1966.

Clark, A. L.: The clinical nursing specialist: one answer to the nursing needs of mothers and children, Child and Family, Summer, 1968.

Dunkley, V. K.: Rooming-in psychotic mother

and healthy baby, Nurs. Outlook **11**:750, October, 1963.

Dwyer, J. M., and Lynch, W. A.: Nursing responsibility for decreasing maternal and perinatal mortality and morbidity, Hosp. Progr. **47**:56, January, 1967.

Greene, J. W.: The nurse midwife, Child and Family, vol. 6, no. 4, Fall, 1967.

Hosford, E.: The maternity cycle, a time of challenge, Bull. Amer. Coll. Nurse Midwifery **12**:45, May, 1967.

Leppert, P.: Chromosomal disorders of the unborn, Bull. Amer. Coll. Nurse Midwifery **13**:14, May, 1968.

Melber, R.: The maternity nurse specialist in a hospital clinic setting, Nurs. Res. **16**: 68, Winter, 1967.

Reiter, F.: The nurse-midwife: clinical nursing specialist, Bull. Amer. Coll. Nurse Midwifery **12**:71, August, 1967.

Rubin, R.: Food and feeding—a matrix of relationships, Nurs. Forum **6**:195, 1967.

Simmons, M. P.: Is this maternity nursing? Nurs. Outlook **14**:66, March, 1966.

Stitt, P.: The family health clinic, Child and Family, Winter, 1965.

Treat, D. B.: Understanding the expectant father, Child and Family, September, 1964.

Wahlstrom, D., and Weston, J. L.: Initiating referrals, Amer. J. Nurs. **67**:332, February, 1967.

Young, E. W.: Prepared childbirth: its impact on nursing, Canad. Nurse **64**:39, January, 1968.

Young, M., et al.: A demonstration of automated instruction for diabetic self-care, Amer. J. Public Health **59**:110, 1969.

Unwed parents

Auerback, A. B.: Parent education groups for unmarried mothers, Nurs. Outlook **14**:38, March, 1966.

Beck, J.: The other face of the problem: the unmarried teen-age father, Today's Health **43**:28, February, 1965.

Beckner, F. J.: How do you respond to the unwed mother, R.N., August, 1970.

Burgess, L. C.: The unmarried father in adoption planning, Children, vol. 15, no. 2, March-April, 1968.

Clark, A. L.: Maturational crisis and the unwed adolescent mother, Nurs. Sci. **2**:113, 1964.

Clark, A. L.: The crisis of adolescent unwed motherhood, Amer. J. Nurs. **67**:1465, July, 1967.

Daniels, A. M.: Reaching unwed adolescent mothers, Amer. J. Nurs., vol. 69, no. 2, February, 1969.

Guttmacher, A.: Unwanted pregnancy: a challenge to mental health, Mental Hyg. **51**: 512, 1967.

Herzog, E.: Unmarried mothers—the service gap revisited, Children, vol. 14, no. 3, May-June, 1967.

Iungerich, Z.: High school for unwed mothers, Amer. J. Nurs. **67**:92, January, 1967.

Murdock, C. G.: The unmarried mother and the school system, Amer. J. Public Health **58**:2217, 1968.

Pannor, R.: The unmarried father, Child and Family, July, 1963.

Reed, E.: Unmarried mothers who kept their babies, Children **12**:118, May-June, 1965.

Sorrel, P. M.: The young unwed mother, Obstet. Gynec. **32**:741, 1968.

Townsend, J.: The unmarried pregnant adolescent's use of educational literature, Nurs. Outlook **15**:48, August, 1967.

Wright, M. K.: Comprehensive services for adolescent unwed mother, Children **13**: 170, September-October, 1966.

Birth defects

Atkinson, H. C.: Care of the child with cleft lip and palate, Amer. J. Nurs. **67**:1889, September, 1967.

Berlow, T. G.: Congenital dislocation of the hip, Nurs. Times **64**:967, 1968.

Bradley, B., et al.: The child with deformed or missing limbs, his problems and prosthesis, Amer. J. Nurs., November, 1962.

Bradley, E. J.: Parents' acceptance of mongolism, Child and Family, Winter, 1965.

Engel, G.: Grief and grieving, Amer. J. Nurs. **63**:93, 1964.

Hirschhorn, K.: L.S.D.—chromosomal damage, Hosp. Practice **4**:98, February, 1969.

Kallaus, J.: The child with cleft lip and palate—the mother in the maternity ward, Amer. J. Nurs. **65**:120, April, 1965.

Owens, C.: Parents' reactions to defective babies, Amer. J. Nurs. **64**:83, November, 1964.

Winick, M.: Birth defects: what is being done about them? Nurs. Outlook **14**:43, January, 1966.

Deviations of mother and newborn

Abortion: the lonely problem, R.N. **33:**34, June, 1970.

American Heart Association, New York City: Heart disease and pregnancy.

Buck, P. S.: The terrible choice: the abortion dilemma, Child and Family, Summer, 1968.

Buxton, L. C.: Induced abortions—one doctor's opinion of abortion laws, Amer. J. Nurs. **68:**1026, May, 1968.

Calliouette, J. C.: Septic AB—pathology and treatment, Amer. J. Nurs., May, 1966.

Carlson, B.: Surgical correction of urethral hymenal fusion, R.N., January, 1968.

Carroll, Rev. C.: Liberalized abortion—a critique, Child and Family, Spring, 1968.

Clark, D., Copeland, W., and Ullery, J.: Prolapse of umbilical cord, Amer. J. Obstet. Gynec., May 1, 1968.

Corcoran, C. J. D.: Abortion: Its humane analysis, Child and Family, Summer, 1968.

Diamond, E. F.: A pediatrician views abortion, Child and Family, Fall, 1968.

Di Palma, J. R.: Drugs for diabetes mellitus, R.N. **30:**71, October, 1967.

Fonseca, J. D.: Induced abortions—nursing attitudes and actions, Amer. J. Nurs., vol. 68, no. 5, May, 1968.

Golub, S.: A new weapon against Rh hemolytic disease, R.N. **3:**38, August, 1968.

Hirschhorn, H.: LSD and chromosomal damage, Hosp. Practice **4:**98, February, 1969.

Jacobson, C., and Barter, R.: Intrauterine diagnosis and management of genetic defects, Amer. J. Obstet. Gynec., Nov. 15, 1967.

Jakobovits, R.: Jewish views on abortion, Child and Family, Spring, 1968.

Larson, G. I.: What every nurse should know about congenital syphilis, Nurs. Outlook **13:**52, March, 1965.

Latham, H. C.: Thrombophlebitis, Amer. J. Nurs., September, 1968.

Leifer, G.: Rooming-in despite postpartal complications, Amer. J. Nurs. **67:**2114, October, 1967.

Martin, M. M.: Insulin reactions, Amer. J. Nurs. **67:**328, February, 1967.

McLaverty, M. P., et al.: Program for toxemia control, Amer. J. Obstet. Gynec. **92:**100, May 1, 1965.

McLenahan, I. G.: Helping a mother who has no 'baby to take home, Amer. J. Nurs., April, 1962.

Porter, D.: Care of puerperal breast, Hosp. Top. **45:**103, March, 1967.

Pringle, J. A.: Respiratory distress unit, Amer. J. Nurs. **68:**2370, November, 1968.

Pritchard, J., and Stone, S.: Clinical and laboratory observations on eclampsia, Amer. J. Obstet. Gynec. **99:**754, Nov. 17, 1967.

Queenan, J. T.: Intra-uterine transfusion for erythroblastosis fetalis, Amer. J. Nurs. **65:**68, August, 1965.

Robertson, J., and Freda, V.: Amniotic fluid analysis in Rh iso-immunization, Amer. J. Nurs. **65:**64, August, 1965.

Rose, P. A.: The high risk mother-infant dyad, Nurs. Forum **6:**94, 1967.

Schneider, W. J., and Boyce, B.: Complications of diuretic therapy, Amer. J. Nurs. **68:**1903, September, 1968.

Slatin, M.: Extra protection for high risk mothers and babies, Amer. J. Nurs., vol. 67, no. 6, June, 1967.

Smith, S., and Scragg, W.: Gestational diabetes, Obstet. Gynec., February, 1968.

Stenchever, M., and Cibils, L.: Management of the Rh-sensitized patient, Amer. J. Obstet. Gynec. **100:**554, Feb. 15, 1968.

Stickle, G.: Defective development and reproductive wastage in the United States, Amer. J. Obstet. Gynec. **100:**442, Feb. 1, 1968.

Ujhely, G. B.: Grief and depression—implications for preventive therapeutic nursing care, Nurs. Forum, vol. 5, no. 2, 1966.

Zuspan, F., and Talledo, E.: Factors affecting delivery in eclampsia, Amer. J. Obstet. Gynec. **100:**672, March 1, 1968.

Gynecology

Brewer, J., and DeCosta, E. J.: Textbook of gynecology, Baltimore, 1967, The Williams & Wilkins Co.

Blanchet, J.: Estrogen and the menopause, Canad. Nurs. **63:**38, February, 1967.

Chalfant, R. L.: Diagnosis and treatment of cancer of uterus, Nurs. Forum **4:** 67, 1965.

Golub, S.: V.D., the unconquered menace, R.N. **33:**38, March, 1970.

Gorlick, M. S.: Hirsutism: its causes and management, R.N. **31:**36, June, 1968.

Gray, M. J.: The use of radiation therapy in gynecologic malignancy, Hosp. Top. **45:** 103, September, 1967.

Gusberg, S. B.: Cancer in situ of the cervix,

treatment as preventive medicine, Amer. J. Nurs. **64:**76, April, 1964.

Hofmeister, J. J., et al.: Suture reinforcement of the incompetent cervix, Amer. J. Obstet. Gynec. **101:**58, May 1, 1968.

Kimbrough, R. A.: Gynecology, Philadelphia, 1965, J. B. Lippincott Co.

Krieger, J. S.: Graded treatment for in situ carcinoma of uterine cervix, Amer. J. Obstet. Gynec. **101:**169, May 15, 1968.

Leegman, S.: Infertility in women, Philadelphia, 1966, F. A. Davis Co.

Lewis, G.: Cancer in situ of the cervix, Amer. J. Nurs. **64:**72, April, 1964.

Mayo, P., and Wilkey, N. L.: Prevention of cancer of breast and cervix, Nurs. Clin. N. Amer. **3:**229, June, 1968.

McEwen, D.: Estrogen replacement therapy at menopause, Canad. Nurse **63:**34, February, 1967.

Miller, N., and Avery, H.: Gynecology and gynecologic nursing, Philadelphia, 1965, W. B. Saunders Co.

Robbins, L., and Walker, E.: Cancer in situ of the cervix—problem of control, Amer. J. Nurs. **64:**80, April, 1964.

Rodman, M. J.: The female sex hormones, R.N. **3:**57, May, 1968.

Smith, M., et al.: The diagnosis of cervical cancer during pregnancy, Obstet. Gynec., February, 1968.

Theobald, G. W.: Reproductive ability in women, Amer. J. Obstet. Gynec. **92:**332, 1965.

Urquhart, A. L.: A study of nursing care of the vulvectomy patient, ANA Clinical Sessions, New York, 1967, Appleton-Century-Crofts.

Wilson, J. R.: Obstetrics and gynecology, St. Louis, 1963, The C. V. Mosby Co.

Preparation for childbearing

Auerback, A.: Parents learn through discussion: principles and practices of parent group education, ICEA, 208 Ditty Bldg., Bellevue, Wash., 1967.

Bing, E.: Six practical lessons for an easier childbirth, ICEA, 208 Ditty Bldg., Bellevue, Wash., 1967.

Birkbeck, A., and Keen, M.: Controlled childbirth, ICEA, 208 Ditty Bldg., Bellevue, Wash., 1969.

Brandner, P.: Childbirth Education Instructor's Manual, ICEA, 208 Ditty Bldg., Bellevue, Wash., 1969.

Chabon, I.: Awake and aware: participating in childbirth, through psychoprophylaxis, ICEA, 208 Ditty Bldg., Bellevue, Wash., 1966.

Chertok, L.: Motherhood and personality, psychosomatic aspects of childbirth, ICEA, 208 Ditty Bldg., Bellevue, Wash., 1969.

Ebner, M.: Physiotherapy in obstetrics, ed. 3, ICEA, 208 Ditty Bldg., Bellevue, Wash., 1967.

Flowers, C.: Obstetric analgesia and anesthesia, ICEA, 208 Ditty Bldg., Bellevue, Wash., 1967.

Haire, D.: Implementing family centered maternity care with a central nursery, ICEA, 208 Ditty Bldg., Bellevue, Wash., 1968.

Hazell, L.: Commonsense childbirth, ICEA, 208 Ditty Bldg., Bellevue, Wash., 1969.

Heardman, H.: Relaxation and exercises for natural childbirth, ICEA, 208 Ditty Bldg., Bellevue, Wash., 1962.

Kitzinger, S.: Experience of childbirth, ICEA, 208 Ditty Bldg., Bellevue, Wash., 1962.

Kitzinger, S.: An approach to antenatal teaching, ICEA, 208 Ditty Bldg., Bellevue, Wash., 1968.

Maternity Center Association, East 92nd St., New York, N. Y.: Preparation for childbearing, 1969.

Richardson, S. F., and Guttmacher, A.: Childbearing: its social and psychological aspects, ICEA, 208 Ditty Bldg., Bellevue, Wash., 1967.

Wright, E.: The new childbirth, ICEA, 208 Ditty Bldg., Bellevue, Wash., 1967.

Periodical journals related to maternal child health

American Journal of Nursing, American Nurses' Association, New York, N. Y.

American Journal of Obstetrics and Gynecology, The C. V. Mosby Co., St. Louis, Mo.

American Journal of Public Health, American Public Health Association, Inc., Albany, N. Y.

Briefs, Maternity Center Association, New York, N. Y.

Child and Family, Abbey Press, Publishing Division, St. Meinrad, Ind.

Children, Children's Bureau, Department of

Health, Education, and Welfare, Washington, D. C.

Journal of Marriage and the Family, Rand McNally & Co., Box 7600, Chicago, Ill.

Nursing Forum, Chicago, Ill.

Nursing Outlook, National League for Nursing, New York, N. Y.

Nursing Science, F. A. Davis Co., Philadelphia, Pa.

Obstetrics and Gynecology, Harper & Row, Publishers, New York, N. Y.

RN Magazine, Oradell, N. J.

The cumulative index to nursing literature, published by the Glendale Sanitarium and Hospital, P.O. Box 871, Glendale, Calif., lists many more nursing and medical journals for research reading.

INDEX

B

500 cc blood

C

D

E

F

G

T